D1679606

Diagnostic Methods in Clinical Cardiology

Distributed to the medical profession
as an educational service —

Compliments of
Ayerst.

Diagnostic Methods in Clinical Cardiology

Edited by

Peter F. Cohn, M.D.
Professor of Medicine and Chief, Cardiology Division, State University of New York Health Sciences Center, Stony Brook

Joshua Wynne, M.D.
Assistant Professor of Medicine, Harvard Medical School; Director, Noninvasive Cardiac Laboratory, Brigham and Women's Hospital, Boston

Little, Brown and Company
Boston

Copyright © 1982 by Peter F. Cohn, M.D., and Joshua Wynne, M.D.

First Edition

All rights reserved. No part of this book may be reproduced in any form or by any electronic or mechanical means, including information storage and retrieval systems, without permission in writing from the publisher, except by a reviewer who may quote brief passages in a review.

Library of Congress Catalog Card No. 81-84193

ISBN 0-316-15033-9

Printed in the United States of America

HAL

For Joan
and
For Charlotte and Canio

Contents

Preface   ix
Contributing Authors   x

1. Value and Limitations of Cardiac Diagnostic Procedures: An Overview   1
   Peter F. Cohn and Joshua Wynne

I. Electrocardiography   3

2. The Resting Electrocardiogram   5
   Gilbert H. Mudge, Jr.

3. Ambulatory Electrocardiographic Monitoring   29
   Elliott M. Antman and Peter F. Cohn

4. Exercise Testing   51
   Peter H. Stone and Peter F. Cohn

II. Echocardiography, External Pulse Recordings, and Related Procedures   81

5. Echocardiography   83
   Thomas A. Risser and Joshua Wynne

6. External Pulse Recordings, Systolic Time Intervals, Apexcardiography, and Phonocardiography   121
   Kenneth M. Borow and Joshua Wynne

III. Radioisotopic Examination of the Heart   163

7. Radionuclide Ventriculography   165
   Marvin A. Konstam and Joshua Wynne

8. Myocardial Perfusion and Infarct Imaging   199
   Edward J. Brown, Jr., and Joshua Wynne

IV. Invasive Procedures   233

9. Bedside Hemodynamic Monitoring, Cardiac Catheterization, and Pulmonary Angiography   235
   Blase A. Carabello and William Grossman

10. Electrophysiologic Studies   271
   Stephen C. Vlay and Peter F. Cohn

V. Additional Diagnostic Procedures   291

11. Nonangiographic Radiologic Examination of the Heart   293
    Donald P. Harrington and J. Daniel Garnic
12. Blood Tests   333
    Samuel Z. Goldhaber and Thomas W. Smith

Index   367

Preface

The purpose of this book is to provide the clinician with a survey of diagnostic methods (exclusive of history-taking and physical examination) that are available for the evaluation of cardiac disorders. Emphasis has been placed not on the technical aspects of most of these procedures but rather on their indications, interpretation (from the clinical point of view), and complications. The introductory first chapter is devoted to an overview, including test sequencing in various disease states. The next five parts deal with specific noninvasive and invasive procedures in considerable detail, but always with the clinician — rather than the specialist — in mind.

Our aim is to provide an integrated approach to the evaluation of cardiovascular disease and to bring some logic to the selection of appropriate tests from an increasingly complex and sophisticated array of possible diagnostic procedures. With the proliferation of noninvasive tests (including electrocardiographic, echocardiographic, and radioisotopic procedures), the clinician is often in a quandary as to which test to order, whether the information it provides is sufficiently reliable and diagnostic, and when to proceed to an invasive procedure such as cardiac catheterization. We have attempted to address these issues and provide guidelines for clinical decision-making without being dogmatic or ignoring controversy. While we have co-authored two-thirds of the chapters, we have tried to avoid a monolithic approach and have encouraged each of our contributors to emphasize areas of uncertainty or disagreement. It is our hope that this text will be a useful guide to the clinician in day-to-day patient care decisions.

It is a pleasure to acknowledge the inspiration, enthusiasm, support, and counsel of our colleagues and cardiology fellows. Special thanks are due to Adele Slatko for her superb administrative and secretarial support, and Lin Richter and Katherine Arnoldi at Little, Brown and Company for their editorial skills.

P.F.C.
J.W.

Contributing Authors

Elliott M. Antman, M.D.
Assistant Professor of Medicine, Harvard Medical School; Director, Samuel A. Levine Coronary Care Unit, Brigham and Women's Hospital, Boston

Kenneth M. Borow, M.D.
Assistant Professor of Medicine, Harvard Medical School; Associate Director, Noninvasive Cardiac Laboratory, Brigham and Women's Hospital; Associate in Cardiology, The Children's Hospital Medical Center, Boston

Edward J. Brown, Jr., M.D.
Assistant Professor of Medicine and Director of Nuclear Cardiology, State University of New York Health Sciences Center, Stony Brook

Blase A. Carabello, M.D.
Associate Professor of Medicine, Temple University School of Medicine; Director of Diagnostic Cardiology, Temple University Health Sciences Center, Philadelphia

Peter F. Cohn, M.D.
Professor of Medicine and Chief, Cardiology Division, State University of New York Health Sciences Center, Stony Brook

J. Daniel Garnic, M.D.
Instructor in Radiology, Harvard Medical School; Cardiovascular Radiologist, Brigham and Women's Hospital, Boston

Samuel Z. Goldhaber, M.D.
Research Fellow in Medicine, Harvard Medical School and Brigham and Women's Hospital, Boston

William Grossman, M.D.
Professor of Medicine, Harvard Medical School; Chief, Cardiovascular Division, Beth Israel Hospital, Boston

Donald P. Harrington, M.D.
Associate Professor of Radiology, Harvard Medical School; Co-Director of Cardiovascular Radiology, Brigham and Women's Hospital, Boston

Marvin A. Konstam, M.D.
Assistant Professor of Medicine and Radiology, Tufts University School of Medicine; Assistant Director, Cardiac Catheterization Laboratory, New England Medical Center Hospital, Boston

Gilbert H. Mudge, Jr., M.D.
Assistant Professor of Medicine, Harvard Medical School; Director, Clinical Cardiology Service, Brigham and Women's Hospital, Boston

Thomas A. Risser, M.D.
Instructor in Medicine, Harvard Medical School; Director, Noninvasive Cardiology Laboratory, The Cambridge Hospital, Cambridge

Thomas W. Smith, M.D.
Professor of Medicine, Harvard Medical School; Chief, Cardiovascular Division, Brigham and Women's Hospital, Boston

Peter H. Stone, M.D.
Instructor in Medicine, Harvard Medical School; Associate Director, Samuel A. Levine Coronary Care Unit, Brigham and Women's Hospital, Boston

Stephen C. Vlay, M.D.
Assistant Professor of Medicine and Director, Coronary Care Unit, State University of New York Health Sciences Center, Stony Brook

Joshua Wynne, M.D.
Assistant Professor of Medicine, Harvard Medical School; Director, Noninvasive Cardiac Laboratory, Brigham and Women's Hospital, Boston

Notice

The indications and dosages of all drugs in this book have been recommended in the medical literature and conform to the practices of the general medical community. The medications described do not necessarily have specific approval by the Food and Drug Administration for use in the diseases and dosages for which they are recommended. The package insert for each drug should be consulted for use and dosage as approved by the FDA. Because standards for usage change, it is advisable to keep abreast of revised recommendations, particularly those concerning new drugs.

Chapter 1

Value and Limitations of Cardiac Diagnostic Procedures
AN OVERVIEW

Peter F. Cohn and Joshua Wynne

Traditionally, physicians have relied on history taking and physical examination for evaluation of patients. Until the latter half of the twentieth century, only a limited number of laboratory tests were available to assist in this clinical assessment. In the last several decades, however, a burgeoning medical technology has altered this general approach and inundated the clinician with new diagnostic procedures. In no field of medicine has this phenomenon been felt more strongly than in cardiology. The array of currently available noninvasive diagnostic procedures is indeed awesome, ranging from simple blood tests to complex systems for imaging the heart. In addition to these noninvasive procedures, the development and refinement of cardiac catheterization and related procedures has provided an invasive "gold standard" with which to measure the noninvasive procedures. How is a clinician to approach these tests? In what order should they be performed? What do their results mean? Are there any dangers in performing them? In succeeding chapters, these issues will be addressed for the specific procedures that are discussed in detail. To provide each patient with effective care, however, the physician must maintain an overview into which these specific considerations fit.

Noninvasive cardiac diagnostic tests are composed of those procedures that rely on the electrocardiogram (such as the resting ECG, the 24-hour ambulatory monitor, and the exercise tolerance test); those procedures involving recording of the pulse tracings, usually along with a phonocardiographic recording; ultrasound, radioisotopic studies, nonangiographic x-ray studies, and serum blood tests. Invasive procedures include hemodynamic evaluations and left ventriculography, pulmonary angiography, and coronary angiography.

We believe that the resting electrocardiogram and chest x-ray belong in the first line of diagnostic tests. What to order next (in addition to the history and physical examination) will depend on what disease is suspected. If, for example, a patient with chest pain has findings suggesting coronary artery disease, an exercise tolerance test is the logical next procedure of choice. When this test cannot be interpreted properly, or when it is not unequivocally positive or negative, some type of radioisotopic study is indicated. Either a myocardial perfusion study or a radioisotopic ventriculogram could be performed, preferably during exercise. Cardiac catheterization is carried out only when these other tests have yielded whatever information they can. When coronary artery disease is acute, as in a suspected myocardial infarction, appropriate serum enzymes must be drawn, "hot spot" radioisotopic perfusion studies performed when indicated, and hemodynamic evaluations obtained in those patients in whom compromise of the left or right ventricle is likely. In this situation, cardiac catheterization is reserved for only those patients who are in shock or impending shock. Other tests that are of value in patients with suspected coronary artery disease are, of course, determination of risk factors, such as glucose intolerance and hyperlipidemia. When valvular heart disease is suspected, the first line of approach after the resting ECG and chest x-ray should include echocardiography, supplemented in some cases by external pulse tracings with phonocardiography. Cardiac catheterization is often performed but not as an initial procedure. If cardiomyopathy is strongly suspected, either echocardiography or a radionuclide ventriculogram should be ordered after the initial work-up. Diseases in which arrhythmias predominate must be evaluated with Holter monitoring or exercise testing.

In all these tests, the clinician must be aware of the value and limitations of the specific procedures, as discussed in the subsequent chapters. Few of these procedures approach 100 percent sensitivity and specificity; their clinical utility depends on the population in which they are being used. Their major value is in combining with one another rather than standing alone. Therefore, the clinician must learn which of these tests are most appropriate for the disease entity in question. Learning when to order which test is almost as important as learning what the results of these tests indicate.

Part I

Electrocardiography

Chapter 2

The Resting Electrocardiogram

Gilbert H. Mudge, Jr.

The resting electrocardiogram (ECG), one of the most common routine diagnostic tests, has become an integral part of any patient evaluation. An average of 1.4 ECGs are obtained for each hospital admission. Because of this ubiquitous nature, it is often awarded a diagnostic precision that is not entirely justified. An imperfect tool, its results can be interpreted to suggest significant cardiac abnormalities when the patient has a normal heart or may be entirely normal when the patient has advanced cardiac disease. This chapter attempts to place the resting ECG into perspective, emphasizing to the clinician who already has a firm working knowledge of electrocardiography both its capabilities and limitations.

A number of constitutional variables can substantially alter a normal ECG, including sex, age, body height and weight, race, and anatomic position of the heart within the chest as well as the conformation of the chest itself. Women may have smaller precordial lead voltage than do men, which may be attributed to a higher content of body fat and breast tissue insulating the precordial exploring electrode [1, 2]. Females likewise have a higher incidence of vertebral osteoporosis, with partial vertebral collapse, which can enhance R-wave voltage in the precordial leads by moving the heart closer to the exploring electrodes. Age is another significant variable in the normal ECG. The precordial lead voltage in the adolescent is usually significantly greater than later in life [3]. Such QRS changes may also be associated with a shift of the QRS axis in the frontal leads toward the left with progressive age [4]. Such shift in axis will also be seen with differences in body habitus. Obese middle-aged patients have a horizontal axis with diminished R-wave and T-wave amplitude, in contrast to the vertical axis associated with normal body weight. Such variations may be due to positional changes of the heart caused by a protuberant abdomen and elevated diaphragm. An otherwise normal ECG may vary according to race. The black population has been found to have a statistically significant shorter QRS interval, larger QRS amplitude, and a more posteriorly directed T-wave vector in the horizontal plane that leads to T-wave inversion in V1–V3, which may be a totally normal variant [1].

Besides such constitutional considerations, variations in the technique of obtaining electrocardiograms may lead to differences in the ECG changes. Some electrocardiographic machines do not respond in the proper frequency to appropriate signals. Significant Q waves seen with one electrocardiographic machine may be incorporated into the R wave by another recording apparatus. The ST segment and height of the T wave can also vary with differences in frequency response and do not reflect changes in the pathologic state. For this reason, subtle changes in the ECG must always be correlated with the clinical condition. Other technical factors, including the use of alcohol solution rather than saline for electrode contact, corroded electrodes, or inadequate contact of the electrodes with the skin may lead to recording falsely low voltage.

Despite meticulous technique, the ECG is also susceptible to day-to-day variations. Such variations in QRS excursion are most often seen in the precordial leads and may vary by as much as 3 to 4 mm [5]. For this reason, some patients may have marginal criteria for left ventricular hypertrophy on one tracing but will not meet those criteria with a subsequent ECG. There is also a natural variation to Q waves, most marked in the inferior leads. Q waves that do not meet criteria for myocardial infarction may be found in the inferior leads on one tracing but absent from the subsequent ECG. Proper evaluation of such small Q waves must include both supine and standing ECGs as well as expiratory and inspiratory tracings.

Variations in the Normal Electrocardiogram

Certain variations in the normal ECG deserve particular emphasis. Incomplete right bundle branch block is found in approximately 2 percent of the normal population and does not represent significant conduction abnormality [6]. The R' wave is thought to represent late, unopposed activation of the crista supraventricularis of the right ventricular outflow tract. In such cases, the R' wave is usually smaller than the R wave, with an amplitude usually less than 4 mm. In patients with significant right ventricular hypertrophy and coexistent incomplete right bundle branch block (see under Right Ventricular Hypertrophy), the R' wave is invariably taller than the R wave.

Another variation in the normal ECG is the S_1, S_2, S_3 pattern. In 20 percent of normal healthy individuals, the bipolar leads may be isoelectric, indicating that the mean vector of depolarization is nearly perpendicular to the frontal plane [6]. Such a finding is also seen in right ventricular hypertrophy, most often due to chronic obstructive pulmonary disease, but in this latter instance, other criteria for right ventricular hypertrophy are usually fulfilled.

Significant variation in T-wave morphology over the right precordial leads with T-wave inversion from V1 to V4 may be seen in normal patients. This is most often seen in healthy young females or the black patient population and can be mistaken for acute anterior myocardial ischemia (Fig. 2-1).

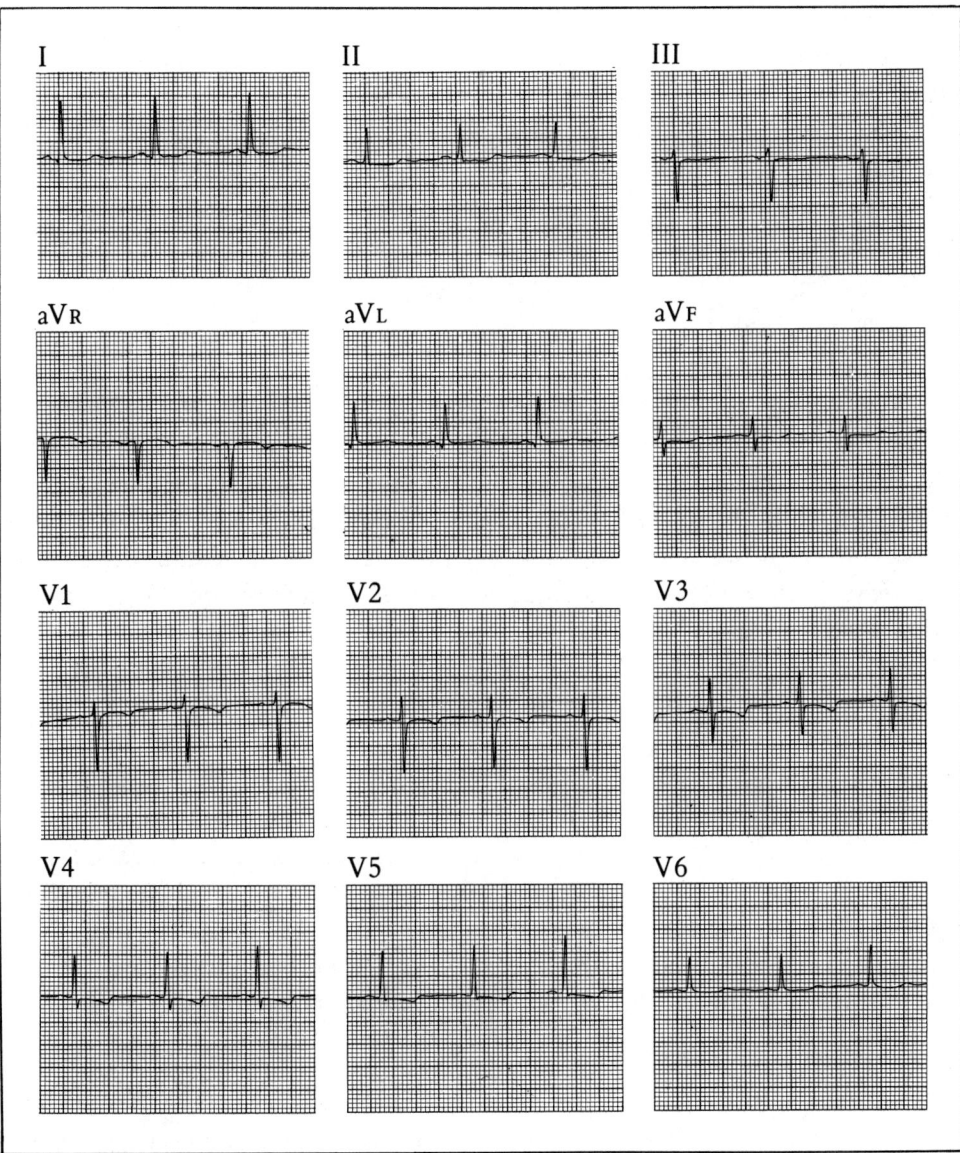

FIGURE 2-1. This ECG shows normal sinus rhythm with normal P–R and QRS intervals and normal QRS morphology. There is T-wave inversion over the anterior precordial leads from V1 to V4 suggestive of myocardial ischemia. This tracing was taken from an asymptomatic 43-year-old female with no evidence for heart disease, with normal coronary angiograms. Such T-wave changes can be a normal variant in the female and black population.

Early repolarization with ST-segment elevation in the anterolateral leads is also a normal variant. There is usually 1- to 2-mm ST-segment elevation, but it can be more pronounced in some individuals, leading to the erroneous diagnosis of either pericarditis or acute myocardial necrosis. In such instances of early repolarization, there is usually a notch at the end of the R wave with an upward concavity to the ST segment (Fig. 2-2). In addition, the T-wave morphology remains distinct and separated from the ST segment. This latter feature is of some help in differentiating the ST segments of acute myocardial necrosis from those of early repolarization.

Atrial Abnormalities

The normal atrial depolarization that originates from the sinus node is a composite of two different depolarizations. The initial right atrial force, directed both inferiorly and anteriorly, is followed by a later left atrial activation, which is directed posteriorly and inferiorly. The net result is to generate a wave of atrial depolarization that in the frontal plane has an axis of approximately 60 degrees, thus parallel to and best visualized in standard lead II; in the horizontal plane this depolarization is visualized as a biphasic configuration in V1. Because of later left atrial activation, a delay in its depolarization may generate electrocardiographic criteria for left atrial enlargement that does not have a true pathologic correlation. Recent studies correlating electrocardiographic criteria for left atrial enlargement with left atrial size and left atrial pressure have shown that in patients with coronary artery disease, the ECG pattern is unrelated to either the pressure or volume overload; an enlarged left atrium correlated with electrocardiographic criteria of left atrial enlargement only in those patients with rheumatic valvular heart disease [7]. Thus, it has been suggested that the term "left atrial enlargement" be replaced by "intraatrial conduction defect." At the present time, such terminology is not uniformly accepted. However, it is probably more appropriate to refer to "atrial abnormalities" rather than "atrial enlargement."

RIGHT ATRIAL ABNORMALITIES

Right atrial abnormalities will enhance the initial component of the P wave, enhancing the anteriorly and inferiorly directed forces without significant prolongation of the P wave. A P wave greater than 2.5 mm deflection in standard leads II, III, and aVF with a normal duration is consistent with right atrial enlargement. In V1, a P wave greater than 1.5 mm deflection is diagnostic of such right atrial abnormalities. However, the correlation between such electrocardiographic interpretation and pathologic findings is particularly poor. In 100 patients with electrocardiographic evidence for right atrial abnormalities, only 49 had right atrial enlargement, with 36 percent having significant left atrial rather than right atrial abnormalities [8]. In this study, criteria for right atrial abnormalities that were met in the right precordial leads were more sensitive for true right atrial enlargement than were those criteria as discussed for lead II.

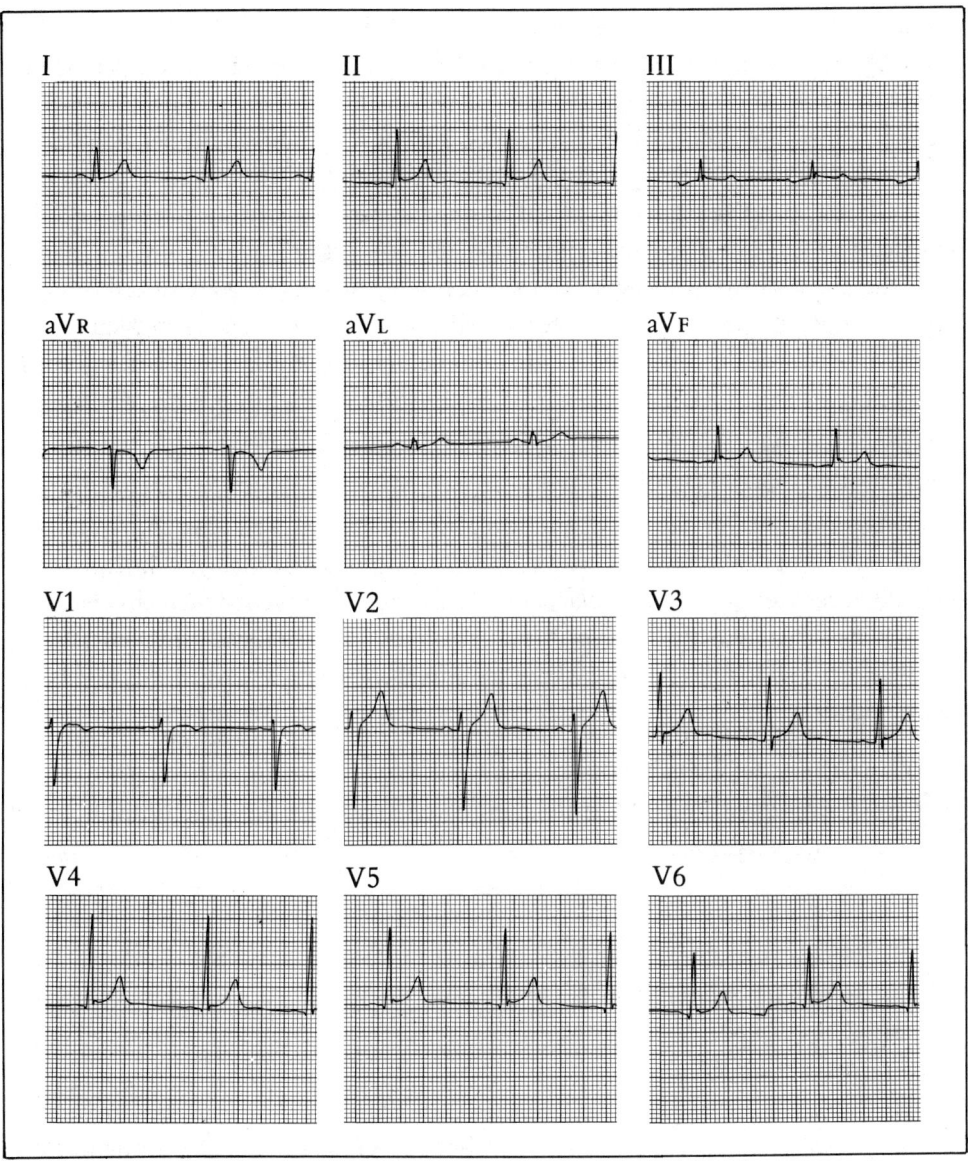

FIGURE 2-2. This tracing shows normal sinus rhythm with normal P–R and QRS intervals and normal QRS morphology. In standard leads II, III, and V3–V6 there is a slight notch at the end of the R wave, with ST-segment elevation. Such changes are characteristic of early repolarization and should not be interpreted as evidence for myocardial ischemia unless such changes correlate with the clinical presentation. The changes of early repolarization are usually most marked in the lateral precordial leads.

LEFT ATRIAL ABNORMALITIES

With either intraatrial conduction defect or left atrial enlargement, there is significant enhancement of the late posteriorly and inferiorly directed forces of left atrial activation. In the frontal lead system, the P wave becomes notched, with prolongation of the P-wave duration to 0.12 second or greater. This is best seen in standard leads I or II. In the horizontal plane, the left atrial abnormality generates a deep negative deflection with an area of 1 mm² (assuming a proper paper speed of 25 mm/sec) as recorded in V1. It should be noted that the negative component to the P wave in the right precordial leads may vary, deepening with progressive left heart failure [9, 10]. This latter criterion, using the P wave in V1, is considered the most sensitive and specific measurement for left atrial abnormalities. The term "P mitrale" is not specific, for the P mitrale pattern has been seen in constrictive pericarditis, myocarditis, atrial ischemia, atrial infarction, or significant atrial fibrosis and does not necessarily imply significant mitral valve disease [11].

Ventricular Hypertrophy

Since the normal left ventricle has three times the muscle mass and thus three times the electrical potential as the normal right ventricle, the normal ECG reflects forces of left ventricular depolarization. Left ventricular hypertrophy accentuates the normally dominant leftward forces, and in right ventricular hypertrophy, normal leftward forces are counterbalanced by enhanced rightward depolarization.

Left Ventricular Hypertrophy

The following have emerged as the standard electrocardiographic criteria for left ventricular hypertrophy.

1. Limb lead criteria
   a. R wave$_I$ + S$_{III}$ greater than 25 mm
   b. R in aV$_L$ greater than 11 mm
   c. R in aV$_F$ greater than 20 mm
2. Precordial lead criteria
   a. S$_{V1}$ or S$_{V2}$ + R$_{V5}$ or R$_{V6}$ greater than 35 mm
   b. Greatest R wave + the greatest S wave greater than 45 mm deflection
   c. R wave$_{V5}$ or R wave$_{V6}$ greater than 26 mm deflection

If one uses these criteria, 70 to 80 percent of true pathologic left ventricular hypertrophy states can be identified by the ECG, with a false-positive rate of approximately 15 percent [12]. Because of this high incidence of false-positive diagnosis, Romhilt and Estes proposed the following point score system in the diagnosis of left ventricular hypertrophy [13]:

1. Amplitude (3 points) (any of the following):
   a. Largest R wave or S wave in the limb leads greater than 20 mm deflection
   b. S wave in V1 or V2 greater than 30 mm deflection
   c. R wave in V5 or V6 greater than 30 mm deflection
2. ST-segment and T-wave abnormalities
   a. Without digitalis (3 points)
   b. With digitalis (1 point)
3. Left atrial abnormality: criteria mentioned above for left atrial abnormality (3 points)
4. Left axis deviation: −30 degrees or more (2 points)
5. QRS duration greater than 0.09 second (1 point)
6. Intrinsicoid deflection in V5 or V6 greater than 0.05 second (1 point)

Left ventricular hypertrophy is considered to be present when the total number of points is 5 or more. This multiple point system has a false-positive diagnosis rate of only 3 percent; unfortunately, it also has a 46 percent incidence of false-negative interpretation.

There are several reasons for the poor correlations between the electrocardiographic diagnosis of left ventricular hypertrophy and cardiac pathology. The distinction at autopsy between a normal and hypertrophied ventricle is often difficult [14]. Measurement of wall thickness at autopsy is imprecise because of loss of muscle tone; total heart or chamber weight depends upon the individual dissection technique. The normal physiologic factors of age, sex, race, and body habitus also affect QRS amplitude and make precise correlation difficult. Other pathologic conditions may mask the voltage generated by left ventricular hypertrophy. Patients with left ventricular hypertrophy and chronic congestive heart failure may develop enough right ventricular hypertrophy secondary to pulmonary hypertension to partially mask the voltage criteria of left ventricular hypertrophy [15]. Myocardial fibrosis, recurrent myocardial infarctions, and interventricular conduction defects may alter QRS amplitude and thus mask the diagnosis of left ventricular hypertrophy. Acute cardiac enlargement with acute congestive heart failure has also been reported to decrease the QRS amplitude, thus masking the conventional criteria for left ventricular hypertrophy [16].

Right Ventricular Hypertrophy

Normal right ventricular depolarization is masked by the more dominant forces of left ventricular depolarization on the normal ECG. Significant right ventricular hypertrophy distorts these forces of left ventricular depolarization, the type of distortion depending in part on the underlying etiology of the hypertrophy. Such distortion is best appreciated if one has an understanding of the vector of depolarization in the transverse or horizontal plane. As shown in Figure 2-3, initial septal depolarization takes place in a left-to-right direction. The forces of depolarization then sweep around to the left, the latter forces directed back posteriorly. In a normal individual, as much as 50 percent of the transverse vector may be directed anteriorly, the balance directed back leftward and posteriorly. This transverse sequence of depolarization is significantly altered in the different forms of right ventricular hypertrophy.

Type A Right Ventricular Hypertrophy
In type A right ventricular hypertrophy, most often seen in patients with congenital heart disease (pulmonic stenosis, tetralogy of Fallot, and Eisenmenger's syndrome) the entire direction of the transverse sequence of depolarization is altered. As shown in Figure 2-3, forces of right ventricular depolarization completely outweigh those of left ventricular activation, swinging the vector of depolarization to the right. This results in a clockwise vector loop. Because of this reversal in direction, a tall R wave will be inscribed in V1, with a deep S wave in V6. The normal location of the septum may be distorted by the enlarged right ventricle, with an abnormal initial leftward septal depolarization generating a small Q wave in V1. Figure 2-4 is an example of type A right ventricular hypertrophy.

Type B Right Ventricular Hypertrophy
As shown in Figure 2-3, this pattern of right ventricular hypertrophy occurs when the enhanced forces of right ventricular depolarization balance left ventricular activation. Thus, most of the vector loop in the horizontal plane is displaced anteriorly, which generates a tall positive R wave equal to or greater than the S wave in V1. To be diagnostic of type B right ventricular hypertrophy, at least 70 percent of the vector must be located anteriorly. This pattern is most often seen in acquired right ventricular hypertrophy, mitral stenosis and atrial septal defect being the paramount clinical examples (Fig. 2-5).

Type C Right Ventricular Hypertrophy
This pattern of right ventricular hypertrophy occurs most frequently in patients with chronic obstructive pulmonary disease. By displacing the left ventricle posteriorly, the enlarged right ventricle, instead of reversing or balancing the vector of left ventricular depolarization, merely accentuates the final posterior direction back to the right. As shown in Figure 2-3, septal depolarization is normal initially, with subsequent leftward shift of left ventricular depolarization. The final forces of ventricular depolarization are shifted far posteriorly and back

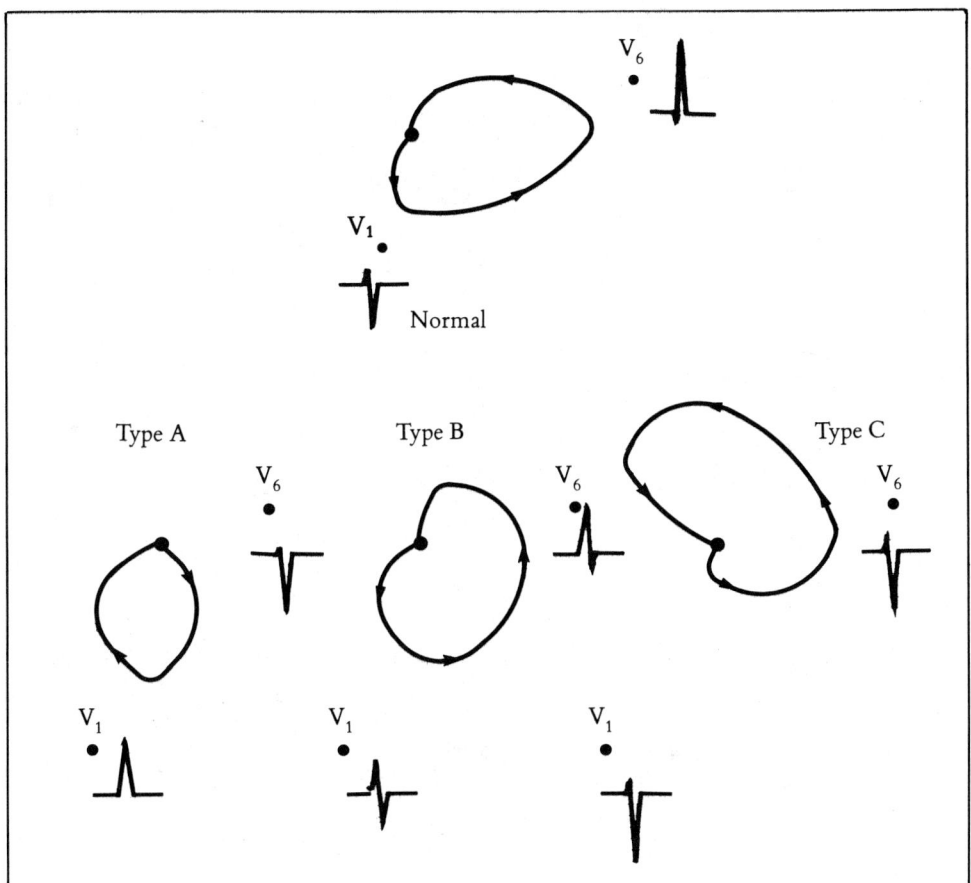

FIGURE 2-3. The three patterns of right ventricular hypertrophy are depicted. The normal horizontal vector of depolarization shows initial septal depolarization in a left-to-right direction, the left ventricular forces then shifting the vector around anteriorly and back to the left, with the major portion of this loop directed posteriorly. In type A right ventricular hypertrophy, the loop is directed entirely rightward in a clockwise fashion. In type B right ventricular hypertrophy, the vector of depolarization is still inscribed in the normal counterclockwise direction, but the hypertrophic right ventricle displaces at least 50 percent of the vector loop anteriorly. In type C right ventricular hypertrophy, the enlarged right ventricular chamber displaces the left ventricle posteriorly, accentuating all the posteriorly directed forces of left ventricular depolarization. (From GH Mudge Jr: *Manual of Electrocardiography*. Boston: Little, Brown, 1981, p 30.)

toward the right. Thus, a normal QRS is inscribed in V1, but a deep S wave is recorded at V6, indicating these late forces moving posteriorly and back to the right. Poor R-wave progression across the anterior precordial leads is characteristic of type C right ventricular hypertrophy (Fig. 2-6).

The changes seen in type A, type B, or type C right ventricular hypertrophy

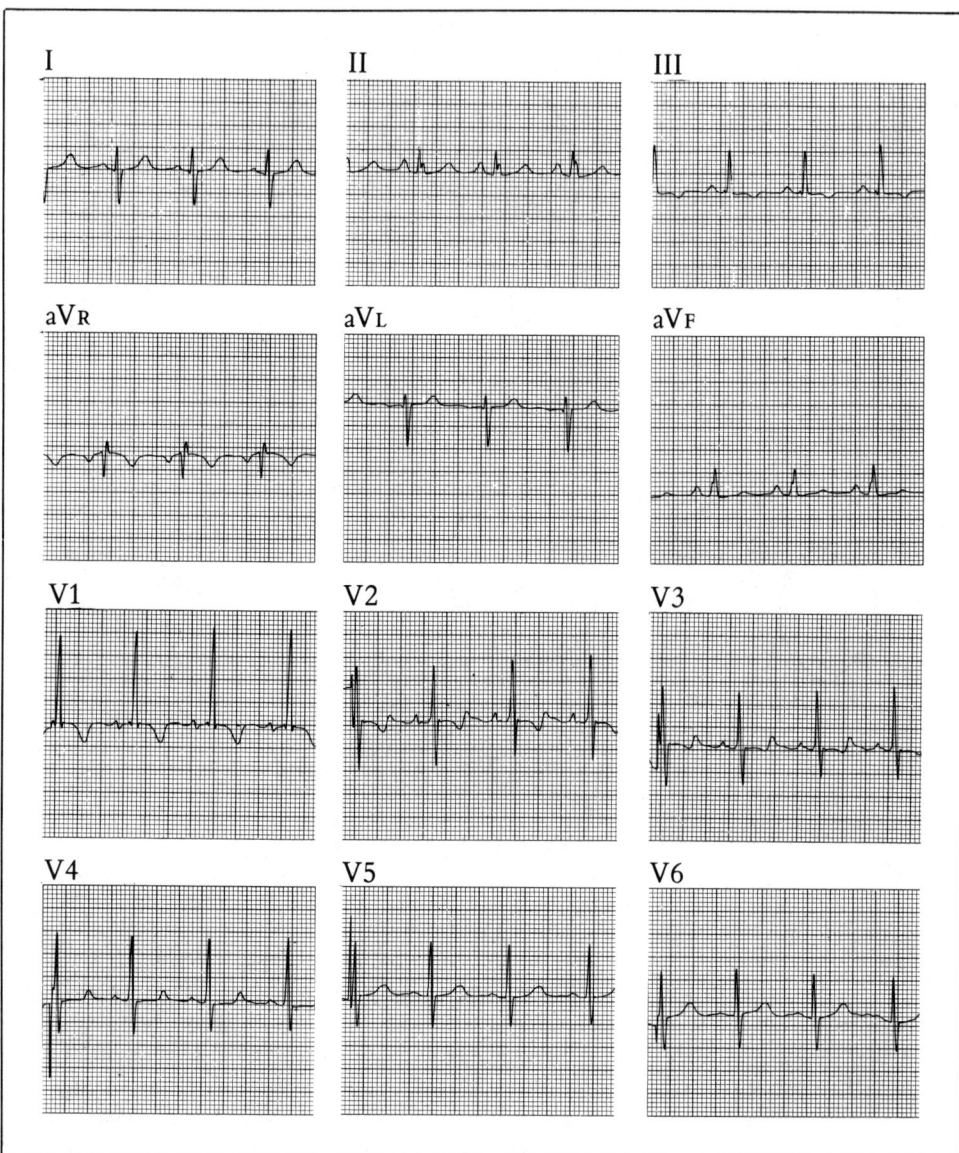

FIGURE 2-4. Type A right ventricular hypertrophy in a patient with pulmonic stenosis. The rhythm is normal sinus, with a normal P–R interval and QRS duration. The axis is directed rightward, and there is T-wave inversion over the right precordial leads. The extremely tall R wave in V1 suggests that the horizontal forces of depolarization are all directed in a clockwise direction toward the right precordial leads, most characteristic of type A right ventricular hypertrophy, which is usually seen in congenital heart disease. (From GH Mudge Jr: *Manual of Electrocardiography*. Boston: Little, Brown, 1981, p 36.)

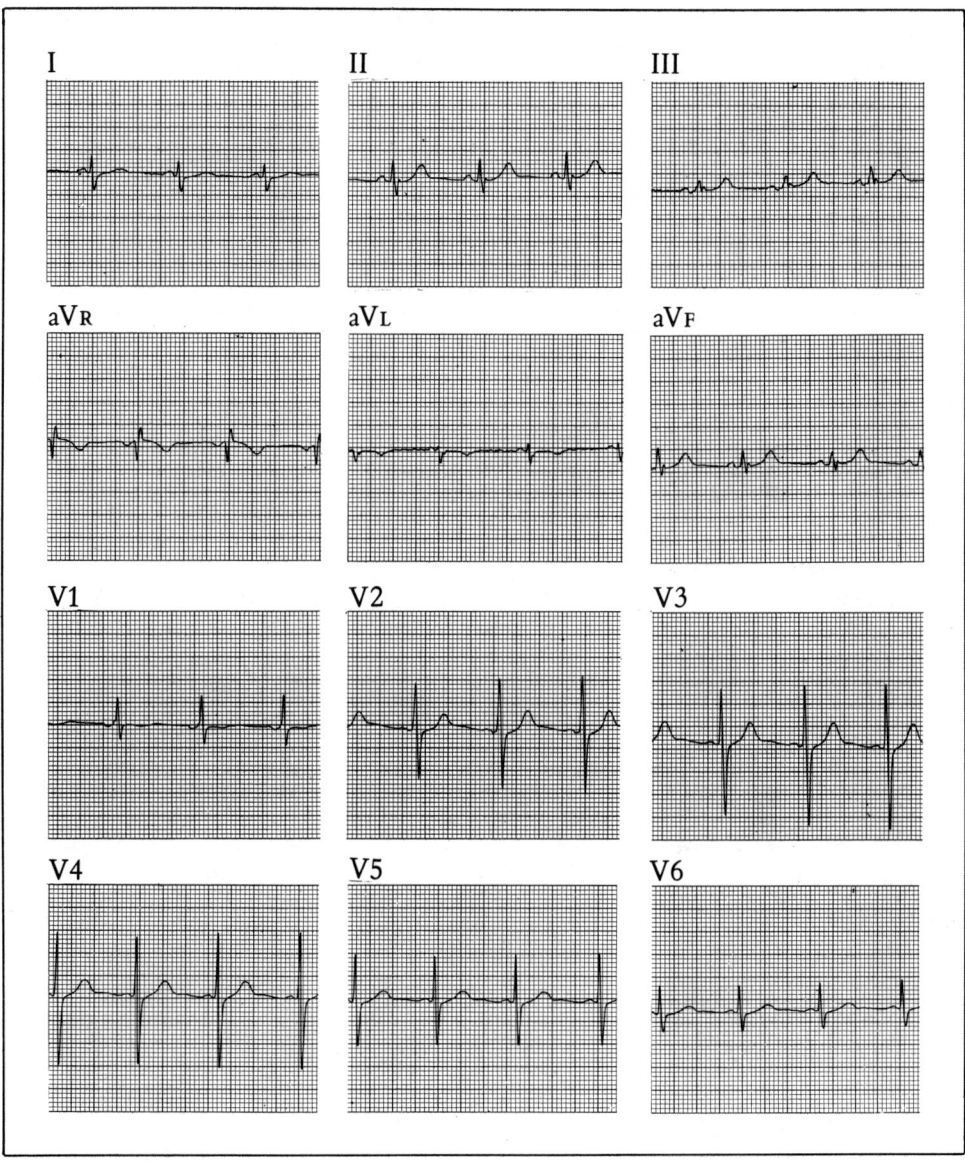

FIGURE 2-5. Type B right ventricular hypertrophy in a patient with atrial septal defect. The rhythm is normal sinus with a normal P–R interval and QRS duration. The axis is +100 degrees. There is an accentuated S wave in V6. The R wave is equal to or greater than the S wave in V1, diagnostic of right ventricular hypertrophy. This prominent R wave in V1 suggests that the anterior forces of depolarization in the horizontal plane are accentuated, most characteristic of type B right ventricular hypertrophy. (From GH Mudge Jr: *Manual of Electrocardiography*. Boston: Little, Brown, 1981, p 33.)

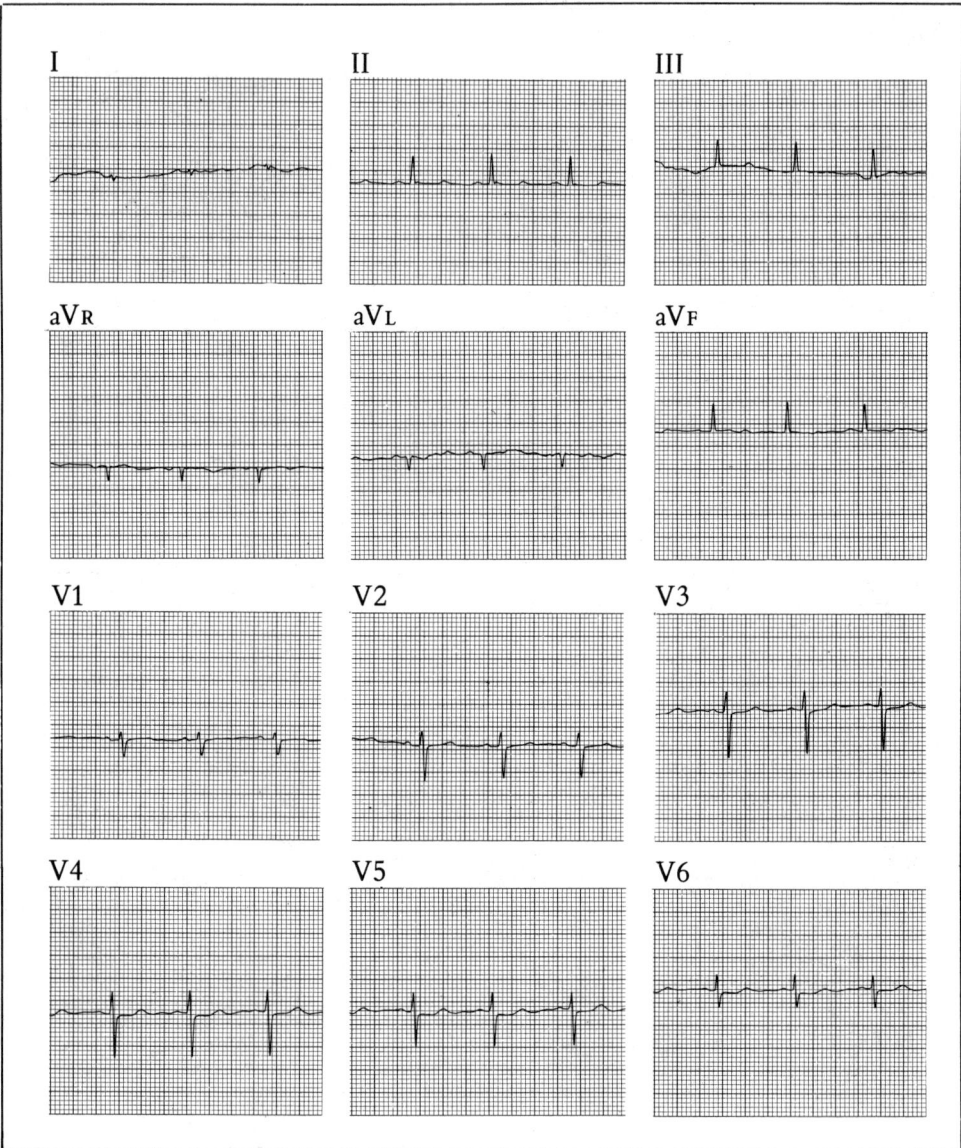

FIGURE 2-6. Type C right ventricular hypertrophy. This characteristic tracing shows normal sinus rhythm with normal P–R interval and QRS duration. The voltage is low. The axis is +90 degrees. There is poor R-wave progression across the anterior precordial leads. The diagnostic feature for right ventricular hypertrophy in this tracing is not alteration in the R/S ratio in V1, but rather the deep S wave in V6, which equals the R wave there. (From GH Mudge Jr: *Manual of Electrocardiography*. Boston: Little, Brown, 1981, p 34.)

involve a distortion in the R/S ratio in either V1 or V6. In type A and type B right ventricular hypertrophy, the R/S ratio in V1 is equal to or greater than 1, while in type C right ventricular hypertrophy, the R/S ratio in V6 is less than 1.

The other major criterion for right ventricular hypertrophy is an axis in the frontal plane of +110 degrees or more positive. Thus, the conventional electrocardiographic criteria for right ventricular hypertrophy include (1) a right axis deviation of greater than 110 degrees, (2) R/S ratio in V1 equal to or greater than 1, or (3) R/S ratio in V6 less than 1.

There are other minor, more subtle diagnostic features of right ventricular hypertrophy. An R wave in V1 greater than 7 mm is secondary evidence for enhanced right ventricular forces. Likewise, a shallow S wave seen in V1 is supporting evidence for right ventricular hypertrophy; an S wave less than 2 mm in deflection is most consistent with right ventricular hypertrophy. Type A or type B right ventricular hypertrophy may generate R′ waves, which do not necessarily indicate right bundle branch block, since the QRS duration is not prolonged. With right bundle branch block, an R′ wave greater than 10 mm in deflection should be considered suggestive of right ventricular hypertrophy, for it represents enhanced and late forces of right ventricular depolarization.

It should be emphasized that the electrocardiographic diagnosis of right ventricular hypertrophy is often subtle. The normal right ventricle is only 3 mm in thickness, and a doubling of right ventricular muscle mass may not be enough to shift forces of left ventricular depolarization both anteriorly and to the right [17]. This is especially true in the adult population with acquired right ventricular hypertrophy, who may never develop the full criteria as listed above. False-negative interpretations can result because of combined left ventricular hypertrophy, right or left bundle branch block, or an anteroseptal myocardial infarction that accentuates the lateral forces of left ventricular depolarization. A false-positive diagnosis of right ventricular hypertrophy may be made in normal young patients with vertical hearts, right bundle branch block, posterior myocardial infarction, dextrocardia, Wolff-Parkinson-White preexcitation syndrome, or a left posterior fascicular block [17].

Combined Ventricular Hypertrophy

Combined ventricular hypertrophy can be recognized when both criteria of right and left ventricular hypertrophy are met. However, it is rare that both criteria are fulfilled, the majority of patients showing nonspecific ST and T-wave changes and the QRS abnormalities balancing themselves out. Only about 17 percent of patients with combined ventricular hypertrophy proved on autopsy have the expected electrocardiographic findings [18].

Acute Pulmonary Embolism

ECG changes in acute pulmonary embolism result from acute dilatation of the right ventricle due to sudden increase in pulmonary arterial pressure. With sudden right ventricular dilatation, the left ventricle rotates posteriorly and back to the right, the heart taking on a more vertical position. The net effect of this will be to shift the mean QRS vector in the frontal plane superiorly, posteriorly, and back to the right, while the QRS vector in the horizontal plane shifts posteriorly. This displacement causes the following classic ECG changes for acute pulmonary embolism [19, 20]:

1. S_1Q_3 or $S_1Q_3T_3$ pattern, which reflects a superior and rightward shift of forces
2. Shift of the QRS axis toward the right
3. Transient complete or incomplete right bundle branch block
4. T-wave inversion over the right precordial leads, representing acute systolic overload of the right ventricle
5. Displacement of the precordial lead transition zone to the left, with development of a QR pattern in V1 and V2

The specificity of such ECG findings in acute pulmonary embolism has been analyzed by the Urokinase-Pulmonary Embolism Trial [21]. These patients had symptoms suggestive of pulmonary embolism for at least 5 days prior to their entry into study, and all had pulmonary arteriography, documenting a filling defect in at least one segmental pulmonary artery. ST-segment depression or T-wave inversion was the most common abnormality noted. The more traditional ECG changes of pulmonary embolism listed above, including right bundle branch block and right axis deviation, were present in only about 30 percent of the patients with massive pulmonary emboli. Six percent of those patients with massive pulmonary emboli had normal ECGs, as did 23 percent of those patients with submassive embolization. One can probably assume that in patients with even smaller pulmonary emboli, the incidence of normal ECGs significantly increases. In light of these conclusions, perhaps the best role for the ECG in this patient population is refining the differential diagnosis between acute myocardial infarction and massive pulmonary embolism [22].

Intraventricular Conduction Defects

Right Bundle Branch Block

The sequence of left ventricular activation remains normal in the presence of right bundle branch block. Hence, the criteria for left ventricular hypertrophy and acute myocardial infarction remain valid with this intraventricular conduction defect. However, the criteria for right ventricular hypertrophy (right axis deviation and alteration of the R/S ratio in V1 or V6) become less specific. With right bundle branch block and a QRS duration of greater than 0.12 second, an R' wave greater than 10 mm deflection should be suspect for right ventricular hypertrophy [23]. The specificity of this criterion has not been adequately tested.

LEFT BUNDLE BRANCH BLOCK

The presence of left bundle branch block indicates an anomalous sequence of left ventricular depolarization; hence, the usual criteria for left ventricular hypertrophy or acute left ventricular necrosis do not hold true. The specificity and sensitivity of voltage criteria in the setting of a left bundle branch block configuration have not been established.

In one instance acute myocardial necrosis can be interpreted with preexistent left bundle branch block configuration. As shown in Figure 2-7, the septum is depolarized in a right-to-left direction in left bundle branch block. This slow right-to-left depolarization generates a slurred R wave recorded in V6 that is characteristic of the intraventricular conduction defect. In a patient with preexistent left bundle branch block, a septal myocardial infarction will significantly alter these right-to-left forces of depolarization. Figure 2-7 shows the changes that result following a septal myocardial infarction. There is no longer right-to-left depolarization of the septum, and the normal early activation of the right ventricle is now unopposed. In V6, this generates a small Q wave representing early, unopposed right ventricular activation before the formation of the slurred R wave, representing delayed left ventricular depolarization. These small Q waves may also be seen in standard lead I and aVL. Thus, in patients with preexistent left bundle branch block configuration, the development of small Q waves in the anterolateral leads indicates that right ventricular depolarization is now unopposed and is electrocardiographic evidence for a septal infarction. Figure 2-8 is an example of anteroseptal myocardial infarction superimposed on left bundle branch block.

Myocardial Ischemia and Necrosis

MYOCARDIAL INFARCTION

With acute myocardial necrosis, the forces of depolarization are no longer generated in the damaged area; thus the remaining forces of ventricular depolarization are accentuated, displacing the mean QRS vector in each lead system away from the zone of necrosis. This generates the abnormal, pathologic Q waves of myocardial infarction. The necrotic area will no longer be capable of depolarization, contraction, or repolarization, but it is always surrounded by an area of ischemic

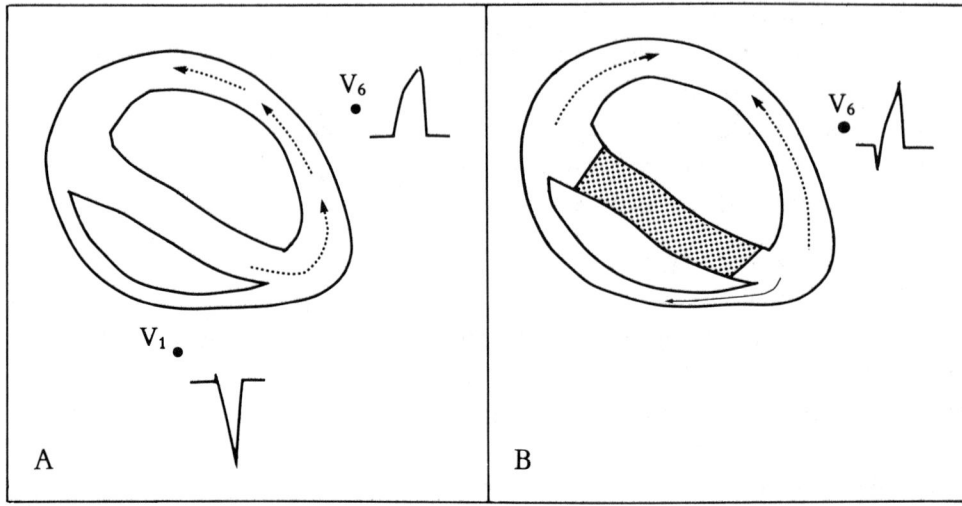

FIGURE 2-7. (A) Normal sequence of left ventricular depolarization in left bundle branch block; the septum is depolarized in a right-to-left direction. This septal depolarization generates a slurred upstroke in V6, characteristic of left bundle branch block and masking normal right ventricular depolarization. (B) Following septal necrosis, right ventricular depolarization is unmasked and appears as a rightward force of depolarization, generating a small Q wave in the lateral precordial leads, representing early right ventricular depolarization before delayed left ventricular activation. The development of a Q wave in the lateral precordial leads (and lead I) representing unmasked right ventricular activation in the setting of preexistent left bundle branch block can be interpreted as evidence for a new septal myocardial infarction.

myocardium, incompletely depolarized with each ventricular activation. Such incomplete depolarization generates ST-segment elevation in that particular area of myocardium overlying acute necrosis and may generate ST-segment depression in those leads that explore a portion of ventricular tissue adjacent to the necrotic area. Because the sequence of ventricular depolarization is altered by acute myocardial ischemia and necrosis, the T waves become inverted or occasionally accentuated.

Generally, significant Q waves should be 0.04 second in duration and have an excursion that is approximately 25 percent of the height of the R wave in the QRS complex. These two criteria are usually adequate for defining a pathologic condition. However, there are minor variations to these criteria that deserve emphasis.

Acute Anterior Myocardial Infarction
A QS or QR complex in V1–V4 that fits the above criteria is diagnostic of an acute anterior myocardial infarction. A decrease in the R-wave excursion over the anterior precordial leads is also consistent with acute anterior necrosis. Reversed R-wave progression, the R wave diminishing from V1 to V4, is often overlooked

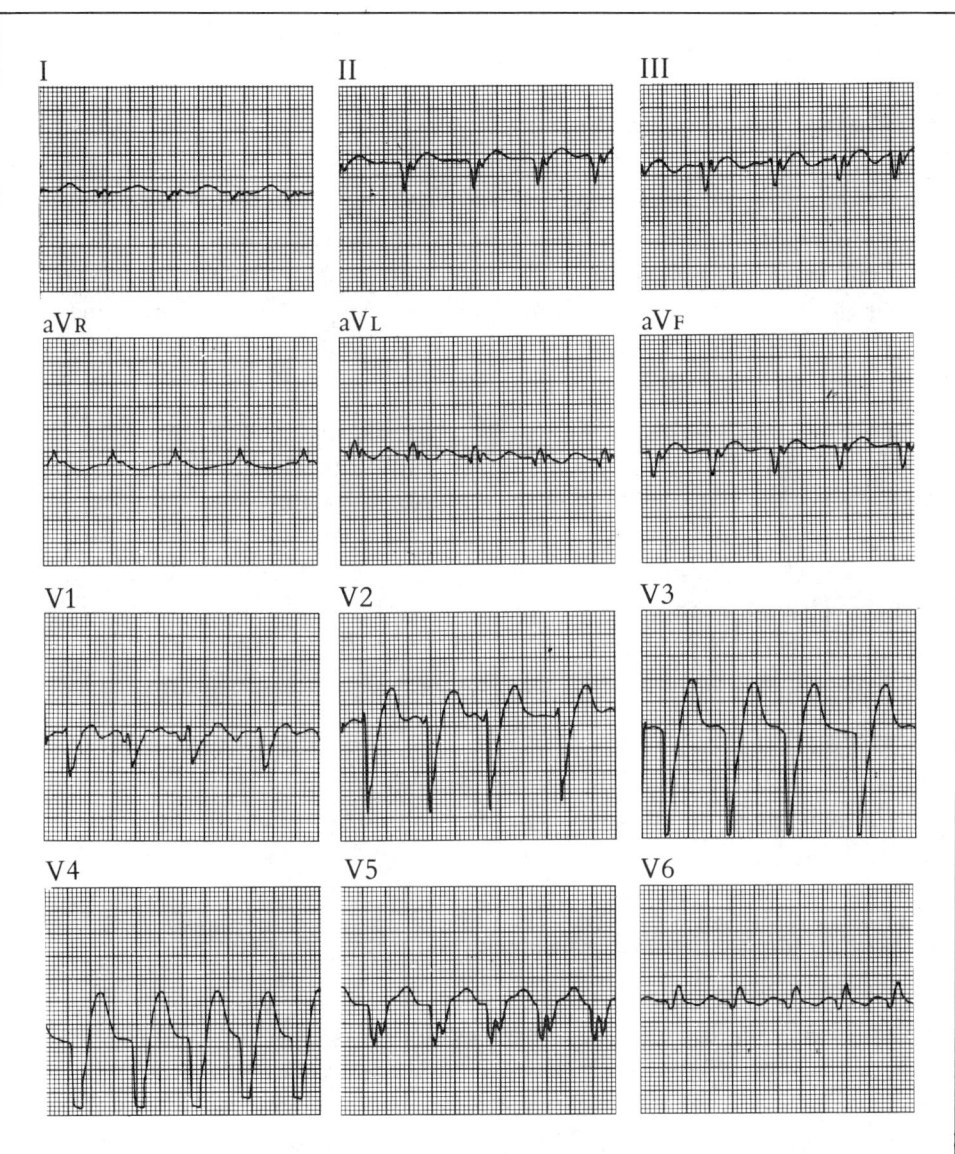

FIGURE 2-8. The rhythm is normal sinus, with normal P-R interval. There is prolonged QRS duration, with delay in ventricular activation time of the left precordial lead indicative of left bundle branch block. In addition, there are Q waves over the lateral precordial leads, indicating early rightward directed forces of ventricular depolarization. This is diagnostic of an anterior septal myocardial infarction in the presence of underlying left bundle branch block.

as a criterion for anterior wall damage. In addition, absent R-wave or poor R-wave progression over the anterior precordial leads may be seen in left ventricular hypertrophy or type C right ventricular hypertrophy. It should be reemphasized that T-wave inversion over the anterior precordial leads may be a normal variant, most often seen in the female and black patient population.

Anterolateral Myocardial Infarction

Significant Q waves in the lateral precordial leads, V4–V6, should be 0.04 second in duration and at least 20 percent of the total amplitude of the QRS complex. These criteria are important, since small, insignificant Q waves may be generated in the normal lateral precordial leads, representing septal depolarization in a left-to-right direction. The same left-to-right septal depolarization forces may also generate a Q wave in aVL and standard lead I. A significant Q wave in aVL should also be 0.04 second in duration but with an excursion that is 50 percent of the subsequent R wave. A significant Q wave in standard lead I should be of similar duration but need be only 20 percent of the R-wave amplitude. Q waves in standard leads I and aVL that do not meet these criteria should not be interpreted as pathologic in origin. A high lateral myocardial infarction should be suspected when there are significant Q waves in the frontal lead system, I and aVL, with no significant changes in the conventional precordial leads. In such an instance, high lateral precordial leads, obtained by moving the entire precordial leads from V1 to V6 up one intercostal interspace, may further define the area of damage.

Inferior Myocardial Infarction

A Q wave in standard lead III may be entirely normal, and thus must always be interpreted in light of ECG changes seen in standard leads II and aVF. The Q wave in these two leads must be 0.04 second in duration and 25 percent of the amplitude of the R wave to be considered significant for myocardial damage.

True Posterior Myocardial Infarction

True posterior myocardial infarctions are the most often overlooked ECG changes. The R wave across the anterior precordial leads is accentuated because of loss of opposing forces of depolarization from the posterior wall, forces of depolarization that move away from the precordial exploring electrodes. The accentuated R wave in V1 or V2 is the mirror image of the Q wave that would be recorded by an exploring electrode located behind the posterior wall of the left ventricle. Therefore, the R wave in V1 or V2 should be greater than the S wave in V1 to be considered diagnostic for true posterior wall damage. These criteria for true posterior wall infarction are invalid if there is coexistent right ventricular hypertrophy.

Abnormal Q waves in general have been correlated with autopsy findings in several studies. Significant Q waves limited either to the anterior precordial leads, V1–V4, or to the inferior leads, standard leads II, III, and aVF, were found to have a false-positive incidence of 46 percent, predictive of myocardial infarction in less than half the patients [24]. Abnormal Q waves appearing in the lateral precordial leads are far more sensitive, with a false-positive incidence of only 4 percent, and significant Q waves that appear in more than one particular area of left ventricular myocardium are equally reliable for documenting the presence of coronary artery disease [25]. Pathologic Q waves have also been correlated with arteriographic findings. Forty-eight patients were studied who had documented inferior wall infarction and total or subtotal obstruction of the right coronary artery with associated inferior wall contraction abnormalities [26]. Fourteen (29 percent) of these patients did not have significant Q waves in any leads, while only seven (15 percent) had diagnostic Q waves in standard leads II, III, and aVF. Lead aVF was felt to be the most reliable lead for the diagnosis of an inferior wall infarction. A significant Q wave in III occurs in 5 to 10 percent of the normal population; inspiratory-expiratory tracings are unreliable in further differentiating the significance of such abnormalities in III [27].

Pathologic Q waves in leads I, aVL, and V5–V6 are more specific for a lateral wall infarction than the anterior or inferior lead system. The one condition to produce pathologic Q waves with a pseudoinfarction pattern is hypertrophic cardiomyopathy, where enhanced forces of septal depolarization in a left-to-right direction generate deep and wide Q-wave deflection.

Pseudoinfarction Patterns

Multiple cardiac anomalies that may mimic acute myocardial necrosis on ECG in the absence of coronary artery disease are listed in Table 2-1 [28, 29]. The more common etiologies deserve emphasis. Left ventricular hypertrophy may generate poor R-wave progression over the anterior precordial leads, suggesting an anterior wall myocardial infarction. Such poor R-wave progression is due to enhanced forces of ventricular depolarization over the lateral wall of the left ventricle. This pseudoinfarction pattern is of particular importance in patients with aortic valve disease, whose initial clinical presentation may include significant anginal pain. Pulmonary emphysema and chronic obstructive pulmonary disease with type C right ventricular hypertrophy may also present with poor R-wave progression. In this instance, the right axis deviation is adequate to differentiate anterior wall myocardial infarction and right ventricular hypertrophy. Pneumothorax is another common etiology of a pseudoinfarction pattern on ECG. Because of displacement of the heart and mediastinum, both the QRS voltage may be reduced and the QRS axis significantly shifted, generating what is interpreted as pathologic Q waves [30]. The ECG changes of acute pulmonary embolism may likewise mask those of acute myocardial necrosis, as previously discussed. Acute increases in intracranial pressure cause widespread ST and T-wave abnormalities [31]. In this instance, the Q–T interval is usually prolonged, with deep T-wave inversion. Figure 2-9 is an example of such changes seen with intracranial hemorrhage.

TABLE 2-1. COMMON CAUSES OF PSEUDOINFARCTION PATTERNS ON ECG

Left ventricular hypertrophy
Chronic obstructive pulmonary disease
Right ventricular hypertrophy
Cor pulmonale
Pneumothorax
Pulmonary embolism
Hypertrophic cardiomyopathy (obstructive and nonobstructive)
Congestive cardiomyopathy
Myocarditis
Amyloid heart disease
Neoplasms of the heart
Leukemic infiltrates in the heart
Left bundle branch block
Left ventricular aneurysm
Left anterior fascicular block
Wolff-Parkinson-White syndrome
Increased intracranial pressure
Hyperkalemia
Trauma
Muscular dystrophy
Friedreich's ataxia

However, in such instances of increased intracranial pressure, pathologic Q waves are rarely formed. Hyperkalemia classically causes peaked T waves, which may incorporate some ST-segment elevation. This can be easily confused with the acute current of injury of myocardial necrosis [32]. Wolff-Parkinson-White (pre-excitation) syndrome can cause pathologic Q waves in both the inferior and anterior leads owing to initial, aberrant forces of depolarization from the accessory bypass tract. When patients with this condition are conducting down the accessory tract, a delta wave is present on the ECG. This makes further conclusions regarding the QRS morphology (infarction and the like) difficult or impossible. Left anterior hemiblock may also mimic an acute anterior myocardial infarction. Because of the initial downward and posterior forces of ventricular depolarization, with later superiorly and laterally directed forces, there may be Q waves or poor R-wave progression recorded over the anterior leads.

ST and T-Wave Changes

While the Q wave is the permanent electrocardiographic marker for cardiac necrosis, changes in the ST segment and T wave provide a better index for the

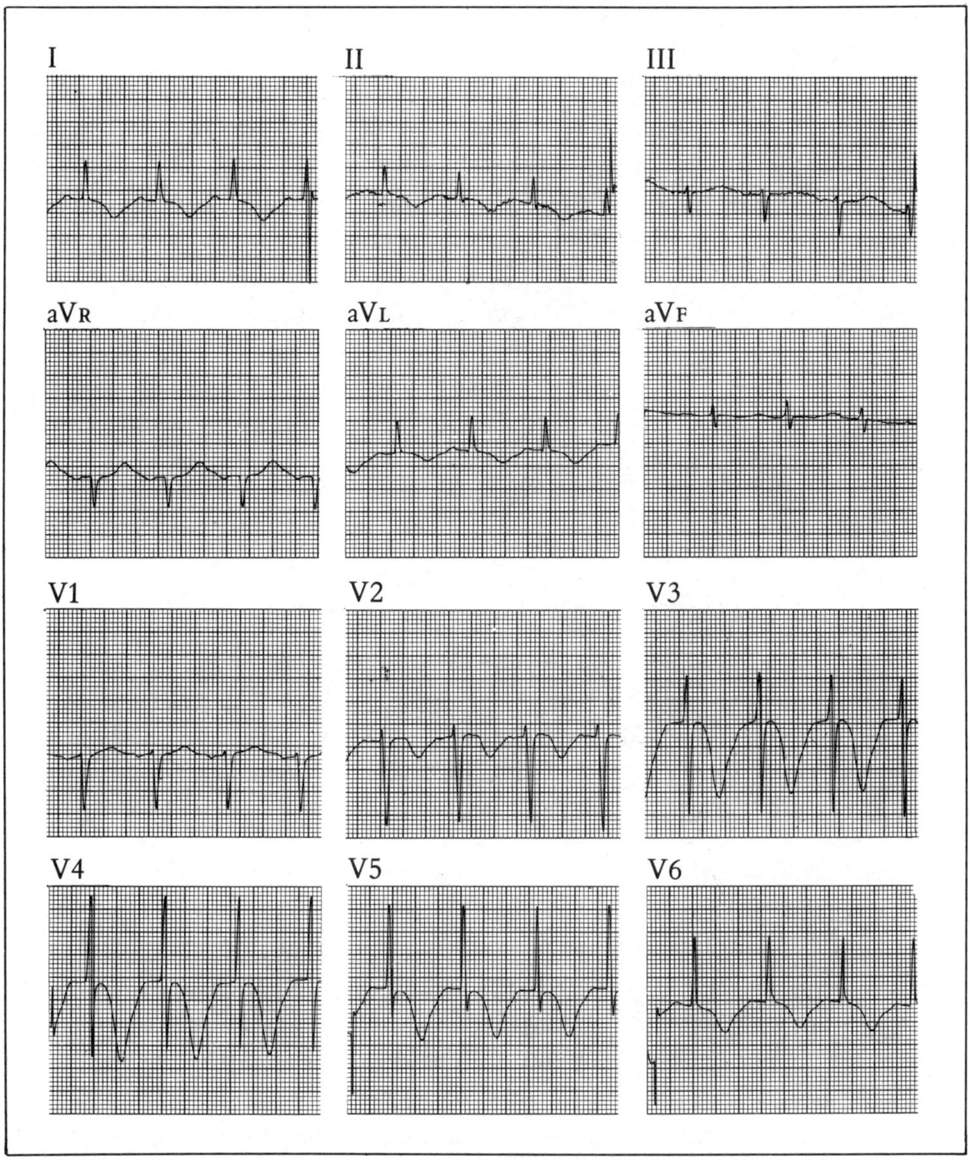

FIGURE 2-9. The rhythm is normal sinus, and the P–R and QRS intervals are normal. The axis is normal and QRS morphology is normal. There is significant Q–T prolongation and deep T-wave inversion over both inferior and anterior leads. Such T-wave inversion might be interpreted as evidence for myocardial ischemia. However, such changes, especially with a Q–T interval prolongation, are also seen with increased intracranial pressure. (From GH Mudge Jr: *Manual of Electrocardiography.* Boston: Little, Brown, 1981, p 165.)

duration of the necrotic process. Peaked and tall T waves may be the initial indication of acute myocardial infarction, the T waves soon incorporated into the ST segment as it too becomes elevated. As the ST segment returns to baseline, the T waves become symmetrically inverted in those exploring electrodes visualizing the damaged area of myocardium. Left ventricular aneurysm should be suspected on the ECG if ST-segment elevation persists for 2 weeks following the acute myocardial infarction [33]. A recent study concluded that 95 percent of patients with inferior wall infarction and 40 percent of patients with anterior wall infarction should have resolution of ST-segment elevation within 2 weeks. Persistent ST-segment elevation was associated with ventricular aneurysm. However, it should be noted that ST-segment elevation is not a particularly sensitive indicator for such left ventricular aneurysms, since many aneurysms documented by pathologic examination do not have corresponding ST-segment abnormalities [34].

Diffuse ST-Segment and T-Wave Abnormalities

ST-SEGMENT ABNORMALITIES

ST-segment depression is nonspecific. While it may be an index of myocardial ischemia or injury, identical ST-segment alterations in the lateral as well as inferior leads can be produced by left ventricular hypertrophy, hyperkalemia, hypokalemia, or hypomagnesemia. Such changes over the right precordial leads are slightly more reliable for specific pathologic conditions, seen with right ventricular hypertrophy and infarction of the true posterior wall.

T-WAVE ABNORMALITIES

T-wave contour is susceptible to many extracardiac factors. T-wave inversion or flattening is nonspecific for ischemic heart disease, but the presence of deep, symmetric T-wave inversion is somewhat more suggestive of the diagnosis. T-wave contour is not only affected by many pathologic cardiac conditions but may also be altered by exercise, hyperventilation, food ingestion, smoking, or significant electrolyte disturbance [35].

The normal amplitude for T-wave excursion has never been firmly established. Precordial T waves that are greater than 10 mm in deflection, however, should be highly suspect for hyperkalemia; they may also be seen in the right precordial leads in patients with left ventricular hypertrophy [36].

References

1. Nemati M, McCaughan D, Doyle J, Pipberger HV: The influence of constitutional variables on orthogonal electrocardiograms of normal women. *Circulation* 56:989, 1977

2. Simonson E, Blackburn H, Puchner TC, Eisenberg P, Ribeiro F, Meja M: Sex differences in the electrocardiogram. *Circulation* 22:598, 1960
3. Manning GW, Smiley JR: QRS voltage criteria for left ventricular hypertrophy in a normal population. *Circulation* 29:224, 1964
4. Simonson E: The effect of age on the electrocardiogram. *Am J Cardiol* 29:64, 1972
5. Willems JL, Poblete PF, Pipberger HV: Day-to-day variation of the normal orthogonal electrocardiogram and vectorcardiogram. *Circulation* 45:1057, 1972
6. Hiss RG, Lamb, LE: Electrocardiographic findings in 122,043 individuals. *Circulation* 25:947, 1962
7. Josephson ME, Kastor JA, Morganroth J: Electrocardiographic left atrial enlargement: Electrophysiologic, echocardiographic and hemodynamic correlates. *Am J Cardiol* 39:967, 1977
8. Chou TC, Helm RA: The pseudo P pulmonale. *Circulation* 32:96, 1965
9. Abraham AS: P wave analysis in myocardial infarction, pulmonary edema, and embolism. *Am Heart J* 89:30, 1975
10. Romhilt DW, Scott RC: Left atrial involvement in acute pulmonary edema. *Am Heart J* 83:328, 1972
11. Surawicz B, Uhley H, Borun R, Laks M, Crevasse L, Rosen K, Nelson W, Mandel W, Lawrence P, Jackson L, Flowers N, Clifton J, Greenfield J, Robles De Medina EO: Task Force I: Standardization of terminology and interpretation. *Am J Cardiol* 41:130, 1978
12. Scott RC: Correlation between the electrocardiographic patterns of ventricular hypertrophy and the anatomic findings. *Circulation* 21:256, 1960
13. Romhilt, DW, Estes EH: Point-score system for the ECG diagnosis of left ventricular hypertrophy. *Am Heart J* 75:752, 1968
14. Dower GE, Horn HE, Ziegler WG: On electrocardiographic-autopsy correlations in left ventricular hypertrophy. A simple postmortem index of hypertrophy proposed. *Am Heart J* 74:351, 1967
15. Ishikawa K, Berson AS, Pipberger HV: Electrocardiographic changes due to cardiac enlargement. *Am Heart J* 81:635, 1971
16. Walker CH, Rose RL: Importance of age, sex, and body habitus in the diagnosis of left ventricular hypertrophy from the precordial electrocardiogram in childhood and adolescence. *Pediatrics* 28:705, 1961
17. Scott RC: Ventricular hypertrophy. *Cardiovasc Clin* 5:220, 1973
18. Chou TC: Electrocardiography: Usefulness and limitations. *Cardiovasc Rev Rep* 2:192, 1981
19. Stein PD, Dalen JE, McIntyre KM, Sasahara AA, Wenger NK, Willis PW: The electrocardiogram in acute pulmonary embolism. *Prog Cardiovasc Dis* 17:247, 1975
20. Szucs MM, Brooks HL, Grossman W, Banas JS Jr, Meister SG, Dexter L, Dalen JE: Diagnostic sensitivity of laboratory findings in acute pulmonary embolism. *Ann Intern Med* 74:161, 1971
21. The Urokinase Pulmonary Embolism Trial. *Circulation* 47 (Suppl II): II-1, 1973

22. Smith M, Ray CT: Electrocardiographic signs of early right ventricular enlargement in acute pulmonary embolism. *Chest* 28:205, 1970
23. Flowers NC, Horan LG: IV. Hypertrophy and infarction. Subtle signs of right ventricular enlargement and their relative importance. In Schlant RC, Hurst JW (eds): *Advances in Electrocardiography,* Vol I. New York: Grune & Stratton, 1972
24. Hilsenrath J, Hamby RI, Hoffman I: Pitfalls in the prediction of coronary artery disease from the electrocardiogram or vectorcardiogram. *J Electrocardiol* 6:291, 1973
25. Horan LG, Flowers NC, Johnson JC: Significance of diagnostic Q wave of myocardial infarction. *Circulation* 43:428, 1971
26. Sheltigar UR, Hultgren HN, Pfeifer JF, Lipton MJ: Diagnostic value of Q-waves in inferior myocardial infarction. *Am Heart J* 88:170, 1974
27. Numbs JW, de Mello V, Roberts R: The effect of respiration on normal and abnormal Q waves. *Am Heart J* 94:579, 1977
28. Hilsenrath J, Hamby RI, Glassman E, Hoffman I: Pitfalls in prediction of coronary arterial obstruction from patterns of anterior infarction on electrocardiogram and vectorcardiogram. *Am J Cardiol* 29:164, 1972
29. Chou T: Pseudo-infarction (noninfarction Q waves). *Cardiovasc Clin* 5:200, 1973
30. Copeland RB, Omenn GS: Electrocardiogram changes suggestive of coronary artery disease in pneumothorax. Their reversibility with upright posture. *Arch Intern Med* 125:151, 1970
31. Cropp GJ, Manning GW: Electrocardiographic changes simulating myocardial ischemia and infarction associated with spontaneous intracranial hemorrhage. *Circulation* 22:25, 1960
32. Levine HD, Wanzer SH, Merrill JP: Dialyzable currents of injury in potassium intoxication resembling acute myocardial infarction or pericarditis. *Circulation* 13:29, 1956
33. Mills RM, Young E, Gorlin R, Lesch M: Natural history of ST segment elevation after acute myocardial infarction. *Am J Cardiol* 35:609, 1975
34. Bodenheimer MM, Banka VS, Helfant RH: Q waves and ventricular asynergy: Predictive value and hemodynamic significance of anatomic localization. *Am J Cardiol* 35:615, 1975
35. Surawicz B: The pathogenesis and clinical significance of primary T-wave abnormalities. In Schlant RC, Hurst JW (eds): *Advances in Electrocardiography,* Vol I. New York: Grune & Stratton, 1972
36. Pinto IJ, Nanda NC, Biswas AK, Parulkar VG: Tall upright T waves in the precordial leads. *Circulation* 36:708, 1967

Chapter 3

Ambulatory Electrocardiographic Monitoring

Elliott M. Antman and Peter F. Cohn

Since its introduction by Holter in 1957 [1], continuous recording of electrocardiographic (ECG) activity over extended periods of time has rapidly become a widely applied clinical tool. Synonymous terms used to describe this technique include ambulatory monitoring, ambulatory recording, ambulatory electrocardiography, Holter monitoring, and Holter recording. The fundamental principle of this test involves *continuous recording* of electrocardiographic information for playback at a later time. It thus differs from *continuous monitoring,* which provides immediate on-line display of the cardiac rhythm, as is commonly found in coronary intensive care units or in exercise testing laboratories.

The most important clinical use of ambulatory monitoring is evaluation of suspected cardiac rhythm disturbances that are thought to play a role in patient symptomatology. Patients may complain of "skipped beats" or "palpitations"; these complaints may be associated with abnormalities of cardiac rate or rhythm or conversely may be psychoneural in origin. By careful correlation of the recorded cardiac rhythm with a simultaneously recorded patient diary, important relationships, or the lack thereof, can be readily determined. In addition, epidemiologic studies have suggested that an important risk factor for sudden cardiac death due to ventricular tachycardia/fibrillation is the frequent occurrence of complex repetitive ventricular premature beats (VPBs)* Ambulatory monitoring is currently being used with increasing frequency for the detection and cataloguing of such complex disturbances of cardiac rhythm.

Optimal Duration of Monitoring
Early coronary care unit experience and studies of patients with chronic stable coronary heart disease indicated that the percentage of patients exhibiting VPBs

---

*Some authors prefer the term ventricular premature depolarizations (VPDs), since electrocardiographic monitoring systems record only electrical events and not contractile events. However, because of the widespread use of the term VPBs in the medical literature, it will be employed for the remainder of this chapter.

TABLE 3-1. Percent of Patients with Coronary Heart Disease Expected to Demonstrate Ventricular Premature Beats with Various Durations of Cardiac Monitoring

Technique	Duration of Monitoring	Patients with VPBs (%)
Standard 12-lead ECG	1 min	10–14
Trendscription	30 min	40
Sedentary Monitoring	60 min	50
Ambulatory Monitoring	24 hr	85–88

VPBs = ventricular premature beats.
Modified from B Lown, TB Graboys: Sudden death: An ancient problem newly perceived. *Cardiovasc Med* 2:219, 1979.

increased with the duration of monitoring. Table 3–1 shows the percentage of patients with coronary heart disease expected to demonstrate VPBs with various durations of cardiac monitoring. In addition to exposing a greater number of patients who exhibit ventricular ectopic activity, monitoring beyond 6 to 12 hours results in a significant improvement in detection of frequent and complex VPBs (i.e., ventricular couplets and salvos of ventricular tachycardia) [2].

Despite these data, some investigators have attempted to determine whether shorter periods of monitoring provide adequate, clinically relevant information because of the large number of patients who require screening for ventricular ectopic activity. Results from the HIP study by Ruberman and coworkers [3] (using one hour of cardiac monitoring in 1739 men with recent myocardial infarction) indicate that a population at risk for sudden cardiac death could be identified without need for long-term monitoring. Those patients who died suddenly exhibited a characteristic VPB profile: the total mortality for patients exhibiting complex ventricular premature beats (multiform, repetitive, and early-cycle VPBs) was nearly 2 times higher than that of patients with simple VPBs (frequent but isolated VPBs) [3].

Similarly, Graboys and Lown have shown that 30 minutes of on-line ECG monitoring (trendscription) in 145 patients with a diversity of cardiac diagnoses (coronary heart disease, valvular heart disease, and primary cardiac arrhythmia) seemed to be a helpful screening technique for identifying about 95 percent of patients in whom extended monitoring would be useful for detailed arrhythmia analysis [4]. Thus, although 30 minutes of on-line ECG monitoring clearly will not detect all patients who exhibit some ventricular ectopic activity, those patients who would exhibit frequent complex VPBs during a 24-hour recording are likely to demonstrate a high degree of ventricular ectopy during a 30-minute monitoring.

Components of an Ambulatory Monitoring System

The original ambulatory monitoring systems devised by Holter consisted of large, cumbersome transmitter devices that emitted a radiotelemetry signal to a nearby oscilloscope. Dramatic improvements and refinements have been achieved since the original recording models. Presently, the cardiac rhythm is recorded onto electromagnetic tape stored either on a cassette or a small plastic reel. The recording apparatus has been reduced in size to a device that can be worn on a belt and is slightly over 2 lb in weight. Improved leads and skin electrodes have resulted in higher fidelity recordings. The recorded tape can now be played back at 60 or 120 times real time with the cardiac rhythm displayed on an oscilloscope in conjunction with an audio signal. A number of computer programs are available for automated arrhythmia detection that simplify the time-consuming task of reviewing a large number of tapes.

It should be noted that whichever of the devices described below is employed, skin resistance must be reduced by abrasion and application of alcohol before multiple gelled adhesive electrodes are positioned on the chest. Either a single-lead or a double-lead system is used (Fig. 3-1). This results in a modified V5 lead or a combination of modified leads V1 and V5.

RECORDERS

A variety of recording devices are available. The most commonly employed is the *continuous recorder* which, once activated, will continuously record all ECG activity until the unit is turned off. Two types of *event recorders* are available. One type can be activated by the patient in response to certain clinical symptoms such as palpitations or lightheadedness. The second type is programmed to monitor the heart beat and record only rhythm disturbances that fall outside the programmed "allowable" range of either the R–R interval or morphology. Because event recorders have had limited clinical exposure, their use will probably be restricted to small numbers of patients. The physician should review the data regarding accuracy of a particular event recorder's arrhythmia detection circuitry before utilizing the device. Since such recorders do not provide a continuous inscription of all QRS complexes that occur during a given monitoring period, it is not possible to directly confirm that all ectopic impulses are in fact detected.

Trendscription, introduced by Lown and associates in 1975 [5], utilizes a continuous on-line printout device. Within the unit a circular drum rotates at a slow speed, and a heated stylus spirals downward and inscribes 1 minute of ECG information on each of 30 lines on the recording paper. An optional, even slower speed recording is available that permits 4 minutes of ECG information to be inscribed on each of 30 lines, providing a total of 2 hours of direct ECG monitoring and printing. An example of such a device is shown in Figure 3-2.

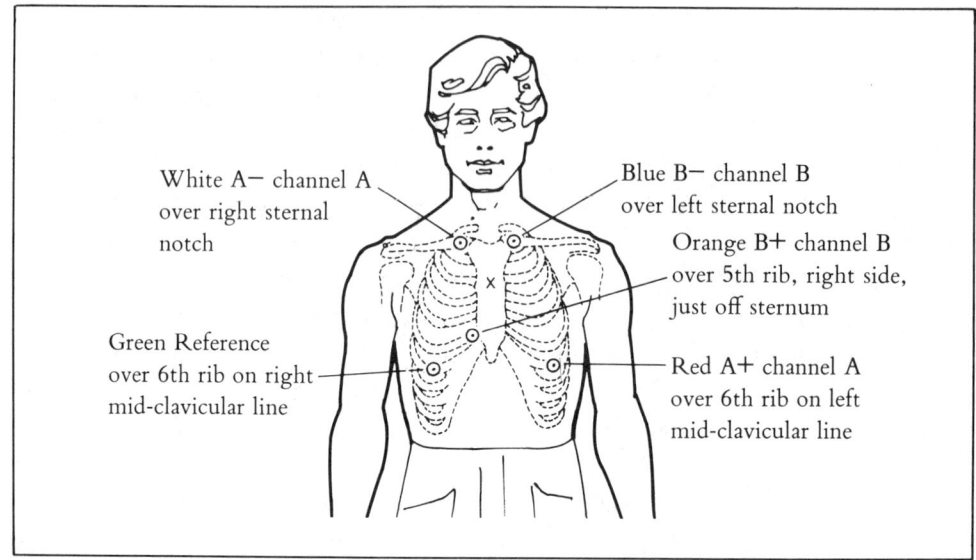

FIGURE 3-1. Electrode placement for double-channel ambulatory recording (Reproduced with permission of Cambridge Instruments, Bedford, MA).

An additional recording system offering important clinical capabilities is *transtelephonic monitoring*. In this case, the patient transmits an ECG signal via a standard telephone line using easily applied ECG limb leads in the form of "bracelets." The transmitted signal can be recorded and printed out directly for review. Such a monitoring system is particularly suitable for evaluation of pacemaker function and stable outpatients with episodic arrhythmias.

SCANNERS

A typical 24-hour Holter recording may contain over 100,000 QRS complexes. High-speed playback devices are used to scan the tape for alterations of heart rhythm. Each ECG complex is superimposed on the immediately preceding complex. If successive complexes are similar, the oscilloscope will present a stationary image. Extrasystoles and changes in heart rhythm are perceived as mismatched complexes, which are readily detected by the human eye even at 30 to 60 times the original recording speed. A simultaneously triggered audio signal will emit characteristic changes in pitch with the appearance of extrasystoles and changes in heart rate or rhythm. Selected samples of ECG recordings can be examined on a standard ECG printout, which is coupled to the oscilloscope.

DATA ANALYSIS AND QUALITY CONTROL

Merely counting all VPBs that occur during a 24-hour period, a simple albeit time-consuming task, is not sufficient to determine the risk of sudden cardiac

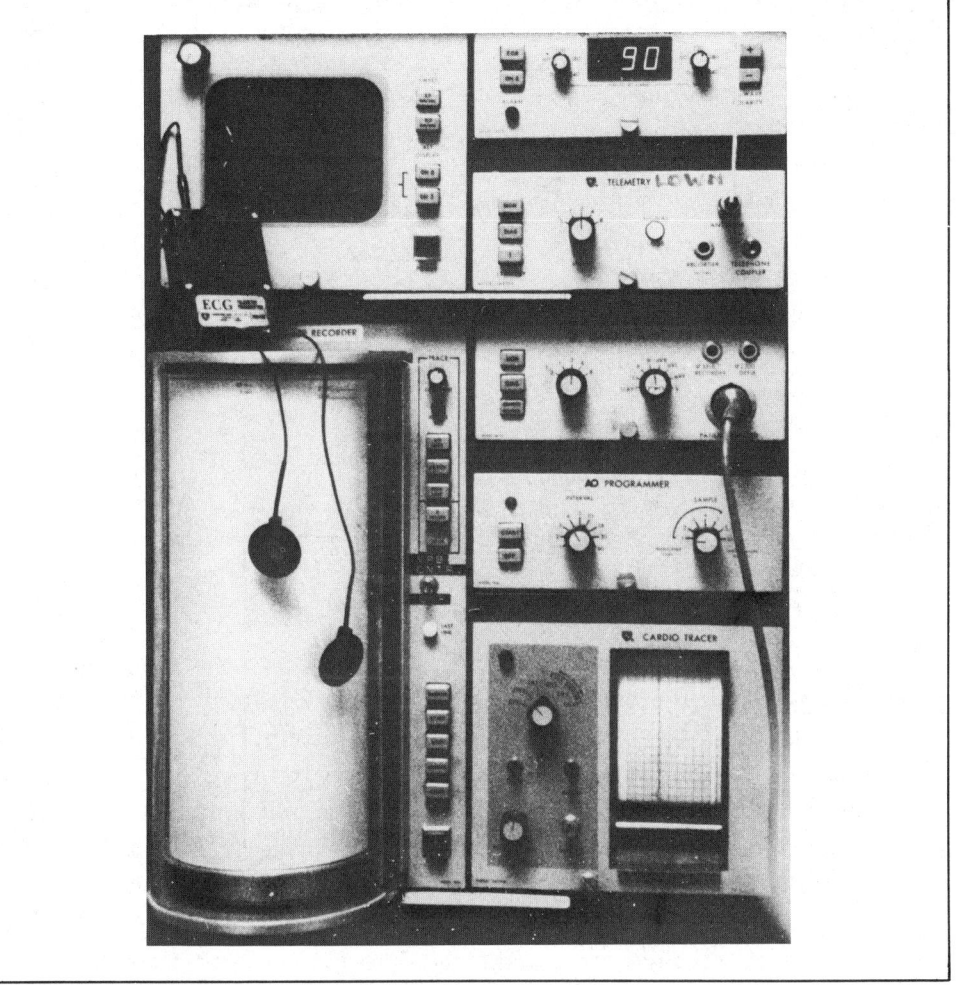

FIGURE 3-2. Trendscription unit consisting of telemetry transmitter, receiver, and rotating drum, which allows direct slow speed recording of rhythm disturbances.

death; the frequency of complex ventricular ectopic activity must also be considered. Therefore, in 1971 Lown and Wolf proposed a grading system for ventricular premature beats [6]. This system, modified since its introduction [7], is outlined in Table 3-2.

Accurate reporting of data requires careful correlation of findings on ECG and patient symptomatology. Suggested techniques for quality control of ambulatory monitoring systems include a complete printout of all ECG data on a fixed percentage of tapes or fixed time periods on a number of tapes with a hand-count of all VPBs compared with that obtained using visual or semiautomated scanning techniques.

TABLE 3-2. Lown Grading System for Ventricular Premature Beats

Grade	Characteristics
0	No ventricular beats
1A	Occasional, isolated VPBs (less than 30/hr) less than 1/min
1B	Occasional, isolated VPBs (less than 30/hr) more than 1/min
2	Frequent VPBs (more than 30/hr)
3	Multiform VPBs
4A	Repetitive VPBs Couplets
4B	Repetitive VPBs Salvos (ventricular tachycardia)
5	Early VPBs (i.e., abutting or interrupting the T wave)

VPBs = ventricular premature beats
From B Lown et al [7].

The features of ambulatory recordings that are theoretically susceptible to computer analysis include R–R interval, QRS amplitude, QRS width, QRS duration, QRS area, and ST–T-wave changes. Although all these features are factored into the clinical evaluation of ectopic beats, computer programs are not available that can duplicate the complex processes used by the human mind in evaluating rhythm disturbances. Computer-based, semiautomated analytic methods are available that utilize software algorithms that compare each beat to "templates" and assist in the recognition of ectopic beats. Most semiautomated systems report an overall error rate compared to real time of approximately 5 to 10 percent in detecting ectopic beat frequency. The accuracy of semiautomated analysis can be improved by introducing technician editing capabilities, but this occurs at the expense of speed of processing. A number of fully automated computer-based systems are being developed that hopefully will reduce the error rate to less than 1 percent.

An example of a semiautomated arrhythmia detection system is the CAMSCAN system,* which detects ectopic beats based upon changes in QRS area and R–R intervals. It is capable of detecting five classes of arrhythmias: isolated VPBs, ventricular couplets, ventricular tachycardia, early cycle VPBs, and "dropped beats." The area of each QRS complex is compared with measurements derived from the average area over the preceding 3 seconds. Although the system works well clinically, it should be understood that the potential for certain false diagnoses is intrinsic to such an algorithm. Figure 3-3 shows an example of two geometric

*Cambridge Instruments, Bedford, MA

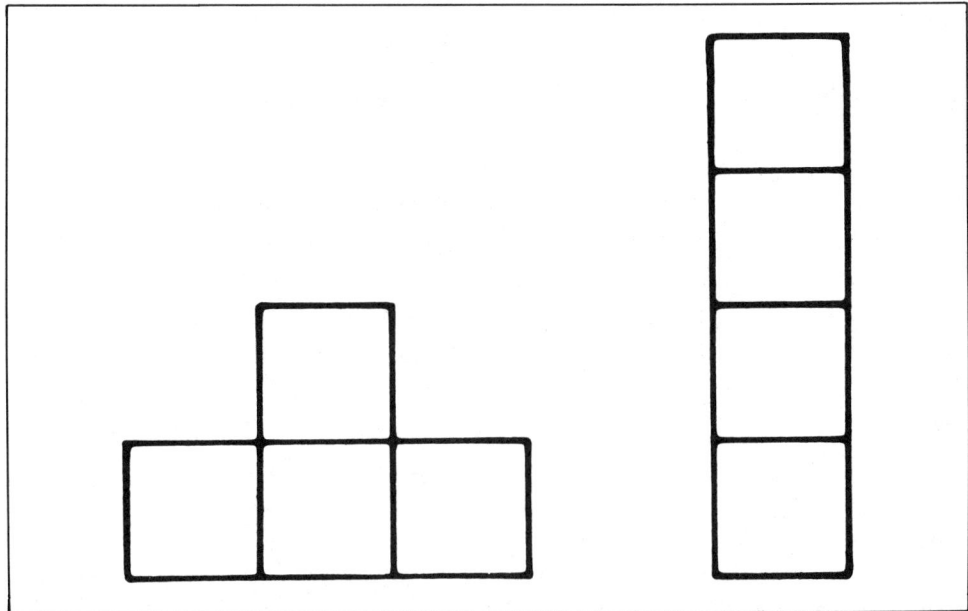

FIGURE 3-3. Two geometric shapes with the same area. High-speed computer measurement of area alone might not correctly identify the shape at the right as being different from the reference complex shown at the left.

shapes with the same area. If the shape at the left were the reference QRS complex, it is possible that high-speed simple area measurement would not identify the shape at the right as morphologically distinct and therefore a probable ectopic impulse.

The potential sources of artifacts during ambulatory recordings can be divided into external and internal sources as follows:

EXTERNAL
1. External electrical interference
2. Muscle artifact
3. Wandering baseline
4. Fading voltage

INTERNAL
1. Mechanical problems (e.g., tape drive)
2. Recording head malfunction

By proper preparation of the skin and positioning of the electrode, cutaneous and muscle sources of artifacts can be minimized. Routine insertion of fresh batteries before each recording and periodic cleaning of the recording heads will help to minimize technical difficulties with the recording apparatus.

Components of Ambulatory Monitoring Report Form

In addition to a list of the patient's diagnoses, medications, and symptoms, a proper ambulatory monitoring report should include a statement as to the underlying rhythm (e.g., sinus, atrial fibrillation) and the range of heart rates observed during the recording session. Abnormalities of atrioventricular conduction should be identified and classified using standard schemes. When dual-channel recordings are obtained, it is sometimes possible to make a diagnosis of intraventricular conduction defects by analysis of QRS morphology and axis.

For many uncomplicated recordings, a simple literal description of the atrial and ventricular arrhythmias detected on the tape suffices for clinical evaluation. However, more complex rhythm disturbances rapidly present an unmanageable mass of data, which is best simplified using a classification scheme. One such scheme utilized at the Brigham and Women's Hospital is shown in Figure 3-4. Atrial arrhythmias are given a letter classification based on the varying mechanisms of supraventricular rhythm disturbances. In addition, the ordering physician is provided with the maximum number of runs of a particular supraventricular arrhythmia which occurred in a given hour, the longest run of supraventricular tachycardia (SVT), and the maximum heart rate observed during the rhythm disturbance.

Ventricular arrhythmias are graded according to the classification devised by Lown and coworkers (see Table 3-2). Implicit in this categorization of VPBs is the belief that high-grade, complex ventricular arrhythmias impart a higher risk for sudden cardiac death. This grading system was initially devised based upon clinical observations of patients with coronary heart disease monitored in a coronary care unit setting. Recently, a number of studies have extended the use of this classification system to ambulatory patients with varying cardiac diagnoses and varying complexity and frequency of ventricular arrhythmias [7]. Data are accumulating from a number of sources to support this clinical practice. A particularly attractive aspect of the grading system is that it provides a shorthand notation that may be rapidly interpreted and lends itself readily for serial comparisons during antiarrhythmic drug trials [7].

Critics of the grading system claim that it deemphasizes the total frequency of ventricular premature beats and makes it difficult to compare ambulatory monitoring recordings on various drug regimens if complete counts of all ventricular extrasystoles are desired [2]. In addition, some workers believe that more importance should be placed upon the "density" of ventricular arrhythmias [8]. Thus, the report should reflect whether the arrhythmias occurred sporadically throughout the monitoring session or were confined to a relatively brief period of marked electrical instability. Despite the above limitations, the Lown grading system is extensively employed clinically and when used appropriately provides an excellent condensation of what otherwise would be an overwhelming pool of data.

```
ATRIAL ARRHYTHMIAS
A) Hours free of arrhythmias_____ B) Hours of occ. APBs_____ C) Hours with frequent APBs_____
D) Hours with runs of SVT_____    Max.# runs/hr._____    Longest run_____ Max. rate_____
E) Hours with flutter       _____ {Max.# runs/hr._____   Longest run_____ Max. rate_____
F) Hours with A. Fib        _____ {Max.# runs/hr._____   Longest run_____ Max. rate_____
VENTRICULAR ARRHYTHMIAS
 O) Hours free of VPBs                _____
1A) Hours with occ. VPBs (≤1/min)_____  (<30/hour)
1B) Hours with occ. VPBs (>1/min)_____  (<30/hour)
2 ) Hours with freq. VPBs (>2/min)_____ (>30/hour)
3 ) Hours with multiformity_____    # of forms    _____
4A) Hours with couplets        _____ Max.#/hr.    _____
4B) Hours with runs of VT _____ Max.# runs/hr._____ Longest run_____ Max. rate_____
5 ) Hours with early cycle VPBs (R on T) _____ Max. per hr._____
```

FIGURE 3-4. Example of report form summarizing atrial and ventricular ectopic activity detected during a 24-hour ambulatory monitoring session. *APBs* = atrial premature beats; *SVT* = supraventricular tachycardia; *A. Fib* = atrial fibrillation; *VPB* = ventricular premature beats; *VT* = ventricular tachycardia.

Another important aspect of the report form is analysis of any ST–T-wave abnormalities that are observed. Diagnosis of rate-related conduction defects or transient myocardial ischemia and evaluation of drug therapy (e.g., digitalis) may sometimes be made by careful review of ECG printouts from the monitoring session. Episodes of palpitations or chest discomfort should be carefully correlated with rhythm disturbances or ST-segment shifts using a timing track keyed to the tape recording.

The advent of dual-channel recordings has greatly enhanced diagnosis of complex cardiac arrhythmias. As shown in Figure 3-5, utilizing orthogonally related leads exposes important axis shifts and alterations in QRS morphology that are particularly helpful in analyzing rhythm disturbances.

Ambulatory Monitoring Studies in "Normal" Individuals

When interpreting the results of an ambulatory monitoring session, clinicians should be aware that on routine monitoring, asymptomatic individuals apparently free of heart disease may show a significant incidence of supraventricular arrhythmias, ventricular arrhythmias, and even conduction defects. Utilizing 6-hour recording sessions, Hinkle and coworkers examined 301 asymptomatic middle-aged men and found 76 percent had supraventricular arrhythmias and 62 percent had some form of ventricular arrhythmia [9]. The incidences of conduction defects were as follows: sinoatrial block 1.4 percent, atrioventricular block 0.7 percent, and intraventricular block 7.7 percent. It may be argued that some of these middle-aged men were likely to have subclinical coronary heart disease.

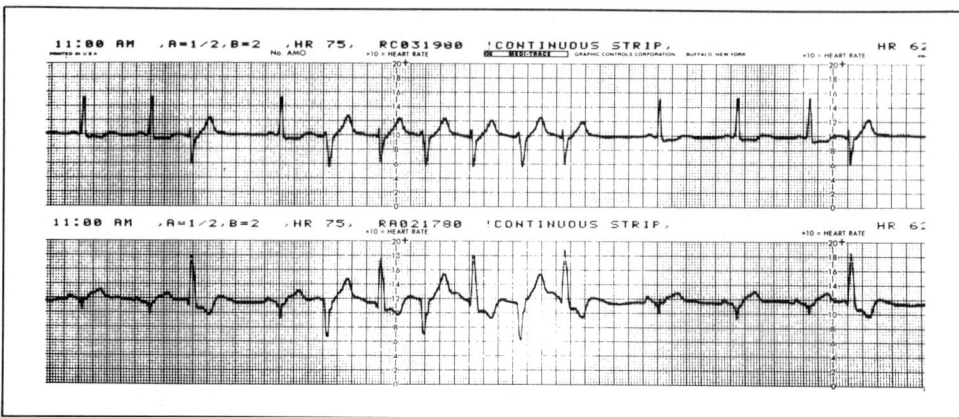

FIGURE 3-5. Dual-channel simultaneous recording of modified V5 (*top*) and V1 (*bottom*) in a middle-aged male with a history of myocardial infarction reveals probable bidirectional ventricular tachycardia. This would have been more difficult to diagnose if only the top channel were recorded.

Winkle has recently summarized the results of 11 studies examining the incidence of ventricular arrhythmias during ambulatory recordings on "normal" subjects [2]. The results of these studies plus two additional series are shown in Table 3-3. These analyses provide an overall guide to the expected frequency of ventricular arrhythmias in a patient population free of clinical evidence of cardiovascular disease. Infrequent VPBs occur commonly, but frequent VPBs are unusual, particularly in younger patients. With increasing age, the frequency and complexity of VPBs increases. As indicated by Winkle, this may represent a function of the normal aging process or an increased prevalence of subclinical heart disease [2].

Several epidemiologic studies in the United States have noted an association of VPBs with an increased risk of cardiac death in patients with coronary heart disease. However, the finding of frequent and complex ventricular ectopic activity in an asymptomatic, apparently healthy individual does not necessarily indicate the presence of significant coronary artery disease. Kennedy and coworkers utilized both noninvasive and catheterization procedures to evaluate a group of asymptomatic subjects who were referred for evaluation of the consistent presence of more than 1 ventricular ectopic beat/min noted on ECG monitoring [10, 11]. Neither the mean ventricular ectopic beat frequency nor the grade of complex ventricular arrhythmias exhibited by the patients served as reliable indicators as to whether the coronary arteriogram would reveal normal coronary arteries, noncritical coronary artery obstructions, or significant coronary artery obstructions. Only six of 25 patients with frequent complex VPBs were found to have significant coronary artery disease, while 14 of 25 patients had normal coronary arteries. The definitive long-term prognosis of such apparently healthy subjects with frequent and com-

TABLE 3-3. Ventricular Arrhythmias on Ambulatory ECG Recordings in "Normal" Subjects

Study	No. of Subjects	Sex	Duration of Monitoring (hr)	Age (yr)	Population	Any VPBs (%)	Frequent VPBs[a] (%)	Multi-focal (%)	R on T (%)	Pairs (%)	Bigeminy (%)	Ventricular Tachycardia (%)	Comments
Gilson[a]	37	M	20+	Average 39	Normal		5						
Gilson[a]	65	M,F	5–15	Most <55	Normal								
Brodsky et al[a]	50	M	24	23–27	Medical students	50	2	0		2	0	2	
Raftery et al[a]	53	M,F	24	20–70	Normal	15	2	2		2		0	
DeMaria et al[a]	40	M,F	10	—	Chest pain with normal coronaries	25							
Verban et al[a]	74	M,F	24	20–80	Normal	76	8	28	5	9	3	1	More frequent in older subjects
Clarke[a]	86	M,F	48	16–65	Normal	73	8	15	2	0	3	2	More frequent in older subjects
Hinkle et al[a]	283	M	6	Median 55	Employed cross-section	62	9	33		13	8	3	More frequent in older subjects
Glasser et al[a]	13	M,F	24	Average 69	Elderly	100	15	8		23		0	
Camm et al[a]	106	M,F	24	>75	Elderly	68	13	22		4	5	6	
Goulding[a]	100	M,F	24	25–74	Normal, half urban, half rural	16	8	1		0		0	
Scott[b]	131	M	48	10–13	Normal	26				<1			
Viitasalo[c]	15	M	4–6	Mean 49	Healthy, active	33	13						
Viitasalo[c]	15	M	4–6	Mean 48	Healthy, sedentary	40	20	7					More frequent in sedentary subjects

[a]Cited by RA Winkle [2].
[b]Scott O, Williams GJ, Fiddler GI: Results of 24 hour ambulatory monitoring of electrocardiogram in 131 healthy boys aged 10 to 13 years. *Br Heart J* 44:304, 1980.
[c]Viitasalo MT, Kala R, Elsalo A, Halonen PI: Ventricular arrhythmias during exercise testing, jogging and sedentary life. *Chest* 76:21, 1979.

plex ventricular arrhythmias has not yet been defined. It would seem, however, that the majority of apparently healthy subjects with frequent and complex ventricular ectopy do not have subclinical coronary artery disease, and therefore a conservative management is indicated.

Reproducibility

Cardiac arrhythmias most often occur sporadically, which may result in variability in arrhythmia frequency over a 24-hour period or when two 24-hour periods are compared. Calvert et al found that in patients undergoing catheterization for known or suspected coronary heart disease, repetitive-form ventricular arrhythmias had a reproducibility of 40 percent when comparing two closely performed 24-hour recordings [12]. Three recent studies utilized a sophisticated statistical analysis of the variability of arrhythmia frequency and complexity on serial ambulatory recordings [13–15]. It was originally suggested that if two 24-hour monitoring periods are compared, a greater than 83 percent reduction in VPB frequency should be observed before declaring a drug to exhibit antiarrhythmic efficacy. Similarly, significant hourly variability in arrhythmia frequency and complexity has been detected in control recordings; this has been felt to mimic either drug-induced suppression or aggravation of ventricular ectopic activity. It should be realized that these more statistically oriented studies on ventricular arrhythmia variability during 24-hour ambulatory recordings have a number of shortcomings. The number of patients studied is small, and the individuals subjected to repeated ambulatory recordings were selected from groups having widely disparate cardiac diagnoses (ranging from no significant heart disease to congestive cardiomyopathy and coronary artery disease). It is not clear that experience gained from a selected group of patients can be extrapolated to individuals with a different clinical profile. In the opinion of some investigators, the patient exhibiting marked variability of ectopic activity often has minimal structural heart disease and may not require antiarrhythmic therapy. By contrast, patients suffering from malignant ventricular arrhythmias and recurrent cardiac arrests usually show little variability in ventricular arrhythmias and should not be subjected to the rigorous statistical standards suggested above. It is necessary to establish for each individual the degree of variability of arrhythmias utilizing control recordings before initiating drug therapy.

Clinical Indications for Ambulatory Monitoring

The clinical indications for obtaining ambulatory monitoring recordings are listed in Table 3-4. An important indication is the *diagnosis of suspected cardiac arrhythmias* based upon reported patient symptomatology. Complaints of lightheadedness or

TABLE 3-4. Clinical Indications for Ambulatory Monitoring

Diagnosis
   Bradyarrhythmias/tachyarrhythmias
   Transient myocardial ischemia
Evaluation of therapy
   Drug efficacy/safety
   Pacemaker function
   Postmyocardial infarction

dizziness may be due to bradyarrhythmias such as profound sinus bradycardia or sinus arrest (Fig. 3-6) or disturbances of atrioventricular conduction leading to pauses in ventricular activity (Fig. 3-7). Alternatively, lightheadedness or palpitations may be due to tachyarrhythmias. Rapid heart action due to supraventricular arrhythmias may result from a poorly controlled ventricular response in atrial fibrillation or flutter or paroxysms of supraventricular tachycardia (Fig. 3-8). Bursts of rapid ventricular tachycardia or ventricular flutter, although occasionally well-tolerated in the young patient without significant heart disease, usually result in hemodynamic compromise with decreased cerebral perfusion and resultant syncope (Figs. 3-9 and 3-10). Accelerating ventricular tachyarrhythmias with early-cycle premature complexes infringing upon the vulnerable period of preceding beats often degenerate into malignant ventricular arrhythmias (Fig. 3-11). Eight patients suffering sudden cardiac death during ambulatory recordings have been described in the literature [2], six of whom were found to have ventricular fibrillation, initiated in all cases by what appeared to be R on T ventricular complexes.

Clinicians should consider ordering ambulatory monitoring sessions for any patients at high risk for potentially lethal cardiac arrhythmias. Table 3-5 provides a partial list of cardiac diagnoses that should alert the clinician to the need for assessment of possible cardiac arrhythmias.

Another important indication for ordering ambulatory monitoring recordings is the *diagnosis of transient myocardial ischemia*. However, it should be recognized that the ECG pattern of the ambulatory monitoring lead equivalent to the standard ECG precordial lead V5 contains a number of peculiarities that can mimic ischemia. These peculiarities include deeper S waves, notches or dips both before and after the T wave, shifts in ST-segment position and T-wave lability as well as variation in the height of the QRS complex. These peculiarities are probably due to a combination of physiologic changes in the patient occurring over a 24-hour period, the variable effects of alterations of patient position on the recorded ECG signal, and in some cases a reduced frequency response of the recording device compared with standard ECG machines.

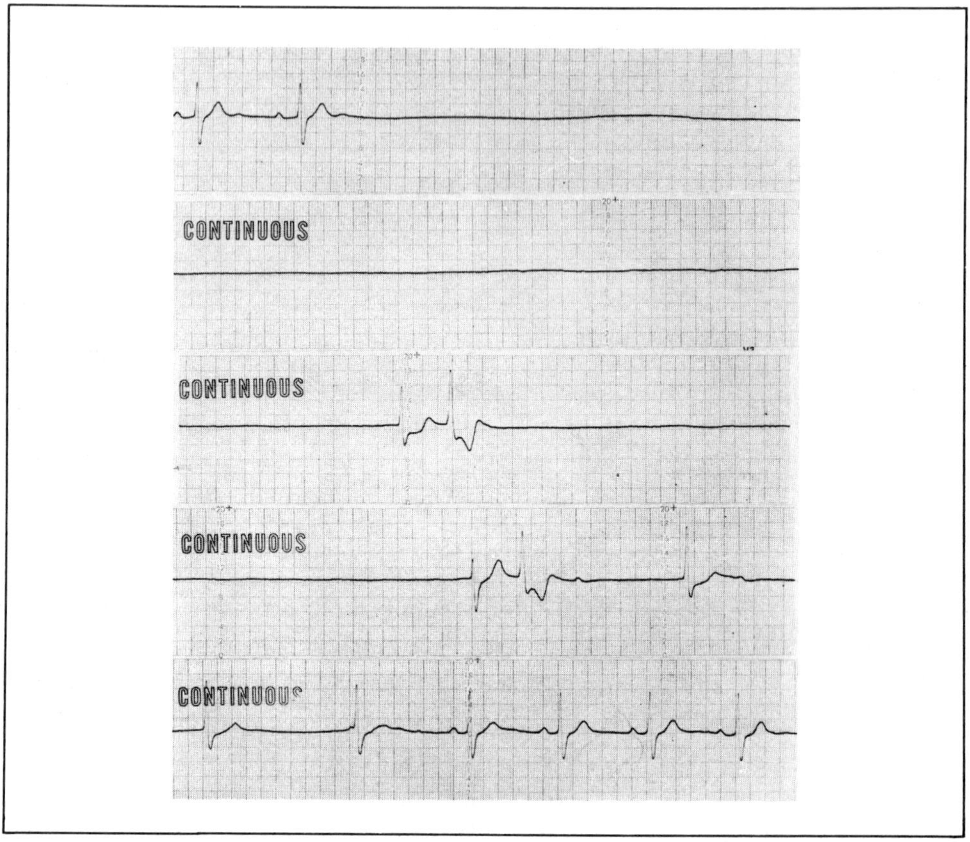

42 / I. Electrocardiography

FIGURE 3-6. The explanation for this patient's syncopal attacks was clearly established by ambulatory monitoring. An episode of profound sinus arrest (approximately 18 seconds) correlated with loss of consciousness.

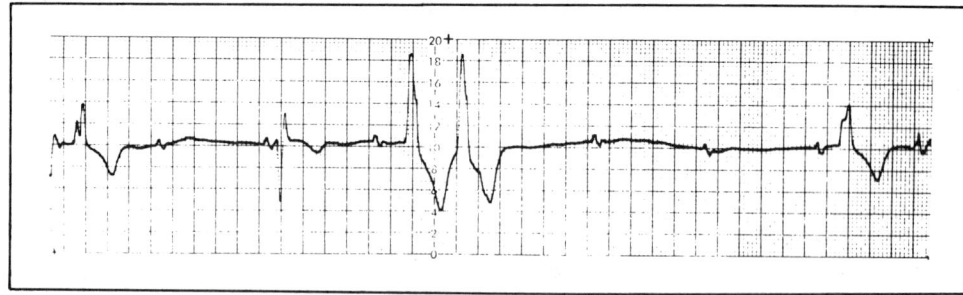

FIGURE 3-7. This patient's lightheadedness was found on ambulatory monitoring to be due to complete heart block with an unstable ventricular escape focus.

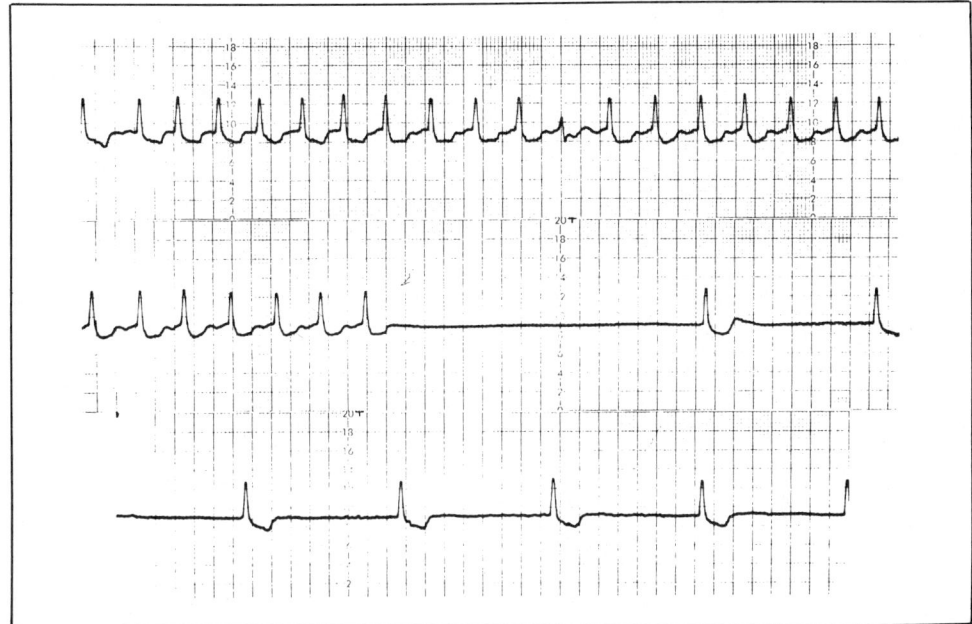

FIGURE 3-8. This elderly patient's complaints of lightheadedness correlated with a repetitive arrhythmia complex consisting of paroxysms of supraventricular tachycardia followed by suppression of sinus node automaticity with a slow junctional escape focus.

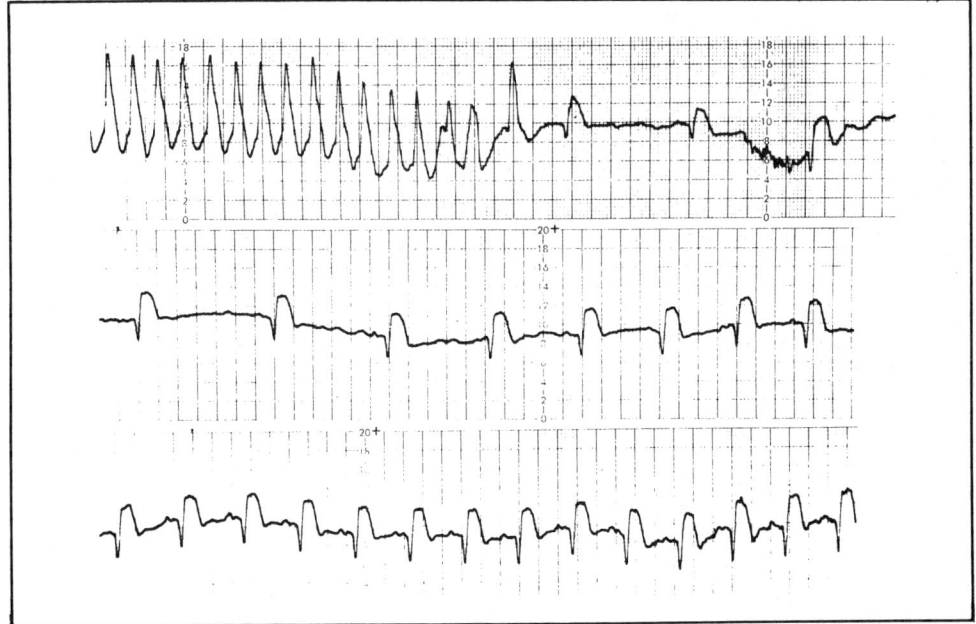

FIGURE 3-9. A rapid paroxysm of ventricular tachycardia (230 beats/min) that terminates spontaneously was recorded in this patient 10 days following acute anterior myocardial infarction. The tachycardia resulted in worsening myocardial ischemia as evidenced by ST elevation and concurrent patient complaints of angina pectoris.

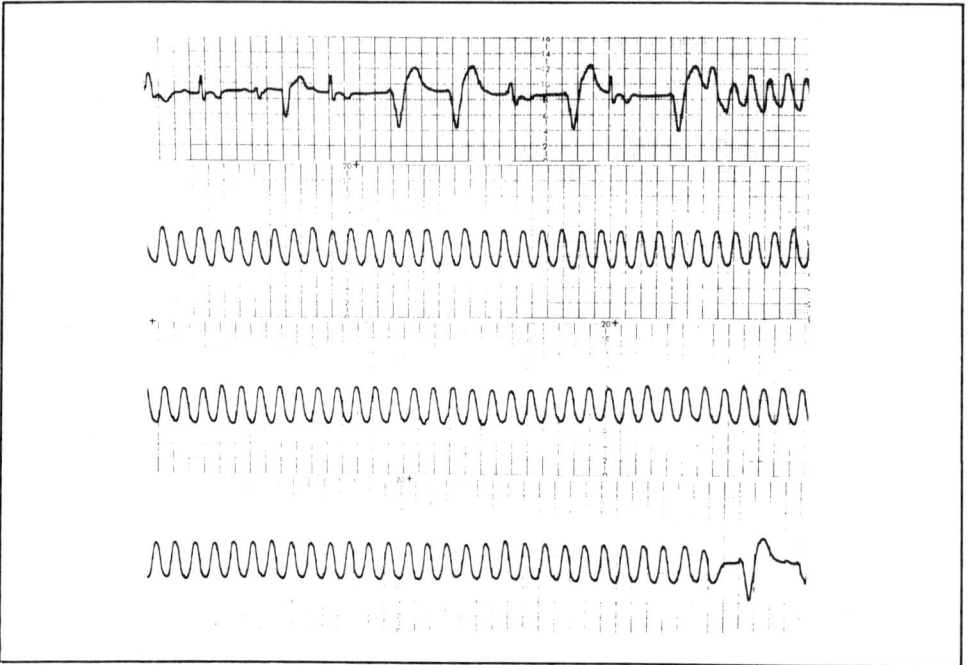

FIGURE 3-10. Conducted sinus beats are seen alternating with demand-mode ventricularly paced beats during the initial portion of continuous rhythm strips. A prolonged episode of ventricular flutter (240 beats/min) that terminates spontaneously was associated with palpitations and presyncope.

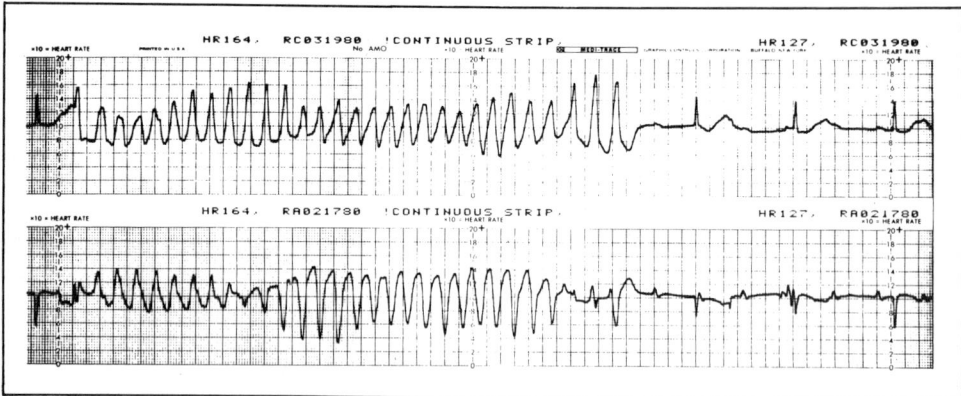

FIGURE 3-11. This elderly patient with severe biventricular failure developed marked Q–T prolongation with quinidine therapy. A nonsustained episode of torsade de pointes was followed by a prolonged episode of ventricular fibrillation from which the patient could not be resuscitated.

TABLE 3-5. Cardiac Diagnoses That Indicate the Need for Ambulatory Monitoring

Myocardial ischemia (angina pectoris, myocardial infarction) with VPBs noted on ECG recordings or exercise testing
Mitral valve prolapse with history of syncope and/or prolonged Q–T interval
Prolonged Q–T syndrome
Cardiomyopathy
History of primary ventricular fibrillation
Preexcitation syndrome
Valvular heart disease with symptoms of palpitations and/or syncope

Ambulatory monitoring offers the clinician the opportunity to perform repeated "exercise tests" on a patient with coronary artery disease as the subject proceeds through his daily activities. Occasionally, although much less frequently than with standard treadmill exercise testing, a patient will demonstrate classical horizontal or downsloping ST-segment depression in association with typical angina pectoris on effort (Fig. 3-12). Other patients will have similar findings, but without pain (e.g., silent myocardial ischemia) [16]. Prolonged slow-speed ECG monitoring by Maseri and coworkers has revealed a surprisingly high frequency of transient ST and T-wave shifts in patients with coronary artery disease which, when combined with hemodynamic monitoring and nuclear medicine techniques, is strongly suggestive of coronary vasospasm [17]. An occasional patient undergoing ambulatory monitoring will reveal spontaneous ST-segment elevation at rest that may or may not occur in association with chest discomfort (Fig. 3-13). Such a spectrum of findings can be considered virtually diagnostic of intense spasm of a major epicardial coronary vessel. One must be careful to differentiate this form of ST-segment elevation from that seen following a tachyarrhythmia, which most likely represents myocardial ischemia due to an increased myocardial oxygen demand (see Fig. 3-9).

An increasingly important indication for ordering an ambulatory recording is *evaluation of drug therapy*. Thus, the clinician may wish to see whether a particular antiarrhythmic drug has either suppressed or aggravated the cardiac arrhythmia for which it is being administered. The technique known as acute drug testing lends itself easily to ambulatory monitoring. This can be performed with a standard continuous Holter recorder described above or with on-line trendscription [7, 18]. The criteria for antiarrhythmic drug efficacy remain controversial. Some investigators stress the need to detect a significant reduction in the number of total ventricular premature beats recorded during 24 hours. Others emphasize elimination of frequent salvos of symptomatic ventricular arrhythmias. One set of criteria incorporating both these features, as described by Lown and associates

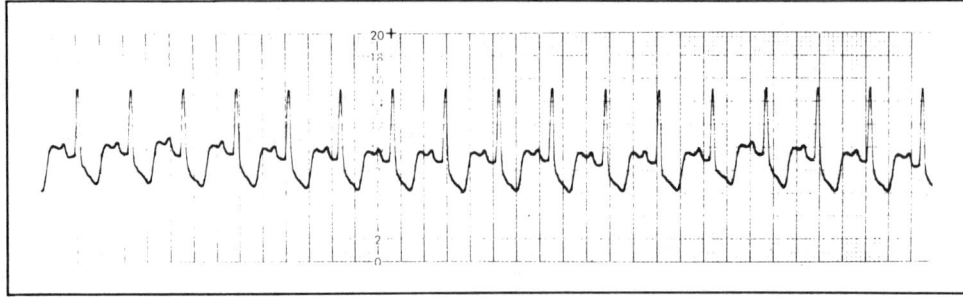

FIGURE 3-12. This episode of exercise-induced sinus tachycardia in a middle-aged male was associated with substernal chest discomfort and ST–T-wave abnormalities typical of myocardial ischemia.

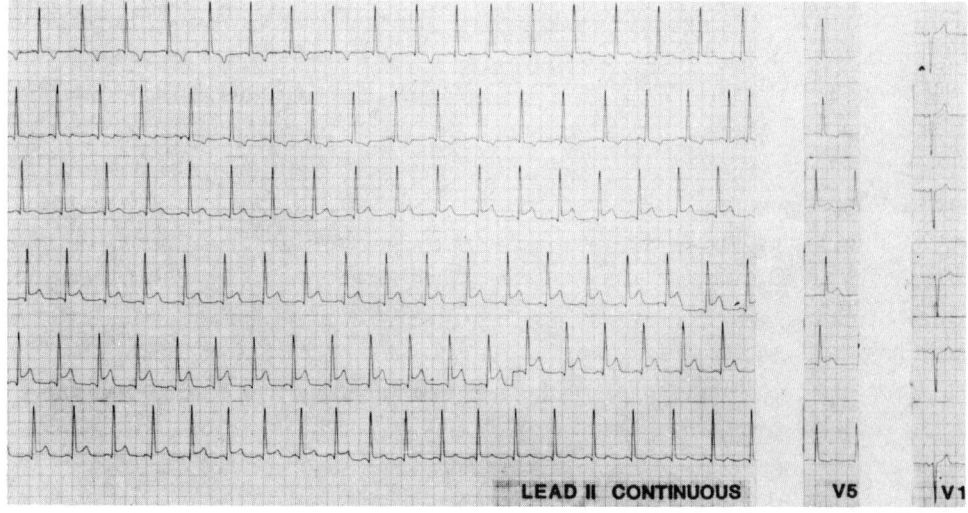

FIGURE 3-13. During prolonged electrocardiographic monitoring, this patient demonstrated transient striking ST-segment elevation that was not accompanied by angina pectoris.

[7], includes the finding of (1) a reduction of at least 50 percent in the number of ventricular premature beats during 24 hours compared with control recordings, (2) a reduction of at least 50 percent in the number of hours during which frequent and multiform ventricular premature beats were observed, and (3) a 90 percent reduction in the frequency of ventricular couplets with complete elimination of ventricular tachycardia.

Another therapeutic modality that can be evaluated with ambulatory monitoring is *pacemaker function*. Utilizing transtelephonic monitoring at scheduled intervals or full 24-hour ambulatory recordings, the clinician may evaluate three fundamental types of pacemaker malfunction. These include failure to sense (Fig. 3-14),

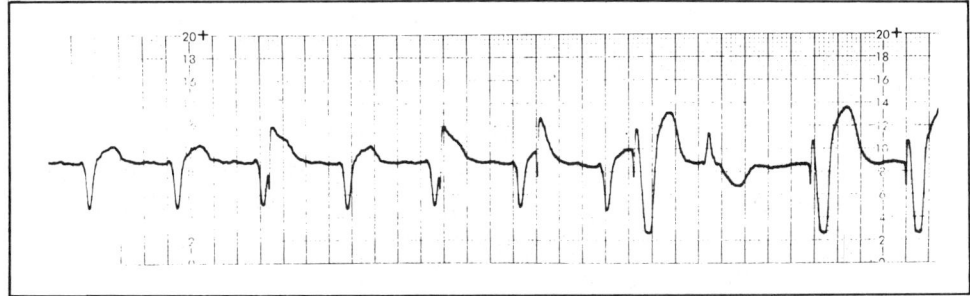

FIGURE 3-14. On several occasions this patient's demand ventricular pacemaker showed evidence of failure to sense conducted sinus QRS complexes, with inappropriate stimulation occurring during the terminal portions of ventricular depolarization.

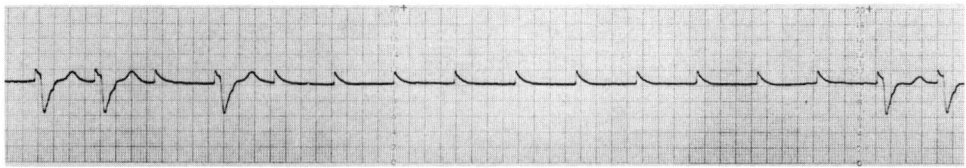

FIGURE 3-15. Two ventricularly paced beats are seen at the left, followed by a single and then a series of 10 pacemaker spikes at a rate of 70 beats/min, which fail to capture the myocardium. Such a finding may be associated with hyperkalemia and/or antiarrhythmic drug toxicity.

failure to capture despite adequate production of pacemaker spikes (Fig. 3-15), or failure to pace at the appropriate rate. It is essential that the characteristics of the individual pacemaker be known when evaluating ECG strips. The features of the many types of pacemakers now available are beyond the scope of this review, but several general facts should be emphasized. Large amplitude pacemaker spikes (greater than 10 mm) usually represent unipolar pacing. The bipolar spikes are often diminutive, and at times it takes an experienced observer to even recognize the presence of ventricular pacing. The chambers paced may include the atrium, ventricle, or both atrium and ventricle (AV sequential pacing); the chambers sensed may be the atrium or ventricle or neither if the device is a fixed-rate pacemaker. Finally, sensing of the appropriate chamber may be used to either inhibit or synchronize pacemaker spikes, thus producing vastly different ECG signals. The specifications of the particular pacemaker implanted in the patient in question should be reviewed before a diagnosis of pacemaker malfunction is made on ambulatory recordings.

Ambulatory monitoring sessions are now being used extensively just prior to hospital discharge in patients recuperating from an acute myocardial infarction as well as at varying intervals during the first year following acute myocardial infarction. Winkle [2] has summarized 11 studies evaluating the prognostic importance of VPBs found on ambulatory recordings in *postmyocardial infarction* patients. It is difficult to compare the various studies due to different endpoints (e.g., total cardiac deaths, sudden cardiac deaths), different durations of ambulatory monitoring (e.g., 1 hour, 24 hours), different classification schemes of ventricular arrhythmias, and different study entry criteria. Nevertheless, it seems clear that there is a relationship between ventricular arrhythmias on ambulatory monitorings and subsequent death (including sudden death) in patients with coronary heart disease, particularly in the early postinfarction period. As we have commented on earlier, a number of studies strongly suggest that even more important than the relative frequency of VPBs is the finding of frequent complex ventricular premature beats [3, 19–21]. In addition, whether ventricular arrhythmias serve as the most important predictor of subsequent mortality or whether they contribute to a high-risk profile in conjunction with other findings (e.g., left ventricular dysfunction, ST-segment depression on exercise testing) has not been completely resolved [2]. At this point, the clinician should understand that the postmyocardial infarction patient who demonstrates ventricular arrhythmias, particularly salvos of repetitive forms and possibly early-cycle VPBs is a candidate for aggressive antiarrhythmic therapy. Some investigators have preliminary data suggesting that abolition of high-grade VPBs can be translated into enhanced patient survival [7].

Studies of populations with coronary artery disease by Calvert et al [12] and Pratt et al [22] have shown that the prevalence and grade of VPBs increases with the number of vessels showing significant luminal obstructions. The presence of elevated left ventricular end-diastolic pressure or left ventricular regional wall motion abnormalities is also associated with increased ventricular ectopic activity. One must recognize, however, that for individual patients the prevalence and grade of ventricular premature beats may not always correlate precisely with the number of coronary vessels involved or with the degree of left ventricular dysfunction.

Studies comparing the sensitivity of ambulatory ECG monitoring and exercise treadmill testing for exposing arrhythmias in patients with coronary heart disease, the mitral valve prolapse syndrome, and hypertrophic cardiomyopathy have all indicated that ambulatory recordings appear to be superior to the standard treadmill test for the detection of ventricular arrhythmias and exposure of complex forms [2, 23]. However, since approximately 10 percent of patients with cardiac disease will demonstrate ventricular arrhythmias *only* on exercise testing, those individuals who are at high risk for sudden cardiac death (e.g., history of primary ventricular fibrillation) are best evaluated by obtaining *both* an ambulatory monitoring session and a screening exercise test. In some individuals, a new procedure, programmed ventricular stimulation (described in Chapter 10), is used as an additional tool for assessing electrical instability and antiarrhythmic efficacy [24].

Future Directions of Ambulatory Monitoring

The success noted above with the ambulatory monitoring of ECG signals has led some investigators to explore the possibility of 24-hour monitoring of blood pressure, respiratory function, electroencephalographic signals, and cyclic changes in the human gastrointestinal tract. Clinicians are thus embarking on a new era of therapy where the effects of pharmacologic interventions on patients can be assessed not merely at a single instant in time (such as a brief office visit) but rather over the dynamic continuum of a 24-hour cycle. An important question for future investigations is whether the most clinically relevant information for long-term follow-up of patients can be provided by intensive monitoring over a 24-hour period or briefer time samples spread out over several days during a given month or year.

Summary

Ambulatory electrocardiographic monitoring refers to long-term recording of an ECG signal for playback and analysis at a later time. It is particularly useful for evaluating known or suspected cardiac arrhythmias, transient myocardial ischemia, antiarrhythmic drug efficacy and pacemaker function. Hopefully, ongoing studies will further define a profile of patients at risk for sudden cardiac death and criteria for therapeutic efficacy of antiarrhythmic agents.

Acknowledgments

The assistance of the members of the Brigham and Women's Hospital Ambulatory Monitoring Laboratory in the preparation of this manuscript is greatly appreciated. The authors wish to thank Andrew White, Pamela Hough, John J. Nosta, and Carol Lochiatto.

References

1. Holter NJ: Radioelectrocardiography: A new technique for cardiovascular studies. *Ann NY Acad Sci* 65:913, 1957
2. Winkle RA: Ambulatory electrocardiography and the diagnosis, evaluation, and treatment of chronic ventricular arrhythmias. *Prog Cardiovasc Dis* 23:99, 1980
3. Ruberman W, Weinblatt E, Goldberg JD, Frank CW, Shapiro S: Ventricular premature beats and mortality after myocardial infarction. *N Engl J Med* 297:750, 1977
4. Graboys TB, Lown B: Abbreviated ECG monitoring for exposing ventricular ectopic activity. *Cardiovasc Med* 4:795, 1979
5. Lown B, Matta RJ, Besser HW: Programmed trendscription: A new approach to electrocardiographic monitoring. *JAMA* 232:39, 1975
6. Lown B, Wolf M: Approaches to sudden death from coronary heart disease. *Circulation* 44:130, 1971

7. Lown B, Podrid PJ, DeSilva RA, Graboys TB: Sudden cardiac death — management of the patient at risk. *Curr Probl Cardiol* 4:7, 1980
8. Bigger JT, Wenger TL, Heissenbuttel RH: Limitations of the Lown grading system for the study of human ventricular arrhythmias. *Am Heart J* 93:727, 1977
9. Hinkle LE, Carver ST, Stevens M: The frequency of asymptomatic disturbances of cardiac rhythm and conduction in middle-aged men. *Am J Cardiol* 24:629, 1969
10. Kennedy HL, Underhill SJ: Frequent or complex ventricular ectopy in apparently healthy subjects. *Am J Cardiol* 38:141, 1976
11. Kennedy HL, Pescarmona JE, Bouchard RJ, Goldberg RJ: Coronary artery status of apparently healthy subjects with frequent and complex ventricular ectopy. *Ann Intern Med* 92:179, 1980
12. Calvert A, Lown B, Gorlin R: Ventricular premature beats and anatomically defined coronary heart disease. *Am J Cardiol* 39:627, 1977
13. Winkle RA: Antiarrhythmic drug effect mimicked by spontaneous variability of ventricular ectopy. *Circulation* 57:1116, 1978
14. Morganroth J, Michelson EL, Horowitz LN, Josephson ME, Pearlman AS, Dunkman WB: Limitations of routine long-term electrocardiographic monitoring to assess ventricular ectopic frequency. *Circulation* 58:408, 1978
15. Michaelson EL, Morganroth J: Spontaneous variability of complex ventricular arrhythmias detected by long-term electrocardiographic recording. *Circulation* 61:690, 1980
16. Cohn PF: Silent myocardial ischemia in patients with a defective anginal warning system. *Am J Cardiol* 45:697, 1980
17. Maseri A, L'Abbate A, Chierchia S, Parodi O, Severi S, Biagini A, Distante A, Marzilli M, Ballestra AM: Significance of spasm in the pathogenesis of ischemic heart disease. *Am J Cardiol* 44:788, 1979
18. Gaughan CE, Lown B, Lanigan J, Voukydis P, Besser HW: Acute oral testing for determining antiarrhythmic drug efficacy. I. Quinidine. *Am J Cardiol* 38:677, 1976
19. Ruberman W, Weinblatt E, Goldberg J, Frank CW: Sudden death after myocardial infarction: Runs of ventricular premature beats and R on T as high risk factors. *Am J Cardiol* 45:444, 1980
20. Moss AJ, Davis HJ, DeCamilla J, Bayer L: Ventricular ectopic beats and their relation to sudden and nonsudden cardiac death after myocardial infarction. *Circulation* 60:998, 1979
21. Schultze RA Jr, Strauss WH, Pitts B: Sudden death in the year following myocardial infarction: Relation to ventricular premature contractions in the late hospital phase and left ventricular ejection fraction. *Am J Med* 62:192, 1977
22. Pratt CM, Foug A, DeMaria AN, Amsterdam EA, Mason DT: Recent advances in the understanding of ambulatory electrocardiography. *Clin Cardiol* 2:56, 1979
23. Kennedy HL, Caralis DG: Ambulatory electrocardiography: A clinical perspective. *Ann Intern Med* 87:729, 1977
24. Mason JW, Winkle RA: Accuracy of the ventricular tachycardia-induction study for predicting long-term efficacy and inefficacy of antiarrhythmic drugs. *N Engl J Med* 303:1073, 1980

Chapter 4

Exercise Testing

Peter H. Stone and Peter F. Cohn

Because physical exercise requires the heart to utilize its reserve capacity for performance, it is an ideal mechanism for objective evaluation of cardiac performance and limitations. At rest the heart may perform adequately and meet the body's requirements for oxygen and other nutrients, but once the system is stressed, latent problems may surface. In order to provide a foundation for the subsequent discussion of the exercise performance of patients with heart disease, it will be helpful to review briefly the normal physiologic response to exercise.

Physiologic Response to Exercise

In contrast to "strength" exercise of the isometric type (e.g., weightlifting), which results in hypertrophy of the muscle cells, "endurance" exercise does not result in muscle hypertrophy or an increase in strength. Instead, it brings about an increase in the capacity for aerobic metabolism. The most accepted physiologic index of total body fitness is the oxygen uptake at maximum exercise, or $\dot{V}O_2$ max [1], which is determined by collecting the expired air at the individual's maximum exercise effort and measuring its volume per minute and the percentage of oxygen extracted. This capacity to take up oxygen is related not only to the effectiveness of the lungs, but also to the ability of the heart and circulatory system to transport oxygen and to the ability of the peripheral tissues to metabolize it. $\dot{V}O_2$ max is a reproducible figure; it increases and decreases directly with the degree of physical conditioning. The uptake of oxygen increases almost linearly with increases in heart rate or cardiac output.

Generally, the increase in $\dot{V}O_2$ max that is observed following endurance exercise results equally from cardiac factors, such as an increase in cardiac output, and from peripheral factors, such as an increase in peripheral tissue extraction of oxygen (i.e., widened arteriovenous oxygen difference) [2] (Table 4-1). The resting cardiac output of a normal adult is about 5.6 L/min, and at maximum exercise, a well trained athlete may increase his cardiac output to about 36 L/min. This dramatic augmentation results from a number of cardiovascular mechanisms, such as an increase in heart rate, stroke volume, and contractility, as well as a marked net decrease in peripheral vascular resistance.

TABLE 4-1. Cardiovascular Responses to Exercise

Cardiac Factors	Peripheral Factors
Increased cardiac output	Decreased peripheral vascular resistance
Increased stroke volume 　Increased venous return 　Increased myocardial contractility	Enhanced capacity for aerobic metabolism
Decreased heart rate at rest and any given work load	

The initial increase in heart rate with exercise is thought to be due to an abrupt inhibition of vagal tone [3]. Evidence in the dog indicates that about 50 percent of the cardiac acceleration is then due to sympathetic drive, primarily beta-adrenergic stimulation. The maximum heart rate attainable is limited by age, although the reason for this limitation is unclear. The heart rate progressively increases with exercise to a predetermined amount, and it then cannot accelerate further. If the individual continues to exercise, however, and the peripheral tissues require more oxygen than the heart is capable of providing, lactate and other metabolites rapidly accumulate and soon render the cardiovascular system incapable of functioning. There is a direct linear relationship between the $\%\dot{V}O_2$ max and the percent of maximum heart rate, and this relationship provides a convenient means of comparing submaximal levels of exercise in a wide range of individuals, regardless of their state of cardiovascular fitness [4].

The stroke volume progressively increases with exercise, but it levels off somewhat before the maximal pumping capacity is achieved. The increased stroke volume is due both to an increase in venous return and to an increase in myocardial contractility. Immediately after the onset of exercise there is a reflex-mediated increase in venous tone that enhances venous return to the heart. In addition, the exercising leg muscles serve as a "pump" that further augments venous return. This increase in venous return causes an increase in myocardial fiber stretch and thereby an increase in contractility and stroke volume through the Frank-Starling mechanism. Circulating catecholamines also serve a major role in increasing contractility. The heart size gets slightly smaller near peak exercise, but because the systolic volume decreases even more than the diastolic volume, stroke volume is maintained. Prolonged endurance conditioning leads to a progressive increase in stroke volume, so that the stroke volume of conditioned athletes may be 50 to 75 percent higher than that of sedentary individuals. This response enables physically conditioned individuals to satisfy the oxygen requirements of the body at a slower heart rate.

In addition to the cardiac responses that enable the heart to pump more blood, there are major peripheral factors that enhance myocardial pump function. First, the increase in cardiac output is facilitated by a marked net decrease in peripheral vascular resistance. This "unloading" allows for a greater increase in cardiac output than would have been possible from increased heart rate and stroke volume alone. Systemic vascular resistance decreases primarily because of vasodilatation in the exercising muscle areas, while a concomitant mild decrease in blood flow to the splanchnic bed (hepatic, visceral, and renal) and nonworking muscles provide a "shunt" to the areas of demand [4]. As a result of the increased cardiac output and decreased systemic resistance, systolic blood pressure increases while diastolic blood pressure changes little or decreases slightly, creating a physiologic situation characteristic of an increased volume load.

The other major peripheral effect of endurance exercise is that of increasing the capacity for aerobic metabolism owing to alterations in the biochemical content of skeletal muscle. When skeletal muscle adapts to endurance exercise it becomes more like cardiac muscle in that its content of mitochondria and its capacity to generate ATP from oxidation of pyruvate and fatty acids increases [2]. Increases in both the size and number of mitochondria are responsible for the increase in total mitochondrial protein. Myoglobin content of skeletal muscle also increases as physical conditioning progresses. Because very little adaptive enhancement of carbohydrate metabolism occurs with exercise training, it appears that physical conditioning shifts the metabolic emphasis toward enhanced utilization of fatty acids, thus bringing about a glycogen-saving effect [5].

A few words about coronary blood flow are important to this discussion, since patients with ischemic heart disease are clearly most compromised by limitations of this factor. Unlike the peripheral tissues, which are capable of increasing their oxygen extraction from the blood in response to exercise, cardiac muscle extracts the maximum amount of oxygen from the blood at rest. The resting arteriovenous oxygen difference across the coronary circulation is therefore much wider than that across the peripheral vascular beds. Since the myocardium cannot increase oxygen extraction during exercise, the only mechanism capable of providing more oxygen to the myocardium is an actual increase in coronary blood flow. In the normal individual, coronary blood flow is "autoregulated" by myocardial oxygen demand, and coronary flow therefore increases in a direct linear fashion as myocardial oxygen demand or consumption increases.

Myocardial oxygen demand or consumption ($M\dot{V}O_2$) is dependent on a variety of factors, many of which can be measured noninvasively. Such measurements are helpful in quantitating the cardiac performance in patients with coronary disease. The principal determinants of $M\dot{V}O_2$ are heart rate, contractility, and ventricular wall tension, the latter in turn determined by the peak ventricular systolic pressure and ventricular volume. Measurement of myocardial oxygen consumption is helpful in evaluating patients with ischemic heart disease since it reflects the limits of the diseased coronary arteries to provide increased flow during stress. Initial estimates of $M\dot{V}O_2$ were made using a "triple product" of heart rate, peak systolic blood pressure, and the systolic ejection time as calculated from the carotid pulse and electrocardiogram. More recent data, however, suggest that the "double product" of heart rate and peak systolic blood pressure alone is a more reliable estimate of $M\dot{V}O_2$ [6, 7].

An understanding of these physiologic responses to exercise are particularly germane for management of the cardiac patient. These physiologic mechanisms indicate how the patient with ischemic heart disease and myocardial dysfunction may be limited in his ability to perform exercise and, equally important, they provide an understanding of the potential role of physical rehabilitation for the cardiac patient. A discussion of cardiac rehabilitation is beyond the scope of this chapter, but in commenting on the role of exercise in the management of patients with coronary disease it is important to mention that exercise testing and conditioning programs form the core of cardiac rehabilitation. Even if the heart is limited in its capacity to perform as a result of coronary disease, physical conditioning may still be of value in rendering the peripheral tissues metabolically more efficient. Conditioning enables the heart to work less hard for any given work load, and the total work load attainable becomes increased. In cardiac rehabilitation programs the exercise laboratory becomes not only the supervised setting in which diagnosis and prognosis is determined for the patient with coronary disease, but it also becomes the practice field for enhancement of work performance. The reader is referred to excellent recent reviews for elaboration on the role of cardiac rehabilitation [8].

Historical Perspective of Exercise Testing

The use of exercise to evaluate patients with suspected coronary artery disease dates back over 50 years. Feil and Siegal [9] were the first to report the use of electrocardiographic (ECG) responses to exercise in 1928. About this time Master [10] introduced a standardized two-step test, which originally was used to observe pulse and blood pressure responses to exercise. A few years later the electrocardiogram was added to the Master two-step test to aid in the evaluation of coronary artery disease [11] and, because of its simplicity and availability, the Master test became a standard for exercise testing for many years. As experience accumulated over the ensuing years, follow-up studies confirmed the prognostic value of abnormal ECG responses to exercise [12], and the exercise stress test achieved a secure role as a vital adjunct in the evaluation and management of patients with coronary disease.

The type of exercise used in stress testing has evolved over the years. Most recently the treadmill and bicycle have been used commonly to provide a more standardized and strenuous exercise at regular stages. Exercise protocols that require leg muscle activity have been chosen because the amount of exercise is more likely to be limited by the cardiac output and not by muscle weakness if the largest and strongest muscles are utilized. In addition, the oxygen demand of active muscle is directly related to muscle mass and metabolic efficiency. Therefore, use of large muscle groups, like those in the legs, is likely to be associated with a higher oxygen uptake. Many stress test physiologists consider the treadmill a preferred means of leg exercise for use in America since most Americans have not developed the muscles used in prolonged bicycle exercise.

Exercise Protocols

Stress testing methodology has recently been extensively reviewed [13]. Figure 4-1 illustrates representative examples of graded multistage treadmill exercise protocols that are commonly employed [14]. When exercise is initiated, the demands of the body usually exceed oxygen intake for a short period and an "oxygen debt" temporarily accumulates. This "oxygen debt" is usually paid back quickly, however, and if the work load remains constant, a steady state of oxygen intake and oxygen consumption is achieved within 2 or 3 minutes. This steady state is characterized by a stable heart rate. If exercise proceeds too rapidly, however, a steady state may not be achieved and the oxygen debt may accumulate excessively. In order to allow the body to balance its oxygen intake and consumption optimally, most exercise protocols increase the work load only at intervals of 2 or 3 minutes. Pollock et al [14] compared the physiologic performance of 51 healthy men using the four protocols illustrated in Figure 4-1 and found that at maximum exercise there was generally no significant difference in $\dot{V}O_2$ max, heart rate, and blood pressure. Because of the more gradual increase in metabolic requirements (METS) observed using the Bruce or Ellestad protocols, however, these two protocols are preferable for routine screening purposes. Most of the recently reported experience using exercise to evaluate patients with ischemic heart disease employs the Bruce protocol; accordingly, most of the subsequent discussion will be based on those data.

Many of the early exercise protocols utilized only a single monitor ECG lead, such as a modified bipolar lead V5, to detect ECG changes characteristic of myocardial ischemia. More recently, however, it has been appreciated that multiple lead systems enhance the sensitivity of the exercise test without reducing the predictive value of a positive test. Chaitman and associates [15] evaluated a variety of single and multiple lead systems with the Bruce treadmill protocol and found that a 14-lead system (three bipolar chest leads plus the 12-lead ECG excluding aVR) increased the ECG sensitivity from 56 to 88 percent as compared to a single bipolar lead system, while maintaining the predictive value of a positive test at greater

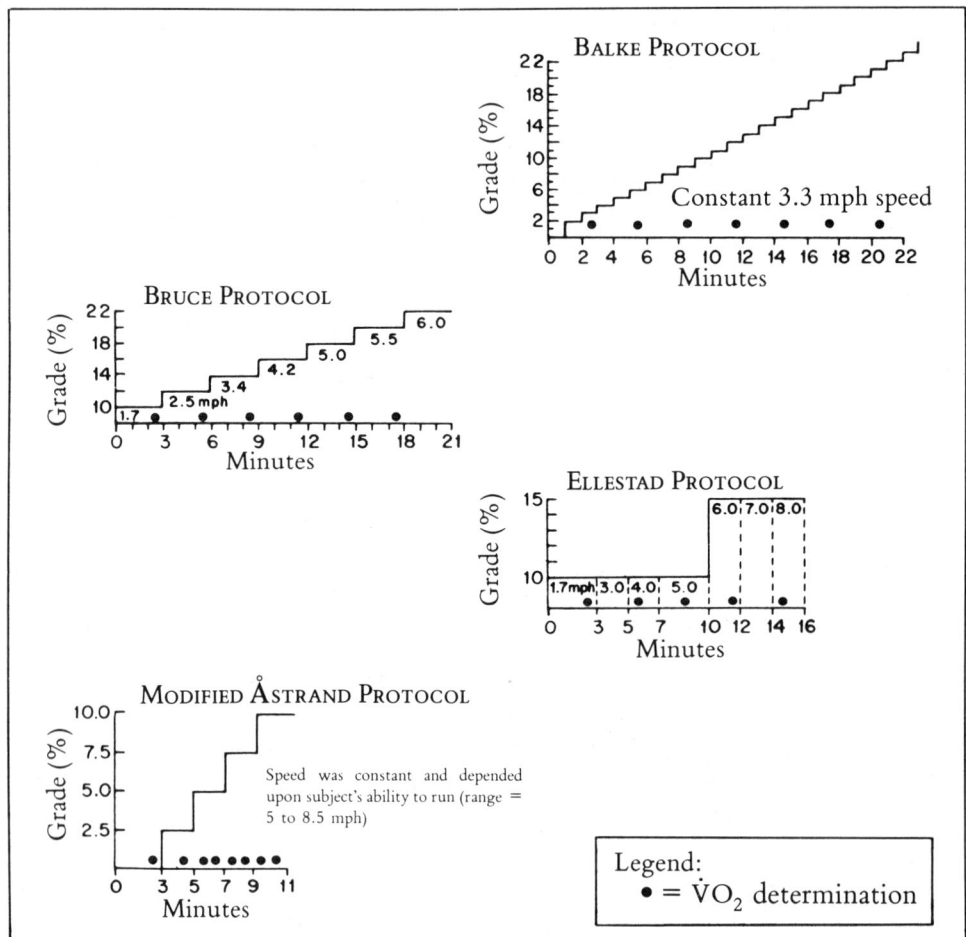

FIGURE 4-1. Work loads employed in a number of popular exercise testing protocols. (From ML Pollock et al [14].)

than 90 percent. The 14-lead ECG was particularly valuable in detecting patients with multivessel coronary disease.

The recommended degree of exercise that a patient should perform on an exercise protocol remains somewhat controversial. A "maximal effort" test is one in which the patient exercises until maximal O_2 consumption ($\dot{V}O_2$ max) is achieved or until limiting symptoms develop. Some investigators consider this degree of maximum effort to be unsafe, although no data exist to support that claim. A "submaximal effort" test, on the other hand, is one in which the endpoint for termination of the study is attainment of an arbitrary heart rate (e.g., 150 beats/min) or greater than 85 percent of a maximal "predicted" heart rate based on exercise tests in healthy individuals. One of the major arguments against the use of submaximal effort tests is that the amount of stress required for different patients to achieve these arbitrary endpoint heart rates may vary considerably. For example, patients with coronary artery disease or those treated with beta-blocking agents may be unable to achieve their "predicted" maximal heart rate. Supramaximal effort, and perhaps even a dangerous degree of exercise, may be required for these patients to attain the heart rate recommended by the predicted guidelines. On the other hand, a very healthy individual may be able to perform substantially more exercise than that recommended by the guidelines, and his or her exercise performance may be inadequately tested. The 95 percent confidence limits around the mean predicted heart rate is ±16 to ±20 beats/min [16], and so a great deal of variation around the mean is normal. Strict adherence to this predicted mean heart rate is therefore neither physiologic nor necessarily safe. The use of a maximal effort test, or symptom-limited exercise, has been shown in the Seattle Heart Watch program to be safe and feasible in widespread use. Performance on these maximal effort tests also correlates well with the accepted physiologic indexes of maximal aerobic capacity, such as a plateau in O_2 consumption ($\dot{V}O_2$ max), elevated lactate levels, and a respiratory exchange ratio above 1 : 15 [17].

Indications for Exercise Stress Testing

In recent years skepticism regarding the exercise test has forced us to reexamine carefully its role in the evaluation of patients with heart disease and thereby to refine our perception of its real value. A more accurate understanding of the stress test has emerged from this controversy. Table 4-2 shows the indications for noninvasive exercise stress testing. Of great value, yet surrounded by great controversy, is the use of the exercise test to aid in the diagnosis of chest pain. More about this controversy will be discussed shortly. Probably the most valuable use of the stress test is to estimate the severity and prognosis of coronary disease and to help provide guidelines for selecting patients who need more extensive diagnostic and therapeutic interventions such as cardiac catheterization and coronary artery bypass surgery. The efficacy of medical or surgical treatment of coronary artery disease can also be evaluated using the stress test. The exercise test may be useful in evaluating the exercise capacity of patients with a wide range of cardiac disease, particularly those with valvular heart disease. In recent years the stress test has been found to be helpful in guiding rehabilitation following a myocardial infarction and, in addition, to provide prognostic stratification of patients postinfarction. The exercise test can aid in the evaluation of cardiac arrhythmias, and it can provide a safety checkup prior to a fitness program. Exercise tests are also used to screen high-risk professionals such as airline pilots. In addition, although contro-

TABLE 4-2. Indications for Exercise Stress Testing

To aid in the diagnosis of chest pain
To determine the severity and prognosis of cardiac disease
To evaluate medical or surgical therapy of cardiac disease
To guide rehabilitation following myocardial infarction
To evaluate cardiac arrhythmias
To provide a safety checkup prior to a fitness program
To screen high-risk professionals
To assess risk factors in asymptomatic patients

versial, the test can be used to assess risk factors in asymptomatic individuals [18, 19].

Exercise testing is contraindicated in patients with certain cardiovascular diseases such as acute myocardial infarction, unstable angina pectoris, acute myocarditis or pericarditis, and decompensated congestive heart failure. In addition, patients with a high degree of resting ventricular ectopic activity or second or third degree AV block should not be exercised. Severe resting hypertension (in the range of >220/150 mm Hg) is a relative contraindication [5], and the hypertension should be better controlled prior to exercise. The presence of aortic stenosis is also a relative contraindication; patients with severe aortic stenosis may be unable to increase cardiac output proportionate to the amount of peripheral vasodilatation that accompanies exercise, and perfusion to vital organs such as the brain and heart may become compromised.

Appropriate Use of the Exercise Test

Before exploring the value of exercise stress testing further, it will be helpful to define some of the terms used, since they will be referred to often (Fig. 4-2). "Sensitivity" refers to the percent of all patients *with* disease who manifest an abnormal test. Sensitivity is determined by calculating the number of true-positive tests divided by the total of true-positive plus false-negative tests. "Specificity" refers to the patients *without* disease who manifest a negative test. Specificity is determined by calculating the number of true-negative tests divided by the number of true-negative tests plus the false-positive tests. "Predictive accuracy" refers to the percent of positive tests that are truly positive and is determined by calculating the number of true-positive tests divided by the number of true-positive tests plus false-positive tests.

It is necessary at the outset to clarify which population of patients can benefit most by the exercise stress test. Much of the recent controversy surrounding exercise testing focuses on the inappropriate use of the stress test. It has recently

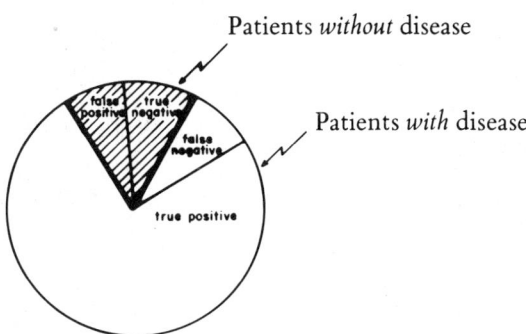

Sensitivity = percent of all patients *with disease* who manifest an abnormal test

$$= \frac{\text{true positive}}{\text{true positive} + \text{false negative}} \times 100$$

Specificity = percent of all patients *without disease* who manifest a negative test

$$= \frac{\text{true negative}}{\text{true negative} + \text{false positive}} \times 100$$

Predictive accuracy = percent of positive tests that are truly positive

$$= \frac{\text{true positive}}{\text{true positive} + \text{false positive}} \times 100$$

FIGURE 4-2. Terms used in exercise stress testing. The open area of the diagram represents patients with coronary artery disease who undergo an exercise stress test and the shaded portion represents patients without coronary artery disease who perform a stress test.

been claimed that exercise testing provides no further insight into the diagnosis of coronary artery disease than that obtained from history and physical examination alone [20]. This leads us to a crucial concept, namely, that the stress test is valuable only when applied to the appropriate patient population. In other words, the predictive accuracy of the exercise stress test is highly dependent on the prevalence of disease in the population tested, the concept formulated in Bayes' theorem of probability. In the example shown in Figure 4-3 [21], 95 percent of *symptomatic* patients whose test was positive had significant underlying coronary disease as determined by angiography, and only 5 percent of tests were falsely positive. Predictive accuracy in this population was therefore 95 percent. On the other hand, of 39 *asymptomatic* subjects with a positive exercise test, only 36 percent had a true-positive response as confirmed by coronary angiography; the remaining 64 percent had either normal coronary arteries or insignificant coronary obstructions. Thus, testing in asymptomatic patients yielded a false-positive incidence of 64 percent. Although the same criterion of 1 mm ST-seg-

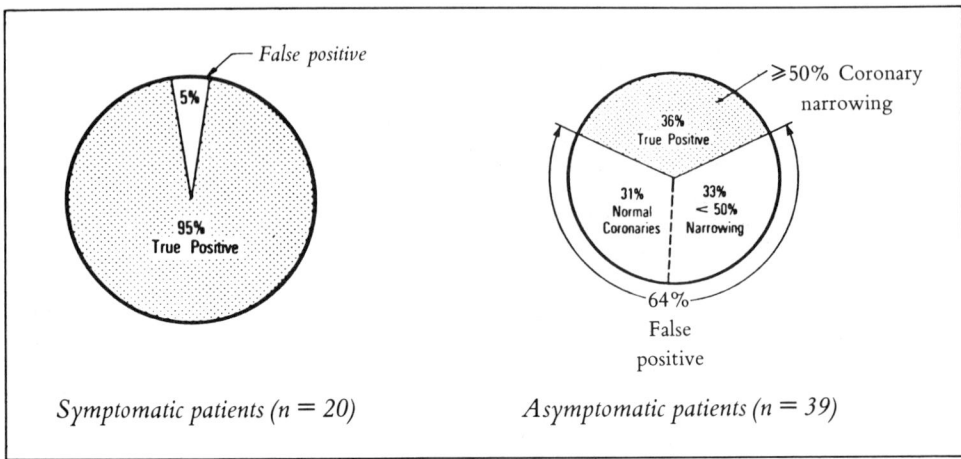

FIGURE 4-3. Predictive accuracy of a positive exercise test in symptomatic vs. asymptomatic patients. A positive test is defined as the development of 1 mm horizontal or downsloping ST-segment depression. (From SE Epstein [21].)

ment depression was used to define a positive test, the predictive accuracy of the test is very different when it is applied to populations with different disease prevalence. The relationship between predictive accuracy and disease prevalence is shown graphically in Figure 4-4. As the disease prevalence increases there is an exponential increase in the predictive accuracy of the test. When the disease is uncommon, the test will not be very accurate; however, the test can become very accurate if the disease prevalence is high.

As shown in Figure 4-5, a whole family of curves relating predictive accuracy to disease prevalence can be calculated based on the various criteria for a positive test. If a relatively small ST-segment depression is used as a criterion to diagnose the presence of coronary disease (e.g., 1 mm of ischemic ST-segment depression), then the predictive accuracy of the test is not helpful until the disease prevalence is quite high. However, if one chooses very stringent criteria for a positive test (e.g., 2.5 mm of ischemic ST-segment depression), then even at a low disease prevalence the stress test may be highly predictive for the presence of coronary disease. As is evident, there is a broad continuum inversely relating specificity and sensitivity, and it is important to interpret the stress test with all of these relationships in mind. It is true that use of the exercise stress test to determine the simple diagnosis of presence or absence of coronary disease is fraught with many complexities. History and physical examination can indeed provide an extremely high index of suspicion for the presence of coronary disease, and in such a clinical setting the exercise stress test may only provide confirmation of that suspicion. However, the greatest value of the stress test is primarily in determining the

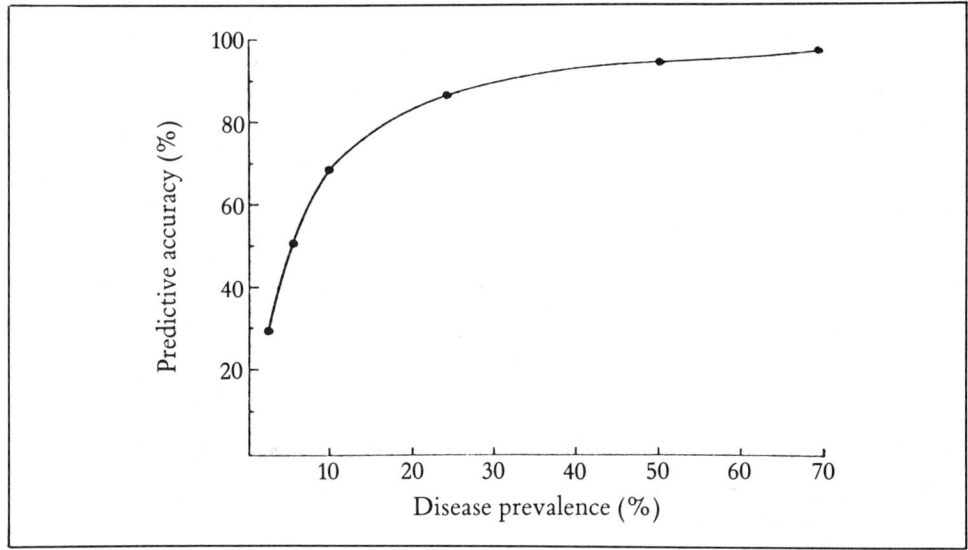

FIGURE 4-4. Influence of disease prevalence on predictive accuracy of a positive test. (From SE Epstein [21].)

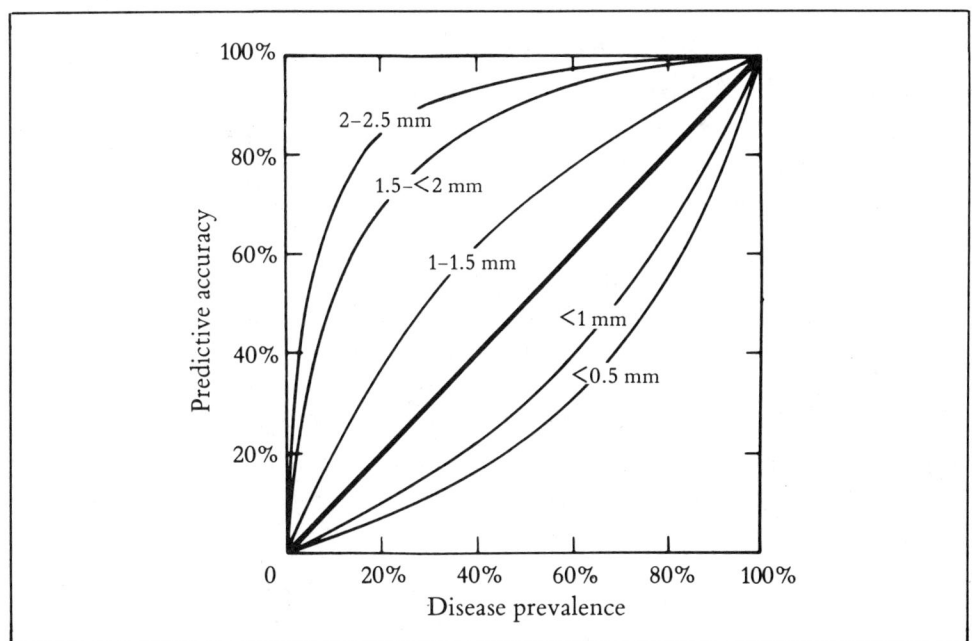

FIGURE 4-5. Family of ST-segment depression curves. (From SE Epstein [21].)

severity of coronary artery disease and the prognosis of patients with *known* coronary disease. Since the prognosis of patients with coronary disease is dependent on the number of coronary vessels involved, as are, in large part, the indications for performing coronary artery bypass surgery, the stress test may be uniquely useful to determine safely and noninvasively which patients are in need of further invasive evaluation and therapy.

Features of the Exercise Test Performance Useful in the Diagnosis of Coronary Disease

The features of the exercise test performance that are most helpful in interpreting the stress test and in determining the severity of coronary artery disease are shown in Table 4-3. These features include the morphology and degree of ST-segment depression, the presence of exercise-induced ST-segment elevation, the time of onset of ischemic ST-segment depression, the duration of the exercise tolerated, the persistence of ST-segment depression in the recovery period, and the development of changes in R-wave amplitude. Exertional hypotension is an ominous indicator of severe coronary artery disease, and the presence of ventricular arrhythmias during the exercise test may reflect multivessel involvement.

EXERCISE-INDUCED ST-SEGMENT CHANGES

Goldschlager and her associates were among the first investigators to clarify the significance of different morphologies of the ST-segment response to exercise [22]. As shown in Figure 4-6, they related the ST-segment morphology to the number of diseased coronary artery vessels in 410 patients. Those patients with either downsloping or horizontal ST-segment depression had an extremely high prevalence of multivessel coronary disease. Patients with slowly upsloping ST segments frequently had significant coronary artery disease, but up to one-third of these patients had normal coronary arteries. Those patients with J-point depression alone without ST-segment depression most often had normal coronary arteries.

Kurita and coworkers in Montreal have evaluated the significance of J-point depression and have demonstrated the importance of determining the degree of ST-segment depression not only at the J-point, but also 0.04 and 0.08 second after the J-point [23]. These investigators related the number of patients with significant coronary disease to the type of J-point depression observed with exercise (Fig. 4-7). They noted that the development of up to 1.4 mm of isolated J-point depression was normal with exercise. This modest amount of J-point depression probably represents the repolarization or "T wave" of atrial depolarization. Isolated J-point depression of 1.5 or 2.0 mm with a rapidly upsloping ST segment was not very sensitive in detecting coronary artery disease: only about 50 percent of these patients had significant coronary obstructions. However, when the J-point was depressed, with ST-segment depression greater than 2.0 mm at 0.08

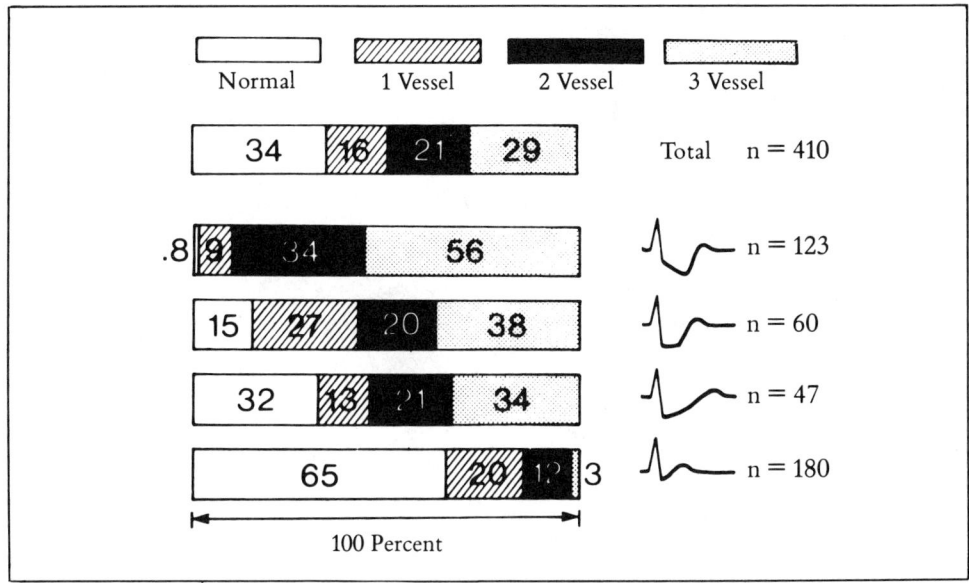

FIGURE 4-6. Relation between the type of ST-segment response and the extent of coronary artery disease. (From N Goldschlager et al [22].)

TABLE 4-3. Cardinal Features of Exercise Test Performance

Morphology and degree of ST-segment depression
Exercise-induced ST-segment elevation
Time of onset of ST-segment depression
Duration of exercise tolerated
Persistence of ST-segment depression in recovery
Changes in R-wave amplitude
Exercise-induced hypotension
Exercise-induced arrhythmias and conduction disturbances

second after the J-point, there was a 94 percent prevalence of coronary artery disease. In comparison, those patients with horizontal or downsloping ST-segment depression had a prevalence of coronary artery disease of about 96 percent. Therefore, J-point depression can be reliable for the diagnosis of coronary disease only if the ST segment remains depressed 0.08 second after the J-point.

The degree of ST-segment depression has great diagnostic significance for the number of coronary arteries involved. Figure 4-8, from the work of Bartel and coworkers [24], correlates the amount of ST-segment change with the number of diseased coronary arteries. There is an almost direct correlation between the degree of exercise-induced ST-segment depression and the extent of coronary disease. Almost 60 percent of patients with a negative test have normal coronary arteries,

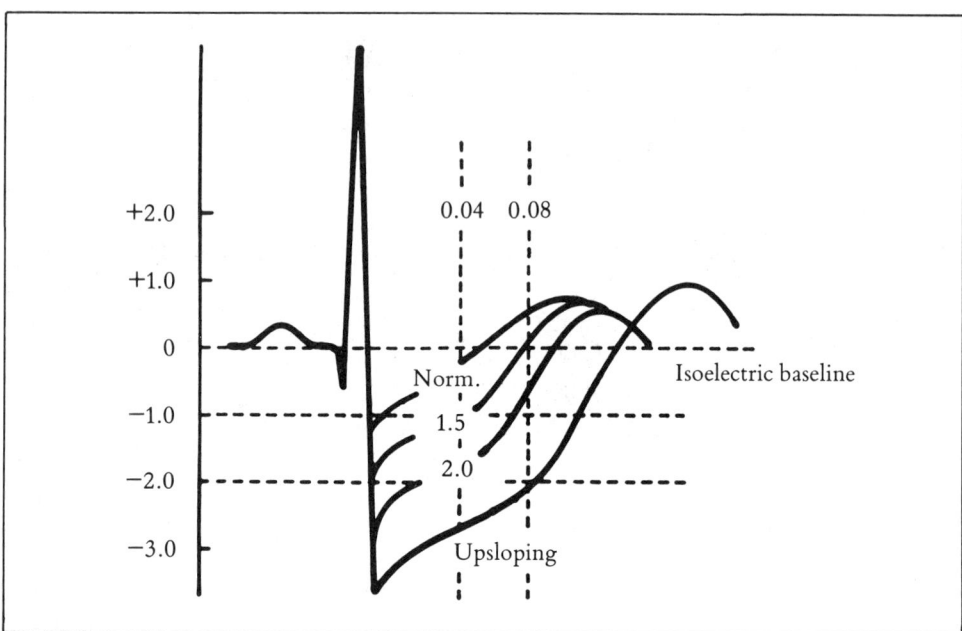

FIGURE 4-7. Types of junctional depression.

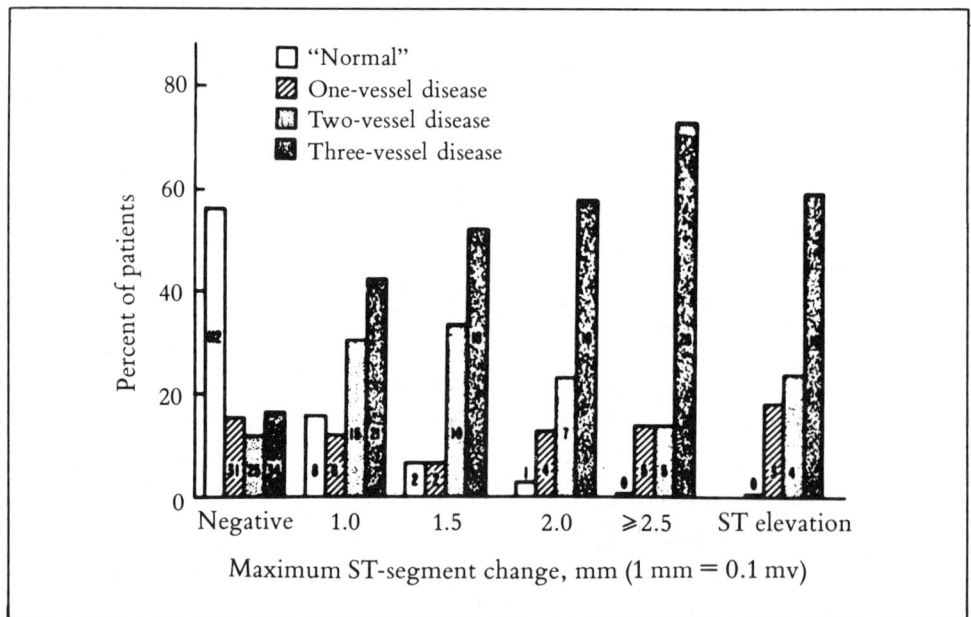

FIGURE 4-8. Maximum degree of ST-segment change related to extent of coronary artery disease. (From AG Bartel et al: Graded exercise stress tests in angiographically documented coronary artery disease. *Circulation* 49:348, 1974, by permission of the American Heart Association, Inc.)

whereas none of the patients with marked ST-segment depression (≥2.5 mm) have normal coronary anatomy. Conversely, relatively few patients with a negative or mildly positive test have multivessel disease, whereas about 90 percent of patients with marked ST-segment depression have multivessel involvement. This treadmill study confirms earlier studies done with the two-step test [25]. Cheitlin et al [26] related the amount of ischemic ST-segment depression to the presence of "critical coronary artery lesions," defined as obstructions in the left main coronary artery, the proximal left anterior descending and the proximal circumflex arteries ("left main equivalent"), or the proximal left anterior descending artery. Among patients with marked ischemic ST-segment depression of greater than 2 mm, almost 25 percent had a left main coronary artery obstruction and another almost 30 percent had a "left main equivalent" lesion. On the other hand, none of the patients with less than 2 mm of ischemic ST-segment depression had left main coronary artery disease. Since coronary artery bypass surgery prolongs life in patients with left main coronary artery disease and perhaps in those with triple-vessel disease as well, patients with marked ST-segment depression should be considered for invasive diagnostic studies to determine their eligibility for coronary artery surgery.

The persistence of ischemic ST-segment depression in the recovery period may also reflect the severity of coronary artery disease (Fig. 4-9). Over 40 percent of patients whose ischemic ST-segment depression resolved within 1 minute of recovery had either normal coronary arteries or single-vessel disease. However, of the patients whose ST depression lasted at least 9 minutes into recovery, 90 percent had multivessel disease [22].

Interestingly, some studies have observed a difference in the predictive value of the exercise test between males and females. The predictive value of a positive ST-segment response to detect the presence of coronary artery disease, for example, is less for females than for males, and the predictive value of a negative test to exclude the presence of coronary disease is greater for females than for males [27]. Furthermore, an analysis of the "nondiagnostic" exercise test, i.e., a test in which the patient cannot achieve the target heart rate and there is less than 1.0 mm of ischemic ST-segment depression, indicated that most of the women who exhibited a nondiagnostic test had normal coronary arteries, whereas most of the men with a nondiagnostic test had coronary artery disease [27]. This suggests that the mechanism for poor exercise performance in the two sexes may be different, i.e., the limitation is usually cardiac in men and extracardiac in women.

The presence of exercise-induced ST-segment elevation may also have great significance in the evaluation of patients with coronary artery disease. Such exertional ST-segment elevation has been correlated with wall motion abnormalities, such as those seen with a ventricular aneurysm following a previous transmural infarction

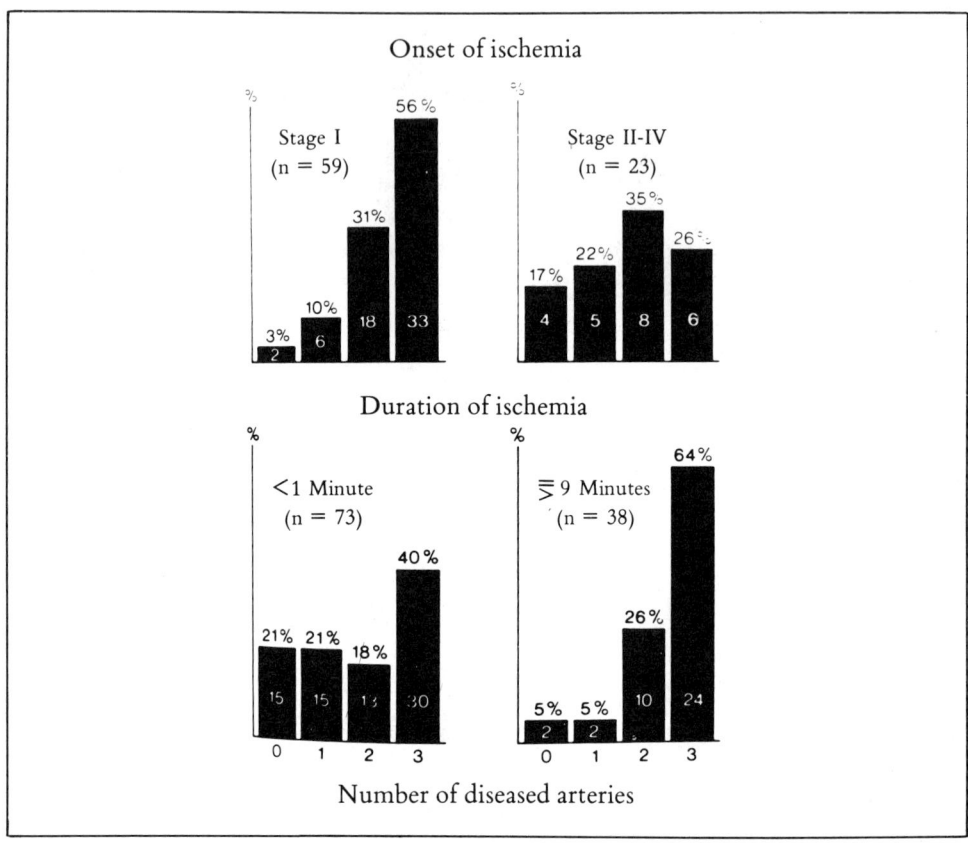

FIGURE 4-9. (*Top*) Relation of appearance time of ischemia to severity of coronary artery disease. (*Bottom*) Relation of duration of ischemic changes in recovery period to severity of coronary artery disease. (From N Goldschlager et al [22].)

[28, 29] or with severe underlying coronary disease [28, 30, 31]. The resting tracing must therefore be carefully examined before interpreting the significance of ST-segment elevation. For example, in Figure 4-10 the resting tracing is normal, and yet with exercise there is marked ST-segment elevation in leads V2–V4. This patient was found to have a severe proximal obstruction of the left anterior descending coronary artery. In contrast, the patient whose ECG is illustrated in Figure 4-11 had a prior transmural infarction in the same area, with exercise-induced ST-segment elevation; the exercise ST-segment elevation may simply represent wall motion abnormalities secondary to the infarction and not necessarily reflect tenuous coronary circulation.

Chahine and coworkers [28] have recently clarified the significance of exercise-induced ST-segment elevation, as shown in Table 4-4. Sixty-four percent of patients with a left ventricular apical aneurysm demonstrated exertional ST-segment elevation. In these patients the wall motion abnormalities from a previ-

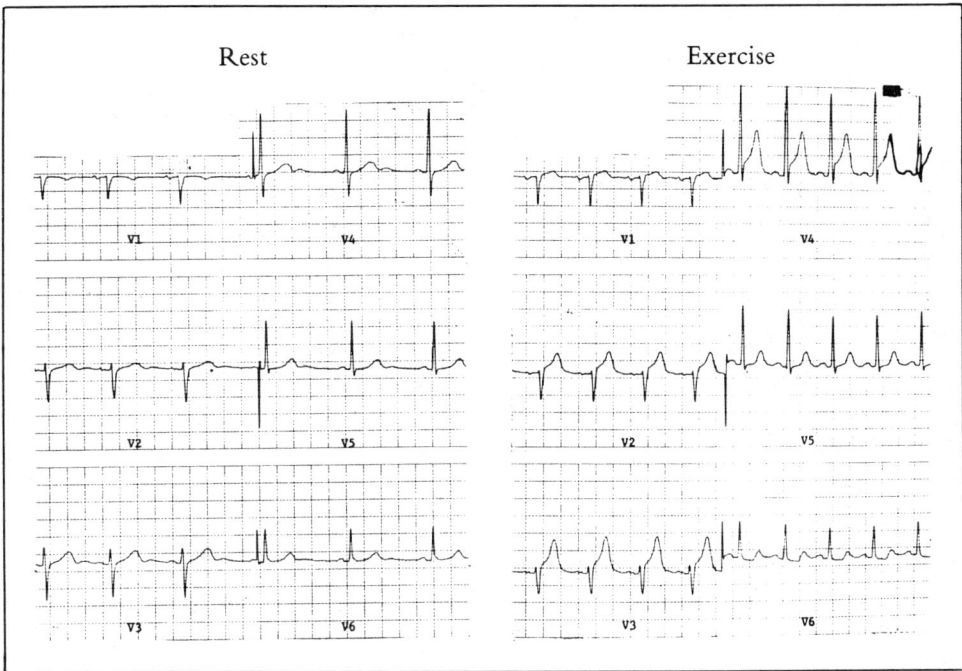

FIGURE 4-10. ST-segment elevation with exercise in the absence of prior myocardial infarction.

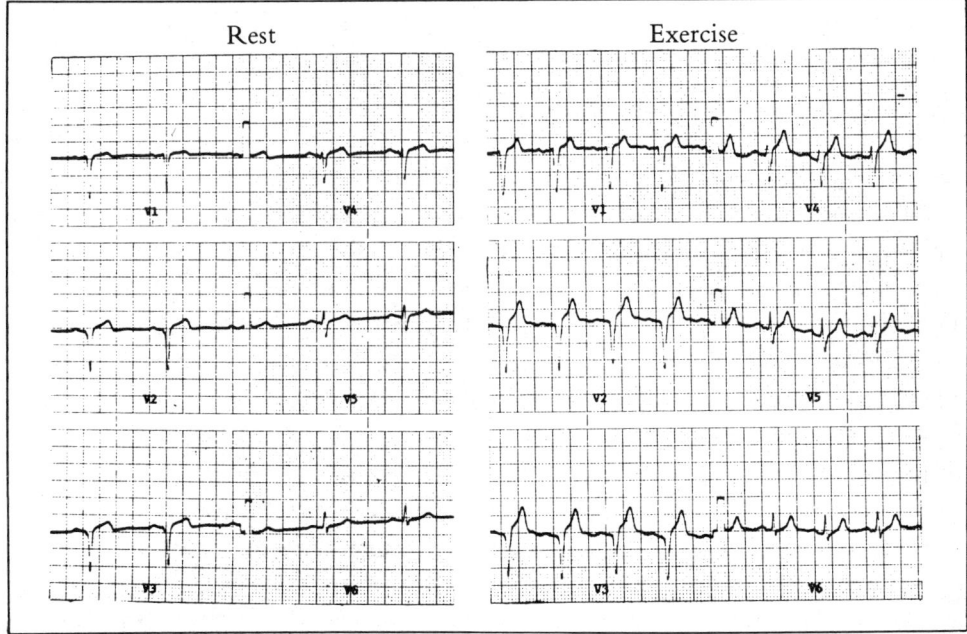

FIGURE 4-11. ST-segment elevation with exercise in the presence of prior myocardial infarction.

TABLE 4-4. Correlates of Exercise-Induced ST-Segment Elevation

	Total	No. of Patients with ST Elevation (%)
Critical proximal LAD obstruction	104	19 (18)
Left ventricular apical aneurysm	28	18 (64)

LAD = left anterior descending coronary artery. Adapted from RA Chahine et al [28].

ous transmural infarction were responsible for the exercise ST-segment elevation. ST-segment elevation is less sensitive, however, for the detection of severe coronary artery disease: only 18 percent of the patients with a critical proximal left anterior descending artery obstruction exhibited ST-segment elevation. In these patients the ST-segment elevation was indicative of severe underlying coronary disease and an area of jeopardized, ischemic myocardium. Thus, in the absence of a known prior transmural infarction or aneurysm formation, ST-segment elevation may be highly indicative of severe underlying coronary disease, and further angiographic investigation may be indicated.

EXERCISE-INDUCED R-WAVE CHANGES

Recently, investigators have evaluated the significance of changes in R-wave amplitude during exercise and, in general, found that they are a useful marker for the identification of patients with ventricular dysfunction and coronary artery disease. On the basis of theoretical considerations, it has been suggested that the amplitude of the R wave on the surface ECG varies directly with ventricular volume [32]. In normal individuals the R-wave amplitude generally decreases [33], presumably owing to the decrease in heart size with exercise. Patients with coronary artery disease often demonstrate exercise-induced ischemia and left ventricular dysfunction with a consequent increase in ventricular volume; one would therefore anticipate that R-wave amplitude would increase in such patients. Bonoris et al [34] found that an analysis of exercise-induced changes in R-wave amplitude enhanced the stress test sensitivity from 48 to 63 percent and specificity from 59 to 79 percent when compared to the conventional analysis of ischemic ST-segment depression. Berman et al [35] also observed that utilizing the sum of R waves in aVL, aVF, and V3–V6 plus the S wave in aVL and V2 improved the accuracy of the exercise ECG in detecting the presence of coronary artery disease beyond the accuracy of the conventional ST segment criteria alone and that these R-wave changes were also a highly significant marker of left ventricular dysfunction. Others, however, report that although changes in R-wave amplitude may increase the sensitivity of the stress test for detection of patients with coronary disease, they also dramatically reduce specificity [36, 37]. Furthermore, one group

[37] found that exercise-induced changes in R-wave amplitude were not closely correlated with either the presence of ischemic ST-segment changes or the extent of coronary artery disease. Although controversial, analysis of R-wave amplitude changes may provide an additional factor to aid in the composite interpretation of the stress test performance.

EXERTIONAL HYPOTENSION

The presence of exercise-induced hypotension often portends severe underlying coronary disease. Morris et al [38] noted that 22 of 279 patients (8 percent) manifested a decrease in systolic blood pressure of 10 mm Hg or more during an exercise treadmill test. The correlation of the severity of coronary disease and exertional hypotension is shown in Table 4-5. Most of the patients who demonstrated this finding had severe triple-vessel or left main coronary artery disease. None of the patients with single-vessel disease developed hypotension.

EXERCISE-INDUCED ARRHYTHMIAS AND CONDUCTION DISTURBANCES

The significance of exercise-induced arrhythmias and conduction disturbances is not entirely clear. Early investigators thought that there was not a very close correlation between the frequency of ventricular ectopic beats at rest, during exercise, or in recovery and the extent of coronary artery disease [39]. However, in more recent studies that correlate angiographic findings with exercise-induced arrhythmias, patients with multivessel disease demonstrated a significantly greater incidence of ventricular ectopic beats both at rest and in the recovery period when compared with patients with only single-vessel involvement [40–42]. In addition, Udall and Ellestad demonstrated that the presence of exercise-induced ventricular ectopic beats adversely affects prognosis both in patients with a positive ST-segment response to exercise and even in those patients with ventricular ectopic beats who do *not* exhibit ischemic ST-segment changes [43]. It should be pointed out, however, that 24-hour ambulatory monitoring (see Chap. 3) is more efficacious than the exercise test in exposing the presence and severity of ventricular ectopic activity in patients with coronary disease [44]. The significance of exercise-induced intraventricular conduction disturbances or atrioventricular block has not been extensively studied, but it is suggested that such phenomena alone do not necessarily indicate the presence of coronary disease [5, 45]. The development of a right bundle branch block conduction pattern does not mask the characteristic ischemic ST-segment depression, especially in the lateral leads, and therefore if ischemic heart disease is the cause of the conduction disturbance, such ischemic changes should be evident in the ST-segment response to exercise. The presence of a left bundle branch block conduction pattern, on the other hand, may indeed mask the ischemic ST-segment response, so that the development of exercise-

TABLE 4-5. Correlation of Severity of Coronary Disease and Exertional Hypotension

	No. of Patients (%)
Single-vessel CAD (90)	0 (0)
Two-vessel CAD (101)	7 (7)
Triple-vessel CAD or LMCAD (88)	15 (17)

CAD = coronary artery disease, LMCAD = left main coronary artery disease. Adapted from SN Morris et al [38].

induced left bundle branch block precludes accurate interpretation of the ST-segment response.

COMBINATION OF EXERCISE PERFORMANCE VARIABLES

Recently, a number of investigators have combined exercise test variables in order to enhance the interpretation of the patient's performance. Shown in Table 4-6, for example, are data that relate both the ST-segment response and the Bruce protocol stage entered to the presence and extent of coronary disease [46]. A positive test was defined as one in which there was at least 1 mm of ischemic ST-segment depression; and a negative test was defined as the achievement of greater than 85 percent of the maximum predicted heart rate without ischemic ST-segment depression. Among the patients with a positive stress test in stage I of the Bruce protocol, 73 percent had triple-vessel disease and 27 percent had significant obstruction of the left main coronary artery. On the other hand, when the stress test was positive to the same degree but the patient was able to exercise to at least stage IV of the Bruce protocol, only 29 percent of the patients had triple-vessel disease and only 5 percent had a left main coronary artery obstruction. Therefore, in addition to the positivity of the ST-segment response, the amount of exercise that the patient can tolerate may indicate the severity of disease. Equally important, of the patients who were forced to stop in stage I because of symptoms even though their ST-segment response was negative, 21 percent nevertheless exhibited triple-vessel disease, and 10 percent had significant obstruction of the left main coronary artery. The development of limiting symptoms alone at such a low level of exercise reflected significant underlying heart disease. On the other hand, extensive coronary disease was very uncommon in patients able to exercise to stage IV with a negative ST-segment response. Goldschlager and her colleagues examined this combination of type and onset of ST-segment deviation even more closely [22]. As shown in Figure 4-9, they noted the exercise stage in which ischemic ST-segment depression first appeared and related that to the number of diseased coronary arteries. Almost 90 percent of patients who developed ischemic ECG signs in stage I had multivessel coronary disease and

TABLE 4-6. Relationship of Exercise Test Stage Entered and ST-Segment Response to Presence and Extent of Coronary Artery Disease

Exercise Test Results (n)	CAD (%)	Triple-Vessel Disease (%)	>50% Obstruction of LMCA (%)
STAGE I			
Positive (51)	98	73	27
Negative (79)	52	21	10
≥STAGE IV			
Positive (104)	77	29	5
Negative (280)	36	9	1

CAD = coronary artery disease, LMCA = left main coronary artery. Adapted from JF McNeer et al [46].

only 10 percent had single-vessel disease. On the other hand, of patients able to exercise to stage III or IV of the Bruce protocol before developing ischemic ECG changes, almost 40 percent had either normal coronary arteries or single-vessel disease. A distinct minority of the patients with late onset ischemia had malignant triple-vessel and left main coronary artery disease.

In a similar manner, Berman and colleagues [27] applied a multivariate approach to the interpretation of the exercise test performance. They found that the predictive value of a positive test improved from 78 percent when ischemic ST-segment depression alone was used to diagnose coronary disease, to 97 percent when any two of the following variables were present in addition to the ischemic ST-segment depression: peak double product less than 23,000, exercise duration less than 6 minutes on the Bruce protocol, and ST-segment depression persisting for more than 3 minutes into the recovery period. These investigators found no added predictive value if angina pectoris developed during the exercise test. Thus silent myocardial ischemia [47] was as likely to be associated with severe coronary artery disease as were ST-segment changes accompanied by test angina pectoris. In contrast, others report test angina pectoris to be more prevalent with severe coronary artery disease [24].

Investigators at Duke University also combined features of the exercise test performance in order to stratify patients prognostically into low-risk and high-risk subgroups [46]. Figure 4-12 shows the 4-year survival for these two groups. The low-risk subgroup includes those patients with either a negative test, an ability to exercise to Bruce stage IV or beyond, or the achievement of a maximum heart rate greater than 160 beats/min. Their 4-year survival is excellent. The high-risk subgroup, on the other hand, are those patients who had a positive ST-segment response and terminated exercise in stage I or II. Their survival is quite poor, and therefore they may be candidates for additional medical or surgical treatment.

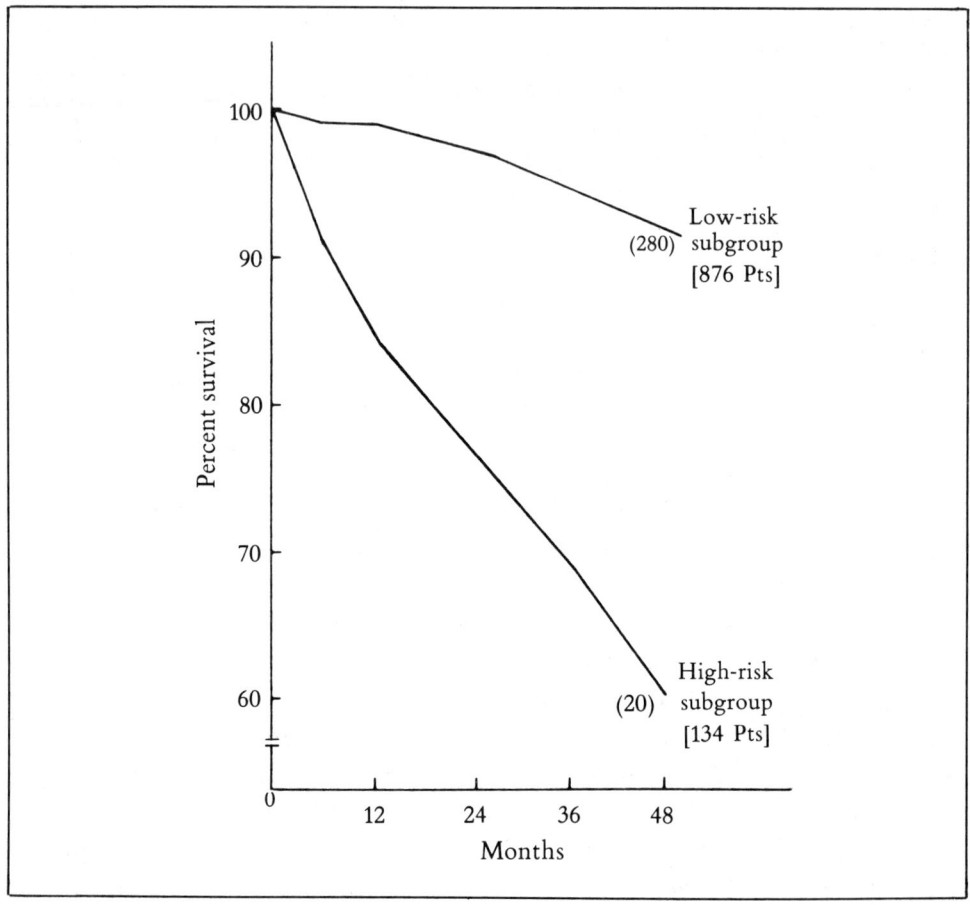

FIGURE 4-12. Cumulative life table survival rates in low-risk and high-risk subgroups. (From JF McNeer et al: The role of the exercise test in the evaluation of patients for ischemic heart disease. *Circulation* 57:64, 1978, by permission of the American Heart Association, Inc.)

Use of the Exercise Test Soon After Myocardial Infarction

The exercise stress test has been used recently to help stratify patients for prognosis soon after an uncomplicated acute myocardial infarction. In appropriately selected patients the exercise test performed prior to hospital discharge can safely identify a subgroup of patients at highest risk for the development of subsequent cardiac events and therefore identify those patients most in need of medical or surgical intervention [48, 49]. Initially the postinfarction exercise tests were performed using an arbitrary maximal heart rate limit of 130 beats/min as the end point of the test in the absence of limiting symptoms. More recent experience, however, indicates that a symptom-limited exercise test can be performed safely within 3 weeks of an uncomplicated infarction, regardless of the heart rate or depth of ST-segment depression, and that the data obtained from this maximal effort test provide more prognostic insight than a heart rate–limited test [49].

The experience of exercise testing in 195 males 3 weeks following an uncomplicated myocardial infarction is summarized in Figure 4-13 [49]. Those patients who had greater than 2 mm of ST-segment depression post infarction had a very high probability of developing a subsequent cardiac event over the ensuing 4 years, regardless of whether they had test angina pectoris. On the other hand, in this population, patients who developed angina pectoris on the stress test, even in the absence of marked ST-segment depression, also had a high probability of developing a subsequent cardiac event, as did those patients who were forced to stop exercise after less than four metabolic equivalent units of exercise (METS). These patients all had a significantly greater incidence of coronary events compared to the 137 other postinfarction patients who did not demonstrate these findings.

Problems with Interpretation of the Exercise ECG

There are some ECG findings on the preexercise tracing that may preclude or obscure the accurate interpretation of the exercise ECG. The presence of left bundle branch block pattern and its associated resting ST–T-wave abnormalities, for example, invalidates the significance of exertional ST-segment depression [5, 50]. On the other hand, although the development of ST-segment depression in the anterior precordial leads in patients with right bundle branch block is not specific for coronary disease, ischemic ST-segment depression in the lateral precordial leads (V4–V6) appears to be highly correlated with the presence of multivessel coronary disease [51]. Since hyperventilation at rest may induce ST-segment changes that mimic those of ischemia even in patients without coronary disease [52], it is important to record an ECG at rest during hyperventilation to ensure that ST-segment changes observed during exercise truly represent ischemia and not simply hyperventilation-induced changes. The presence of left ventricular hypertrophy also increases the incidence of false-positive ST-segment responses to exercise, and a diagnosis of coronary artery disease cannot be validly applied in that setting [53]. A very high incidence of false-positive ST-segment responses are also reported in the syndrome of mitral valve prolapse, although the mechanism remains unknown [54]. Digitalis is well known not only to accentuate ischemic ST-segment changes induced by exercise but also to produce ST-segment depression even in the absence of coronary artery disease [5]. If a patient on digitalis therapy is exercised to maximum heart rate and has no ST-segment deviation, significant coronary disease is unlikely. If ST-segment depression occurs in a patient on digitalis therapy, however, no diagnostic inference can be made. Patients with the Wolff-Parkinson-White preexcitation syndrome who conduct through the anomalous pathway during exercise consistently exhibit ST-segment depression that mimics

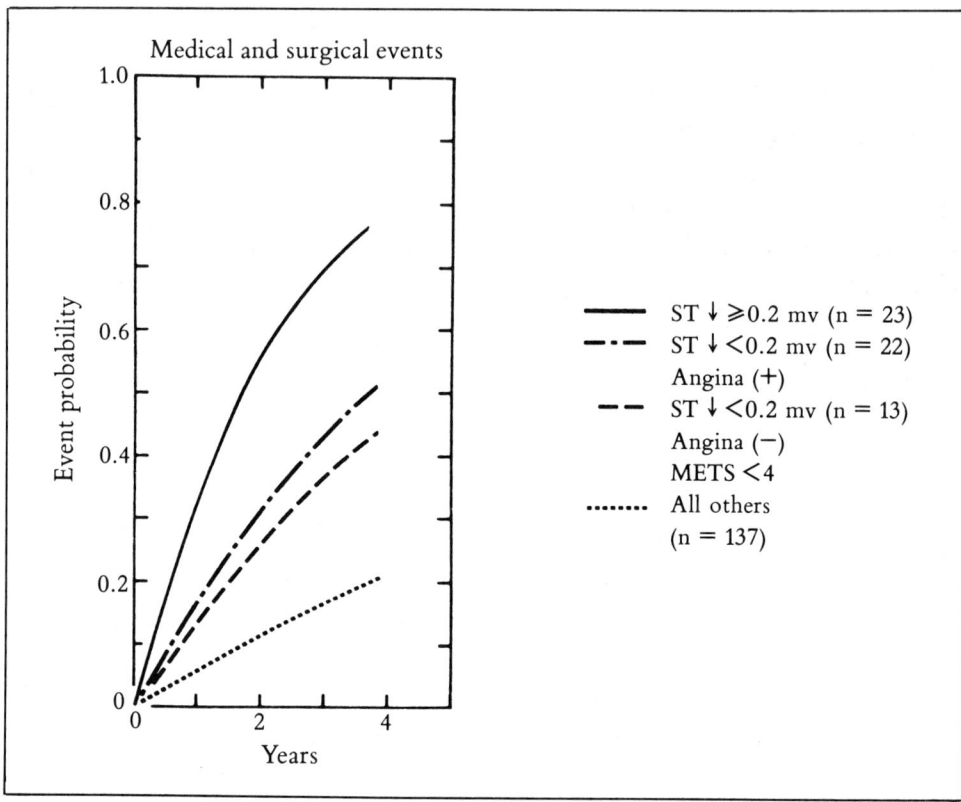

FIGURE 4-13. Probability of subsequent cardiac events in 195 men after myocardial infarction, defined as myocardial infarction, sudden death, cardiac arrest, or coronary artery bypass surgery. (From DM Davidson and R DeBusk: Prognostic value of a single exercise test 3 weeks after uncomplicated myocardial infarction. *Circulation* 61:236, 1980, by permission of the American Heart Association, Inc.)

myocardial ischemia [55]. However, patients with the preexcitation syndrome who conduct through the anomalous pathway at rest often develop partial or total normalization of the QRS complex during exercise as a result of enhanced atrioventricular nodal conduction.

The presence of an abnormal resting ECG was initially considered a relative contraindication for exercise testing, since the control abnormalities might obfuscate the development of ischemic ST-segment deviations. Cohn and his associates [56], however, noted that even in the presence of nonspecific ST-T abnormalities 86 percent of patients with at least 0.5 mm of additional ischemic ST-segment depression following a submaximal Master two-step exercise test had significant coronary disease. In addition, each of the patients with ischemic ST-segment depression greater than 2 mm had multivessel involvement. Using a maximal effort

Bruce treadmill protocol, Linhart and Turnoff [57] also found that an additional 1 mm of ST-segment depression superimposed on nonspecific ST–T-wave abnormalities resulted in a sensitivity of 76 percent and a specificity of 79 percent.

Complications of Exercise Testing

A survey of 73 medical centers, summarizing the experience with approximately 170,000 tests, was reported in 1971 and indicated a mortality rate of about 1 per 10,000 (0.01 percent) and an approximately 4 per 10,000 (0.04 percent) risk of morbidity [58]. In 1980 Stuart and coworkers reported a survey of 444,396 treadmill tests, 44,460 bicycle stress tests, and 25,592 Master tests performed at 1,375 medical centers [59]. Even though use of the exercise test had become more widespread since the 1971 survey, the test remained a safe, noninvasive technique: Complications reported included 3.5 infarctions, 48 serious arrhythmias, and 0.5 death per 10,000. McHenry [60] has recently emphasized that by careful attention to blood pressure and cardiac rhythm during exercise, many of the morbid and fatal events may be avoided. It appears that the incidence of exercise complications can be greatly minimized by careful monitoring of the patient's condition during the exercise performance and that with the appropriate degree of caution the risks of serious complications in exercise stress testing are reasonable.

Summary

In summary, a few principal concepts have been emphasized in this discussion of exercise stress testing. First, the test must be applied to an appropriately selected group of patients. If it is applied to a group where the presence of coronary artery disease is very unlikely, the test must be interpreted with an appropriate degree of caution. Second, the exercise test is perhaps most helpful in estimating the *severity* of disease and, therefore, its prognosis. Its value in the simple identification of patients with coronary disease may be controversial. The exercise test interpretation of the degree and significance of a patient's coronary artery disease is based not only on careful scrutiny of the exercise ECG, but also on the combination of ECG variables and a variety of clinical performance variables. With this noninvasive and inexpensive test patients at high risk for the development of subsequent cardiac events can be identified and can be appropriately screened for more invasive diagnostic and therapeutic interventions.

References

1. Taylor HL, Buskirk E, Henschel A: Maximal oxygen intake as objective measure of cardiorespiratory performance. *J Appl Physiol* 8:73, 1955

2. Holloszy JO: Adaptations of muscular tissue to training. *Prog Cardiovasc Dis* 18:445, 1976
3. Fagraeus L, Linnarsson D: Autonomic origin of heart rate fluctuations at the onset of muscular exercise. *J Appl Physiol* 40:679, 1976
4. Dehn MM, Mullins CB: Physiologic effects and importance of exercise in patients with coronary artery disease. *Cardiovasc Med* 2:365, 1977
5. Ellestad MH: *Stress Testing. Principles and Practice.* Philadelphia: FA Davis, 1980
6. Bing RJ: Cardiac metabolism. *Physiol Rev* 45:2, 1965
7. Gobel FL, Nordstrom LA, Nelson RR, Jorgensen CR, Wang Y: The rate-pressure product as an index of myocardial oxygen consumption in patients with angina pectoris. *Circulation* 57:549, 1978
8. Pollock ML, Schmidt DH (eds): *Heart Disease and Rehabilitation.* Boston: Houghton Mifflin, 1979
9. Feil H, Siegel M: Electrocardiographic changes during attacks of angina pectoris. *Am J Med Sci* 175:225, 1928
10. Master AM, Oppenheimer EJ: A simple exercise tolerance test for circulatory efficiency with standard tables for normal individuals. *Am J Med Sci* 177:223, 1929
11. Master AM, Jaffe HL: The electrocardiographic changes after exercise in angina pectoris. *J Mt Sinai Hosp* 7:629, 1941
12. Robb GP, Marks HH: Latent coronary artery disease: Determination of its presence and severity by the exercise electrocardiogram. *Am J Cardiol* 13:603, 1964
13. Sheffield LT, Roitman D: Stress testing methodology. *Prog Cardiovasc Dis* 19:33, 1976
14. Pollock ML, Bohannon RL, Cooper KH, Ayres JJ, Ward A, White SR, Linnerud AC: A comparative analysis of four protocols for maximal treadmill stress testing. *Am Heart J* 92:39, 1976
15. Chaitman BR, Bourassa MG, Wagniart P, Corbara F, Ferguson RJ: Improved efficiency of treadmill exercise testing using a multiple lead ECG system and basic hemodynamic exercise response. *Circulation* 57:71, 1978
16. Bruce RA, Kusumi F, Hosmer D: Maximal oxygen intake and nomographic assessment of functional aerobic impairment in cardiovascular disease. *Am Heart J* 85:546, 1973
17. Clarke LJ, Bruce RA: Exercise testing. In Cohn PF (ed): *Diagnosis and Therapy of Coronary Artery Disease.* Boston: Little, Brown, 1979, p 81
18. Bruce RA, DeRouen TA, Hossack KF: Value of maximal exercise test in risk assessment of primary coronary heart disease events in healthy men. *Am J Cardiol* 46:371, 1980
19. Cohn PF: Asymptomatic coronary artery disease. Pathophysiology, diagnosis, management. *Mod Concepts Cardiovasc Dis* 50:53, 1981
20. Weiner DA, Ryan TJ, McCabe CH, Kennedy JW, Schloss M, Tristani F, Chaitman BR, Fisher LD: Exercise stress testing. Correlations among history of angina, ST-

segment response and prevalence of coronary artery disease in the coronary artery surgery study (CASS). *N Engl J Med* 301:230, 1979
21. Epstein SE: Controversies in cardiology II. Value and limitations of the electrocardiographic response to exercise in the assessment of patients with coronary artery disease. *Am J Cardiol* 42:667, 1978
22. Goldschlager N, Selzer A, Cohn K: Treadmill stress tests as indicators of presence and severity of coronary artery disease. *Ann Intern Med* 85:277, 1976
23. Kurita A, Chaitman BR, Bourassa MG: Significance of exercise-induced junctional S-T depression in evaluation of coronary artery disease. *Am J Cardiol* 40:492, 1977
24. Bartel AG, Behar VS, Peter RH, Orgain ES, Kong Y: Graded exercise stress tests in angiographically documented coronary artery disease. *Circulation* 49:348, 1974
25. Cohn PF, Vokonus PS, Most AS, Herman MV, Gorlin R: Diagnostic accuracy of two-step post-exercise ECG. Results in 305 subjects studied by coronary arteriography. *JAMA* 220:501, 1972
26. Cheitlin MD, Davia JE, deCastro CM, Barrow EA, Anderson WT: Correlation of "critical" left coronary artery lesions with positive submaximal exercise tests in patients with chest pain. *Am Heart J* 89:305, 1975
27. Berman JL, Wynne J, Cohn PF: A multivariate approach for interpreting treadmill exercise tests in coronary artery disease. *Circulation* 58:505, 1978
28. Chahine RA, Raizner AE, Ishimori T: The clinical significance of exercise-induced ST-segment elevation. *Circulation* 54:209, 1976
29. Manvi KN, Ellestad MH: Elevated ST segments with exercise in ventricular aneurysm. *J Electrocardiol* 5:317, 1972
30. Longhurst JC, Kraus WL: Exercise-induced ST elevation in patients without myocardial infarction. *Circulation* 60:616, 1979
31. Fortuin NJ, Friesinger GC: Exercise-induced S-T segment elevation. *Am J Med* 49:459, 1970
32. Brody DA: A theoretical analysis of intracavitary blood mass influence on the heart-lead relationship. *Circ Res* 4:371, 1956
33. Simoons ML, Hugenholtz PG: Gradual changes of the ECG waveform during and after exercise in normal subjects. *Circulation* 52:570, 1975
34. Bonoris PE, Greenberg PS, Christison GW, Castallanet MD, Ellestad MH: Evaluation of R wave amplitude changes versus ST segment depression in stress testing. *Circulation* 57:904, 1978
35. Berman JL, Wynne J, Cohn PF: Multiple-lead QRS changes with exercise testing. *Circulation* 61:53, 1980
36. Gillespie JA, Bodenheimer MM, Fouche CM, Banka VS, Helfant RH: Limitations in use of change in R wave amplitude with stress electrocardiogram to improve detection of coronary heart disease (Abstract). *Circulation* 58(Suppl II):II-199, 1978
37. Wagner S, Cohn K, Selzer A: Unreliability of exercise-induced R wave changes as indexes of coronary artery disease. *Am J Cardiol* 44:1241, 1979

38. Morris SN, Phillips JF, Jordan JW, McHenry PL: Incidence and significance of decreases in systolic blood pressure during graded treadmill exercise testing. *Am J Cardiol* 41:221, 1978
39. Lamb LE, Hiss RG: Influence of exercise on premature contractions. *Am J Cardiol* 10:209, 1962
40. Helfant RH, Pine R, Kabde V, Banka VS: Exercise-related ventricular premature complexes in coronary heart disease. *Ann Intern Med* 80:589, 1974
41. Goldschlager N, Cake D, Cohn K: Exercise-induced ventricular arrhythmias in patients with coronary artery disease. Their relation to angiographic findings. *Am J Cardiol* 31:434, 1973
42. McHenry PL, Morris SN, Kavalier M, Jordan JW: Comparative study of exercise-induced ventricular arrhythmias in normal subjects and patients with documented coronary artery disease. *Am J Cardiol* 37:609, 1976
43. Udall JA, Ellestad MH: Predictive implications of ventricular premature contractions associated with treadmill stress testing. *Circulation* 56:985, 1977
44. Ryan M, Lown B, Horn H: Comparison of ventricular ectopic activity during 24-hour monitoring and exercise testing in patients with coronary heart disease. *N Engl J Med* 292:224, 1975
45. Sandberg L: Studies in electrocardiogram changes during exercise tests. *Acta Med Scand* 169(Suppl 365):1, 1969
46. McNeer JF, Margolis JR, Lee KL, Kisslo JA, Peter RH, Kong Y, Behar VS, Wallace AG, McCants CB, Rosati RA: The role of the exercise test in the evaluation of patients for ischemic heart disease. *Circulation* 57:64, 1978
47. Cohn PF: Silent myocardial ischemia in patients with a defective anginal warning system. *Am J Cardiol* 45:697, 1980
48. Theroux P, Waters D, Halphen C, Debaisieux JC, Mizgala HG: Prognostic value of exercise testing soon after myocardial infarction. *N Engl J Med* 301:341, 1979
49. Davidson DM, DeBusk R: Prognostic value of a single exercise test 3 weeks after uncomplicated myocardial infarction. *Circulation* 61:236, 1980
50. Whinnery JE, Froelicher VF, Stewart AJ, Longo MR, Triebwasser JH, Lancaster MC: The ECG response to maximal treadmill exercise of asymptomatic men with LBBB. *Am Heart J* 94:316, 1977
51. Tanaka T, Friedman MJ, Okada RD, Buckels LJ, Marcus FI: Diagnostic value of exercise-induced S-T segment depression in patients with RBBB. *Am J Cardiol* 41:670, 1978
52. Lary D, Goldschlager N: Electrocardiographic changes during hyperventilation resembling myocardial ischemia in patients with normal coronary arteriograms. *Am Heart J* 87:383, 1974
53. Harris CN, Aranow WS, Parkes DP: Treadmill stress test in left ventricular hypertrophy. *Chest* 63:353, 1973
54. Devereux RB, Perloff JK, Reichek N, Josephson MG: Mitral valve prolapse. *Circulation* 54:3, 1976
55. Strasberg B, Ashley WW, Wyndham CRC, Bauernfeind RA, Swiryn SP, Dhingra

RC, Rosen KM: Treadmill exercise testing in the Wolff-Parkinson-White syndrome. *Am J Cardiol* 45:742, 1980
56. Cohn PF, Vokonas PS, Herman MV, Gorlin R: Post exercise electrocardiogram in patients with abnormal resting electrocardiograms. *Circulation* 43:648, 1971
57. Linhart JW, Turnoff HB: Maximum treadmill exercise test in patients with abnormal control electrocardiograms. *Circulation* 49:667, 1974
58. Rochmis P, Blackburn H: Exercise tests. A survey of procedures, safety and litigation experience in approximately 170,000 tests. *JAMA* 217:1061, 1971
59. Stuart RJ, Ellestad MH: National survey of exercise stress testing facilities. *Chest* 77:94, 1980
60. McHenry PL: Risks of graded exercise testing. *Am J Cardiol* 39:935, 1977

Part II

Echocardiography, External Pulse Recordings, and Related Procedures

Chapter 5

Echocardiography

Thomas A. Risser and Joshua Wynne

In the two decades since its introduction into clinical cardiology, the growth of echocardiography as a key clinical procedure has been nothing short of spectacular. Echocardiography is presently available in every major medical center and most medium- and large-sized community hospitals. This safe, painless technique presently plays a role in the evaluation of virtually all forms of heart disease and in many conditions is the diagnostic procedure of choice. A working knowledge of the uses and pitfalls of this technique is essential to every physician who treats patients with heart disease.

Principles of Ultrasound

Ultrasound is defined as sound energy with a frequency above the upper limit of human perception, 20,000 Hz (hertz, cycles/sec). By and large, however, the frequency of diagnostic medical ultrasound lies between 1.9 and 5.0 MHz (megahertz, million cycles/sec). Higher frequencies yield better resolution images but penetrate tissue only short distances. Lower frequency sacrifices some image resolution for the advantage of better tissue penetration. Hence, high frequencies are used in pediatrics, where the sound beam need penetrate only a few centimeters to image the heart. Lower frequencies are used in adults, particularly in those who are corpulent or who have hyperinflated lungs due to chronic pulmonary disease. Commercially available echocardiographic machines will accept transducers of varying frequencies; the transducer can be changed in seconds merely by plugging in the cord of the desired one in place of its predecessor.

Ultrasound waves are reflected off of structures when the wave strikes an interface between two tissues of differing acoustic impedance, which is the product of tissue density times the velocity of sound in that tissue. The amplitude of the reflected echo is proportional to the magnitude of acoustic impedance mismatch. Hence the interface of blood and endocardium produces a relatively weak echo, but the interface of posterior pericardium and air-filled lung behind it reflects a very strong echo. The other key factor in echo formation is the angle with which the echo beam strikes the surface of the target from which it is reflected. The strongest echoes are formed when the angle approaches 90 degrees.

Despite 25 years of clinical use, no tissue damage has been demonstrated to result from diagnostic ultrasound, partly owing to its short duration of pulse propagation. Typical commercial M-mode echocardiographic machines emit a sound pulse of approximately 1 μsec duration, which is repeated every millisecond. Hence, 1000 pulses are emitted per second, but pulses are present only about one-thousandth of the time during an examination. That is, the transducer "talks" 1000 times/sec, but it "listens" 1000 times longer than it "talks." A negligible quantity of heat is generated in this setting. In contrast, therapeutic ultrasound, or so-called diathermy, employs continuous sound waves of much greater amplitude that generate heat deep in tissues, and, in excessive dosage, can cause severe tissue damage.

The functional portion of ultrasound transducers is the piezoelectric crystal, a device that converts electrical energy into sound waves (transmit mode) and in turn converts the reflected sound waves from mechanical energy back to electrical energy (receive mode). The transducer is coupled to the chest wall with a special bubble-free gel. Since virtually all cardiac structures are located within 20 cm of the usual transducer locations, and since the velocity of sound in tissue averages 1540 m/sec, the sound beam can make a "round trip" in less than 300 μsec. Thus, a "listening time" of 999 μsec between 1-μsec transmissions occurring every 1 msec is feasible.

The advantages of ultrasound as an imaging medium include portability; relatively brief acquisition time; painlessness; and, most importantly, harmlessness, such that sequential studies can be performed without hazard to the patient. Disadvantages of ultrasound include the need for a skilled technician; moderate expense, both for the imaging system and the technician's salary; and, most importantly, the inability of the echo beam to penetrate bone or air. In some patients with lung disease or skeletal deformities, technically adequate studies cannot be obtained.

Instrumentation

The reflected echocardiographic (echo) signal is displayed in a number of different formats: (1) A-mode; (2) B-mode; (3) M-mode; (4) two-dimensional, also called cross-sectional, sector scan, and real-time. *A-mode* (for amplitude) echo was the earliest format for echo display. One axis represents distance from the transducer, and the other represents the amplitude of echoes received from any given depth (Fig. 5-1). This format is still displayed in most M-mode echo machines and is used principally to adjust gain settings, since gain changes, especially local gains which affect only a limited depth range, are easily appreciated in the A-mode format.

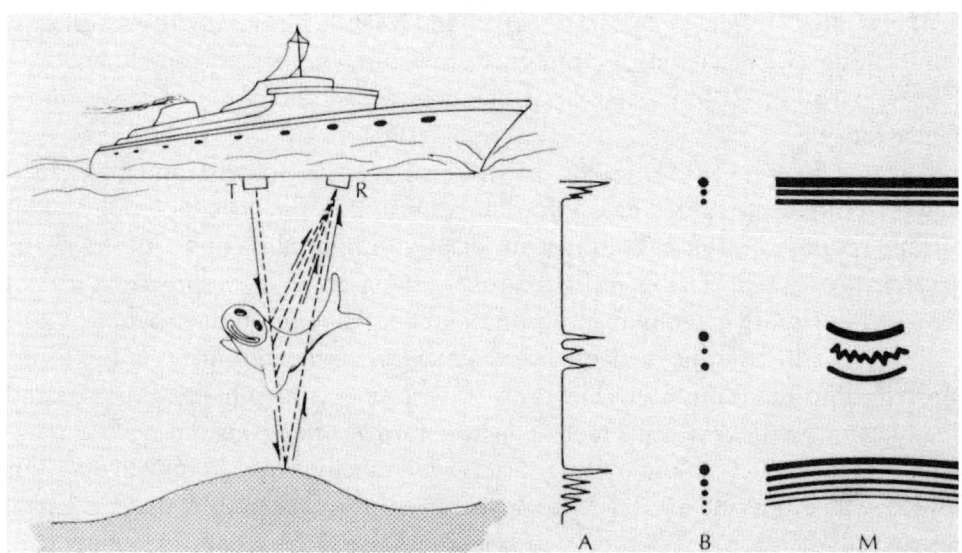

FIGURE 5-1. Imaging modes in echocardiography. A sonar system illustrates propagation of a single pulse of ultrasound from a transmitter (*T*) and reflections from a moving fish and the ocean bottom to a receiver (*R*). A-mode display (*A*) features oscilloscopic baseline deflections, the amplitude of which varies with the intensity of the signal. In B-mode (*B*), spikes are converted into dots that vary in brightness according to echo strength. When these dots are swept across a recording medium, motion derived from transit of ship or from targets within the beam is presented as a variation in the position of reflectors as they change with time and is designated M-mode (*M*). The information contained in these modes is one-dimensional in nature. (Reprinted with permission from R Gramiak and SA Borg: Abdominal ultrasound in surgical patients. In C Rob et al [eds]: *Advances in Surgery,* Vol 2. Copyright 1977 by Year Book Medical Publishers, Inc, Chicago.)

B-mode (for brightness) scan is usually displayed so that strength of the echo signal is represented by the brightness of that echo at any given distance from the transducer (see Fig. 5-1). A static two-dimensional echocardiogram can be generated via B-mode format by moving the transducer in either an arc of rotation or sliding it along the skin. A system of sensors in a mechanical arm that holds the transducer detects the nature and extent of movement of the transducer in B-mode scanning systems used, for example, in abdominal ultrasound imaging, and a composite image is generated based on sensed transducer position as echo signals are received. B-mode scanning systems are commonly used for noncardiac structures; however, static B-mode scanning is not useful for cardiac imaging because a composite view requires a few seconds to produce, during which time the heart continues to move and blurs the composite image.

M-mode (for motion) echo consists of a static B-mode format in the vertical axis, representing distance from the transducer, and time on the horizontal axis, as in Figures 5-1 and 5-2. M-mode echo is the most widely used form of echocardiography today.

The past 5 years have witnessed the striking evolution and dissemination of the newest echo imaging format, two-dimensional (2-D) echocardiography. This technique consists of near-simultaneous display of multiple echo beams in arcs as wide as 90 degrees. The effect is that of a tomogram, i.e., a narrow "slice" of tissue whose width is set by the transducer arc; depth is set on the machine with a variable switch; and thickness of slice is a fixed pattern determined by the focusing built into the transducer. Thirty to 60 such images are obtained each second and, when viewed, result in a motion picture format permitting flicker-free imaging of cardiac structure and motion. Studies are usually recorded on videotape for subsequent review and analysis. The advantage of this technique is that the lateral relationship of cardiac structures to one another can be readily demonstrated, whereas in M-mode the relationship must be inferred. The disadvantages of this format include substantially higher cost of equipment and the need for a bulkier transducer, rendering imaging from windows between the ribs more difficult. Also, because of the need to generate the 30 to 60 sweeps/sec of the two-dimensional arc to produce a flicker-free picture, resolution in this format is not as fine as with M-mode. Accordingly, all 2-D systems preserve M-mode capability — the two formats are complementary, not exclusive.

All M-mode and 2-D systems incorporate an on-line cathode ray tube (similar to a television screen) display. However, examinations can be stored on Polaroid photographs, paper printout, video tape, and video disk. Although initially measured simply with calipers, increasingly sophisticated devices are becoming available to assist in echo analysis, ranging from simple mechanical-arm digitizers to complex light-pen systems with software packages to calculate dimensions, areas, volumes, ejection fractions, and other functional parameters.

An altogether different ultrasound technique that nonetheless falls in the realm of echocardiography is Doppler ultrasound. This technique, which is only beginning to be sufficiently refined as to be clinically useful, utilizes the frequency shift of rebounding sound waves as an index of the velocity of the interface that reflected it. Doppler signal can be transmitted either continuously or in pulses. The pulsed technique is gaining the most popularity. The Doppler signal can also be "range-gated" such that information analyzed can be restricted to that obtained at a given depth. Hence, by placing the gated Doppler beam at a chosen region determined by M-mode or 2-D echo, flow characteristics at that particular locus can be determined. The potential clinical applications are wide and include (1) measuring flow through the great vessels, yielding cardiac output and an index of shunt magnitude, (2) determination of the presence and magnitude of valvular regurgitation,

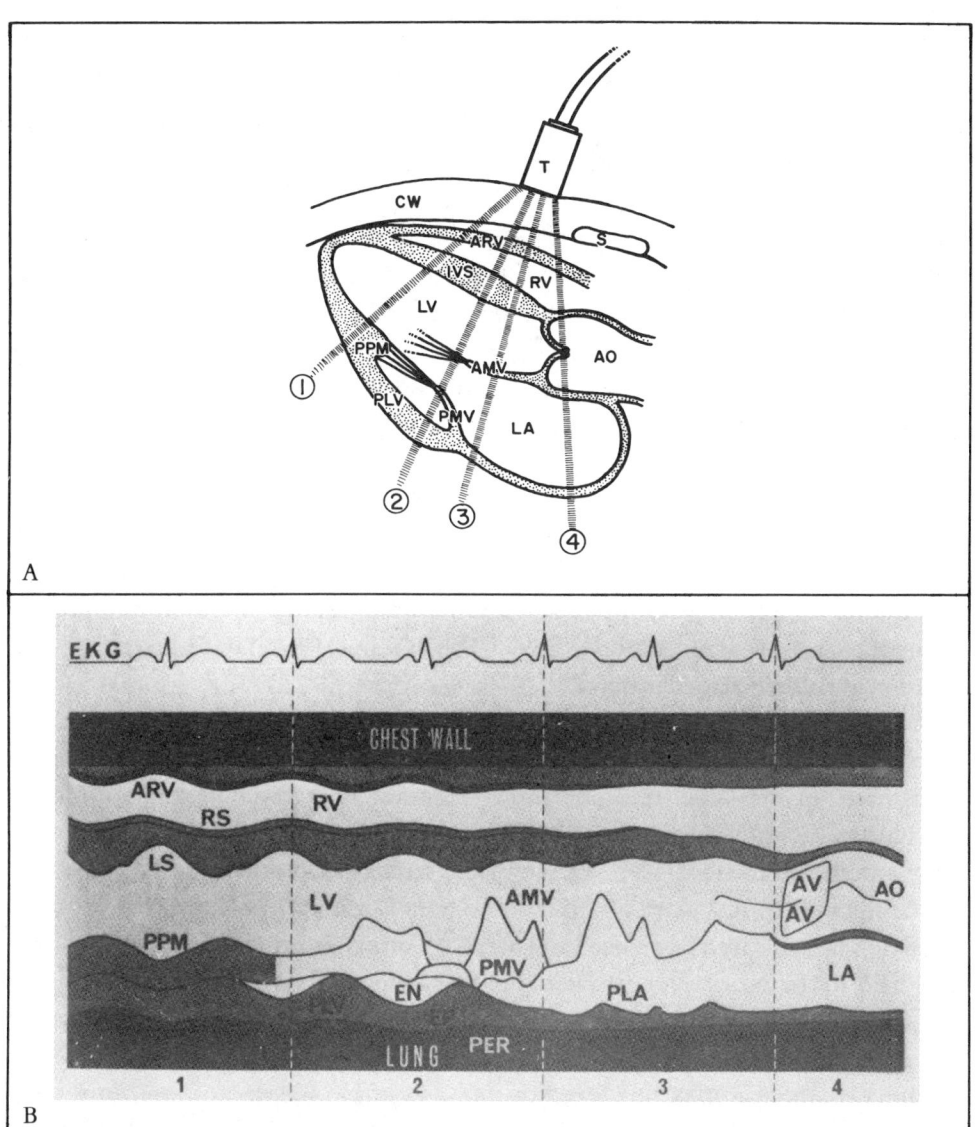

FIGURE 5-2. (A) Cross-section of the heart showing the structures through which the ultrasonic beam passes as it is directed from the apex toward the base of the heart. (B) Diagrammatic presentation of the M-mode echocardiogram as the transducer is directed from the apex (1) to the base of the heart (4). The areas between the dotted lines correspond to the transducer position as depicted in (A). AMV = anterior mitral valve leaflet, AO = aorta, ARV = anterior right ventricular wall, AV = aortic valve, CW = chest wall, EN = endocardium of the left ventricle, EP = epicardium of the left ventricle, IVS = interventricular septum, LA = left atrium, LS = left septum, LV = left ventricle, PER = pericardium, PLA = posterior left atrial wall, PLV = posterior left ventricular wall, PMV = posterior mitral valve leaflet, PPM = posterior papillary muscle, RS = right septum, RV = right ventricular cavity, S = sternum, T = transducer. (Reprinted with permission from H Feigenbaum: Clinical applications of echocardiography. *Prog Cardiovasc Dis* 14:531, 1972.)

and (3) identifying the presence of turbulent flow, indicative of obstruction to flow. Several commercial manufacturers are now incorporating gated pulsed Doppler in their 2-D systems, and the technique is rapidly developing increased capability. We can anticipate an expanding role for this newest of echocardiographic techniques. Because it is not yet part of the standard echocardiographic examination, the technique will not be discussed further in this chapter.

All 2-D transducers fall into one of three major categories: linear array, mechanical, and phased array. Linear-array transducers consist simply of multiple parallel M-mode transducers built into a single frame. Each transducer functions independently, and the resultant image consists of multiple side-by-side B-mode images. Because this necessarily large, cumbersome transducer cannot be fit between the ribs as can the other 2-D transducer types, image dropout occurs in the transducers over the ribs, and an inadequate image is generated. Linear-array transducers are no longer used in adult echocardiography; however, because the nonossified ribs of children do conduct echo beams, these transducers are still occasionally used for pediatric studies.

Mechanical transducers consist of one to four M-mode transducers mounted on an axle and driven through an arc by an electric motor mounted inside the transducer head. Phased-array transducers may contain 32 or more separate immobile transducers mounted in the 2-D transducer head. These transducers are electronically stimulated to transmit in varying time sequences so as to "steer" the resulting compound sound waves.

Advantages of mechanical heads over phased-array transducers include enhanced near-field resolution, fewer artifactual echoes, and somewhat lower cost. Advantages of phased-array transducers include the absence of audible noise or vibratory sensation produced by the transducer. Furthermore, certain phased-array systems feature a cursor that may be moved on the 2-D image screen to allow simultaneous display on another screen of the M-mode echo along that cursor. Mechanical transducer systems may incorporate a cursor system, but when the M-mode along the cursor is displayed, the 2-D image is lost, since the motion of the transducer must be stopped to allow a fixed location M-mode to be obtained.

The Echocardiographic Examination

The standard M-mode echocardiographic examination consists of views of five principal regions: the aortic root with aortic leaflets and the left atrium posterior to these structures; the mitral valve at the leaflet tips; the left ventricle at the level of the chordae tendineae; the tricuspid valve; and the pulmonic valve (see Fig. 5-2). This standard examination frequently can be performed without moving the transducer from a single location on the chest wall. The examiner begins by attempting to image the heart from several left parasternal intercostal locations, looking for the best "window." Optimally, the transducer should be perpendicular to the chest wall when imaging the mitral valve. From the mitral valve position, the transducer is angulated cephalad and medially to image the aortic valve and root; caudad and laterally to image the left ventricle; medially and inferiorly to visualize the tricuspid valve; and superiorly and laterally to image the pulmonic valve. In addition to careful views of these structures, a "sweep" at a low recording speed (12.5–25.0 mm/sec) is performed over about 10 seconds from left ventricle through the mitral valve to the aortic valve to examine the relationship of structures in one view to those in the other views (see Figs. 5-2 and 5-3). Other less common M-mode echo transducer locations include the supraclavicular fossa, the suprasternal notch, and the epigastrium. Recommendations for locations and techniques of M-mode measurements have been published and are widely utilized [1] (Fig. 5-4). The normal dimensions of cardiac structure in children are normalized for body surface area. Unfortunately, there is no consensus on this issue in adults — each laboratory establishes its own policy. A table of normal values appears in Table 5-1.

In a two-dimensional echo examination, imaging is performed along three principal tomographic planes: long axis of the heart, short axis of the heart, and apical four-chamber axis, as shown in Figures 5-5 and 5-6. The long-axis plane sections the heart from the left hip to the right shoulder, slicing through the aortic root and body of the left ventricle. Multiple short-axis views may be obtained by rotating the transducer 90 degrees and imaging sections perpendicular to the long axis. The transducer is placed over the cardiac apex for the four-chamber view as well as the apical two-chamber view, or so-called right anterior oblique equivalent view. The standard two-dimensional echo examination consists of six principal views: the parasternal long-axis view; parasternal short-axis views at the levels of the aortic valve, the mitral leaflets, and the papillary muscles; the parasternal view of the right ventricular inflow tract; and the apical four-chamber view. As many as 20 separate views have been described for the two-dimensional echocardiographic examination [2]. Standards for nomenclature have been suggested but are not universally utilized [3].

Diseases Assessed by Echocardiography

THE MITRAL VALVE

The Normal Mitral Valve

Because the normal mitral valve, which produces a very distinctive "M" shape on the M-mode echocardiogram, is relatively easy to find with the M-mode transducer, it is the usual orientation point for initiation of M-mode examinations

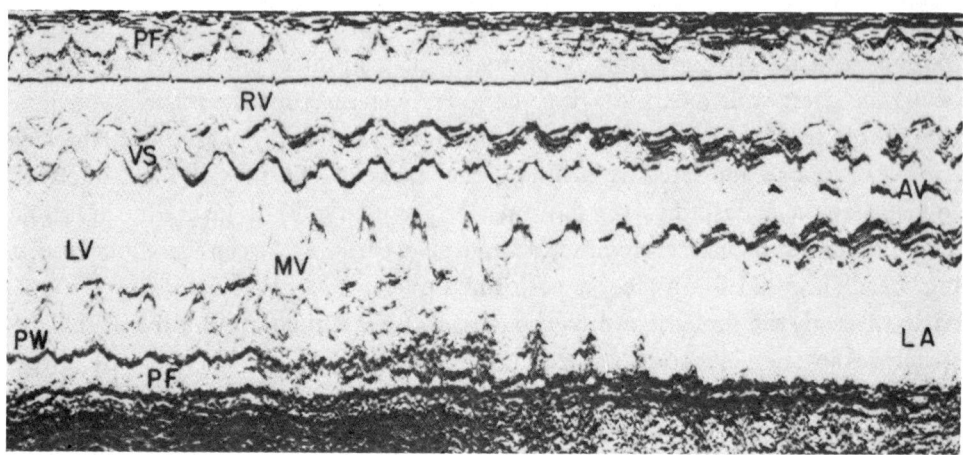

FIGURE 5-3. Continuous M-mode scan from the body of the left ventricle to the base of the heart in a patient with moderate pericardial effusion. At the ventricular level, moderate anterior and posterior echo-free spaces can be seen. As the beam is tilted toward the aortic root with the left atrium behind, the echo-free space disappears behind the left atrium. The motion of the right ventricular anterior wall, ventricular septum, and left ventricular posterior wall is normal. AV = aortic valve, LA = left atrium, LV = left ventricle, MV = mitral valve, PF = pericardial fluid, PW = posterior wall of the left ventricle, RV = right ventricle, VS = ventricular septum. (From F Lemire et al: *Mayo Clinic Proc* 51:13, 1976.)

(Fig. 5-7A). Diastole occurs at the D point where the valve first opens, with the anterior leaflet moving toward the transducer (i.e., moving upward on the paper printout), corresponding to the period of rapid ventricular filling. The valve reaches a maximal excursion at the E point, and then begins to close spontaneously, reaching a mid-diastolic closure point at F, during which time slow ventricular filling is occurring. Depending on the heart rate, the valve may then have several small undulations, which are called *h* waves. However, at faster heart rates, the *a* wave due to atrial systole follows the F point relatively quickly, resulting in a narrow letter "M" configuration. At the onset of systole, the mitral valve is already spontaneously closing from the A point. The anterior and posterior leaflets coapt at the C point. In the presence of bradycardia, the E point and A point may be separated so far that they do not appear related, and the letter "M" is not apparent. It is important to recognize this pattern, as it is quite normal in the presence of bradycardia. Normal values for mitral valve measurements are displayed in Table 5-1. The normal long axis two-dimensional view of the mitral valve is seen in Figure 5-7B.

Mitral Stenosis

Mitral stenosis is characterized on M-mode echocardiography by (1) leaflet thickening; (2) diminished excursion, that is, a diminished D–E height; (3) diminished

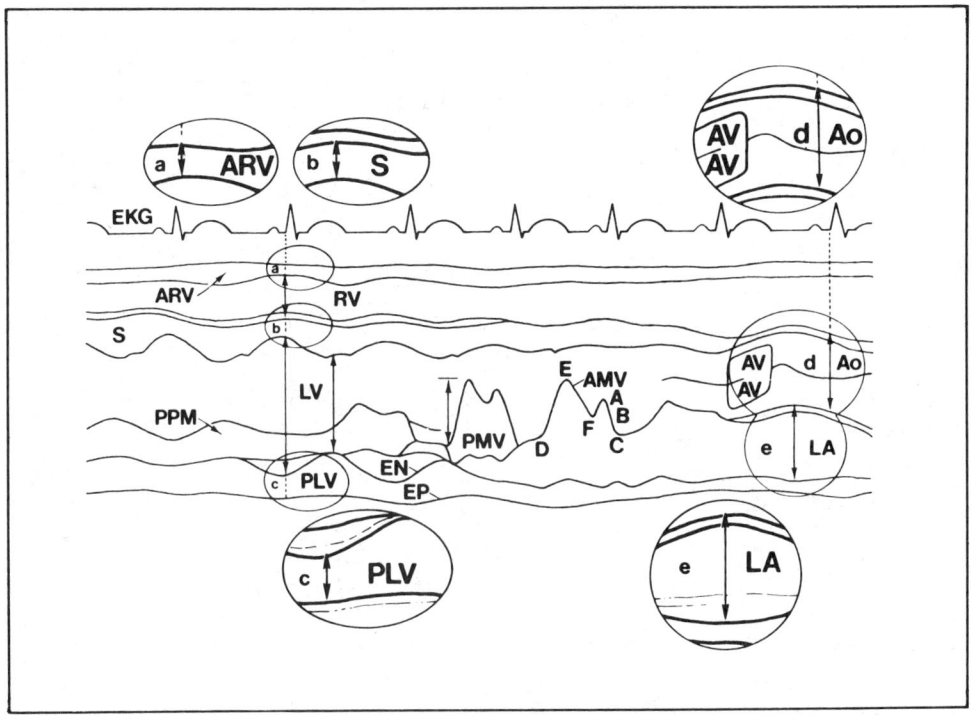

FIGURE 5-4. Diagrammatic echocardiographic sweep shows recommended criteria for measurement superimposed upon the structures. Diastolic measurements are made at the onset of the QRS complex of the ECG; cavities and walls are measured at the level of the chordae tendineae below the mitral valve. The leading edge method (elliptical inserts *a, b, c, d,* and *e*) as well as measurements using the thinnest continuous echo lines are illustrated. *A, B, C, D, E,* and *F* = points of mitral valve motion, *AMV* = anterior mitral valve leaflets, *AO* = aorta, *ARV* = right ventricular anterior wall, *AV* = aortic valve, *EN* = endocardium, *EP* = epicardium, *LA* = left atrium, *LV* = left ventricle, *PLV* = posterior left ventricular wall, *PMV* = posterior mitral valve leaflets, *PPM* = papillary muscle, *RV* = right ventricle, *S* = septum. (From D Sahn et al: The Committee on M-mode Standardization of the American Society of Echocardiography. *Circulation* 58:1072, 1978, by permission of the American Heart Assocation, Inc.)

mid-diastolic closing velocity, that is, a decreased E–F slope; (4) concordant diastolic motion of the two mitral leaflets, such that the normal initial posterior movement of the posterior mitral leaflet at the onset of systole is instead an anterior motion. The stenotic posterior leaflet may move posteriorly in mid diastole but only after being partially dragged anteriorly by the larger anterior leaflet to which it is fused (Fig. 5-8). Two-dimensional echo in mitral stenosis is also characteristic (Fig. 5-9). In the long-axis parasternal view, the leaflets are seen to move in a doming fashion, such that the tips do not separate significantly, although the leaflets do descend somewhat into the left ventricular cavity. Doming

TABLE 5-1. Adult Normal Values

			Normalized to Body Surface Area	
Findings	Range	Mean	Range	Mean
CHAMBER SIZE				
RV, supine (cm)	0.7 – 2.3	1.5	0.4–1.4	0.9
RV, left lateral (cm)	0.9 – 2.6	1.7	0.4–1.4	0.9
LV, supine (cm)	3.7 – 5.6	4.7	2.1–3.2	2.6
LV, left lateral (cm)	3.5 – 5.7	4.7	1.9–3.2	2.6
LA (cm)	1.9 – 4.0	2.9	1.2–2.2	1.6
Ao root (cm)	2.0 – 3.7	2.7	1.2–2.2	1.5
WALL THICKNESS				
Posterior LV wall (cm)	0.6 – 1.1	0.9		
Interventricular septal wall (cm)	0.6 – 1.1	0.9		
MOTION				
Posterior LV wall amplitude (cm)	0.9 – 1.4	1.2		
Posterior LV wall thickening (%)	39.0 –82.0	60.0		
Interventricular septal wall amplitude				
Mid (cm)	0.3 – 0.8	0.5		
Apical (cm)	0.5 – 1.2	0.7		
Interventricular septal wall thickening (%)	18.0 –53.0	35.0		
Aortic valve cusp separation (cm)	1.5 – 2.6	1.9		
Vcf (circ/sec)	1.02– 1.94	1.3		
%ΔD	29.0 –45.0	37.0		

RV = right ventricle, LV = left ventricle, LA = left atrium, Ao = aortic, Vcf = mean velocity of circumferential shortening, %ΔD = percent fractional shortening.

is a distinctive feature of stenosis in all four cardiac valves. Thickening of the leaflets is also readily appreciated in mitral stenosis, as is a reduction in the rate of return of the leaflets back toward the valve plane in early diastole, which is the counterpart of the E–F slope of M-mode. The short-axis 2-D view in mitral stenosis can be used to measure the area of the valve orifice. It is crucial that the echocardiographic view selected for planimetry be located at the level of the leaflet

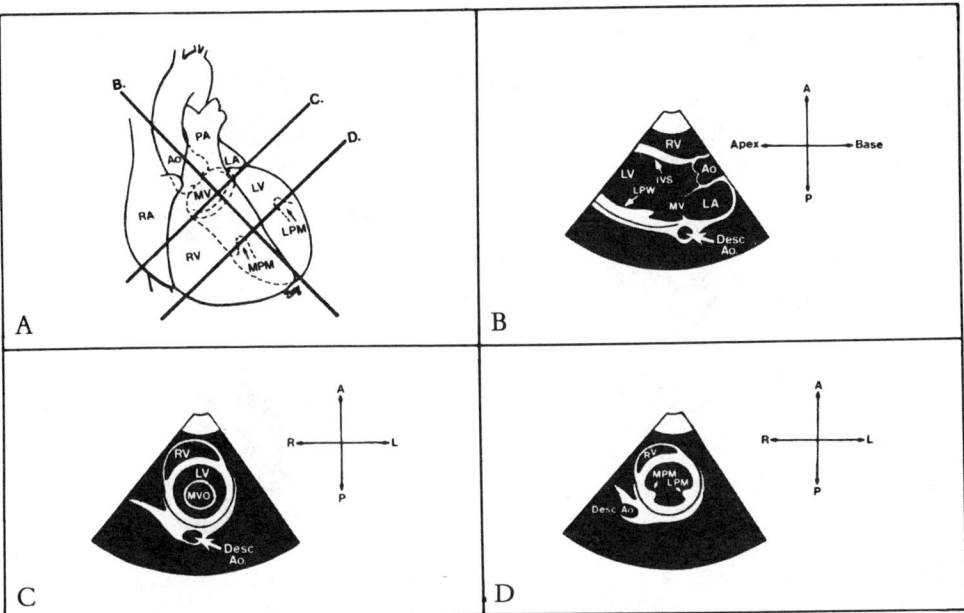

FIGURE 5-5. (A) Drawing of the heart demonstrating three ultrasonic planes. Line *B* represents the plane of the long axis of the left ventricle and is parallel to a line joining the patient's right shoulder to the left flank. Lines *C* and *D* represent short-axis planes of the heart at the level of the mitral valve (*MV*) and papillary muscles (*LMP* and *MPM*), respectively, and are at right angles to the long-axis plane. (B) Long-axis view of left ventricle. The aorta (*Ao*) is to the right and the apex of the left ventricle (*LV*) is to the left of the image. The right ventricle (*RV*) is anterior, and the left atrium (*LA*) is posterior. The anterior and posterior mitral leaflets of the mitral valve (*MV*), interventricular septum (*IVS*), left ventricular posterior wall (*LPW*) and descending aorta (*Desc. Ao.*) are seen. (C) Cross-sectional view of the left ventricle at the level of the mitral valve. The right ventricle (*RV*) is anterior and to the left of the left ventricle (*LV*). The left ventricle appears as a circular structure. The mitral valve orifice (*MVO*) has a "fishmouth" appearance during diastole. (D) Cross-sectional view of the left ventricle at the level of the papillary muscles. The anterolateral papillary muscle (*LMP*) and the posteromedial papillary muscles (*MPM*) project into the left ventricular cavity at approximately the 4 o'clock and 8 o'clock positions. *A* = anterior, *L* = left, *P* = posterior, *PA* = pulmonary artery, *R* = right, *RA* = right atrium. (From MN Kotler et al: *Am J Cardiol* 45:1061, 1980.)

tips, since that is the location of the smallest aperture. This echo-derived value for valve orifice area correlates closely with catheterization-determined valve areas computed via the Gorlin equation. Many institutions now undertake mitral valve commissurotomy or replacement in mitral stenosis on the basis of the two-dimensional echo and clinical findings alone, without resorting to cardiac catheterization.

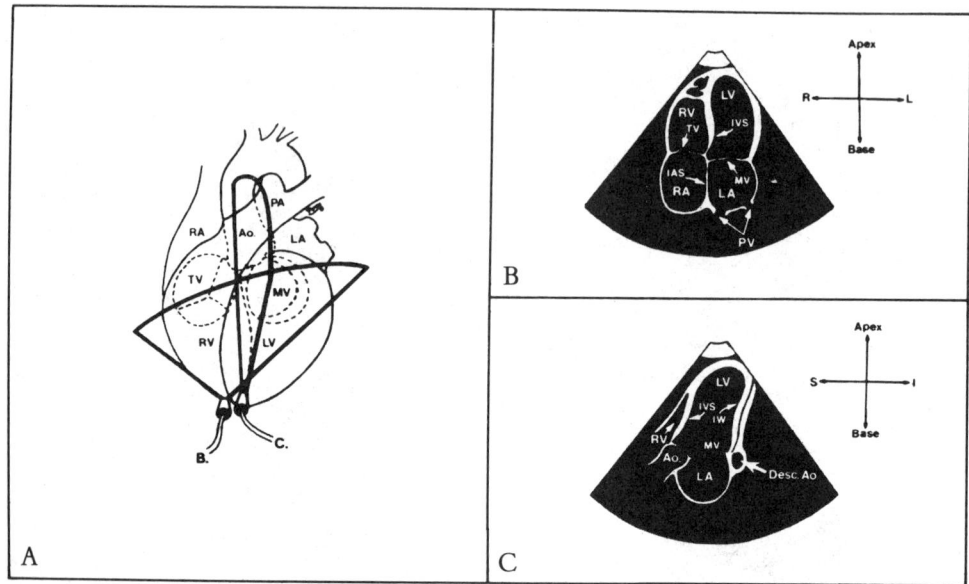

FIGURE 5-6. (A) Drawing of the heart demonstrating the apical or four-chamber view (position B) and the apical two-chamber right anterior oblique view of the left ventricle (position C). The transducer is placed at the apex of the heart and angulated toward the base of the heart. (B) Apical or four-chamber view of the heart. The interventricular septum (*IVS*) separates the right and left ventricles (*RV, LV*). The interatrial septum (*IAS*) separates the right and left atria (*RA, LA*). The attachments of the tricuspid valve (*TV*) and mitral valve (*MV*) are seen. The pulmonary veins (*PV*) may be seen entering the left atrium. The apex of both ventricles is situated anteriorly and the base of the heart posteriorly. (C) Apical two-chamber or right anterior oblique view of the left ventricle. The beam is parallel to the plane of the ventricular septum. The left ventricle and apex are anterior and to the right and the aorta (*Ao*) is posterior and to the left. The inferior wall (*IW*) of the left ventricle is best seen in this view. *Desc. Ao.* = descending aorta, *I* = inferior, *L* = left, *PA* = pulmonary artery, *R* = right, *RA* = right atrium, *S* = superior. (From MN Kotler et al: *Am J Cardiol* 45:1061, 1980.)

The Mitral Valve and Aortic Regurgitation

In aortic regurgitation, the regurgitant jet of blood commonly strikes the anterior mitral leaflet. The echocardiographic result of that impingement is high-frequency fluttering, or vibration, of the leaflet during diastole (Fig. 5-10). The presence of high-frequency diastolic flutter is highly predictive for the presence of aortic regurgitation. However, high-frequency diastolic flutter of the anterior leaflet has also been seen in high-flow states such as chronic renal failure with anemia. The absence of anterior leaflet diastolic flutter does not rule out aortic regurgitation, since the regurgitant jet may be directed more medially. In fact, the interventricular septum may exhibit high-frequency diastolic flutter when the jet is directed at the high septum (see Fig. 5-10). In one study, 66 percent of patients with aortic

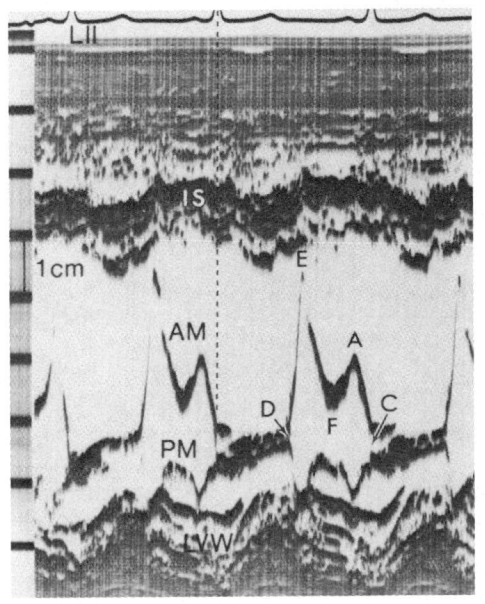 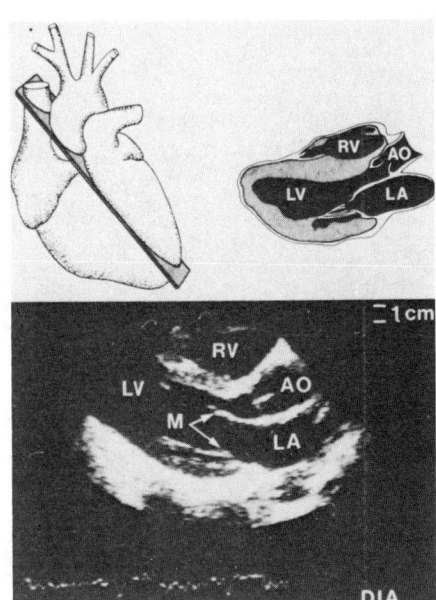

A   B

FIGURE 5-7. (A) M-mode echocardiogram of the normal mitral valve evinces the characteristic "M" shape beginning at the D point and moving through the E, F, A, and C points. The anterior leaflet (*AM*) and posterior leaflet (*PM*) move in a mirror-image fashion, but the anterior leaflet excursion is much greater than that of the posterior leaflet. The dashed vertical line depicts the onset of ventricular systole at the peak of the R wave of the electrocardiogram (standard lead II). *IS* = interventricular septum, *LVW* = left ventricular posterior wall. One-centimeter calibration markers are shown to the left of the figure. (From AN DeMaria: The mitral echogram. In DT Mason [ed]: *Advances in Heart Disease*, Vol 2. New York: Grune & Stratton, 1978, p 22.) (B) *Top*, Long-axis plane of a two-dimensional echocardiogram (*left*) with a schematic illustration of the cardiovascular structures from which ultrasonic signals are obtained in this plane (*right*). In this view the beam is oriented from the patient's right shoulder to the left iliac crest. *Bottom*, Diastolic (*DIA*) two-dimensional echocardiogram obtained in the long-axis plane in a normal subject. In diastole the mitral valve leaflets (*M*) are in the open position (*arrows*), whereas in systole (not shown) the aortic valve leaflets are open and the papillary muscle may be seen. *AO* = aorta, *LA* = left atrium, *LV* = left ventricle, *RV* = right ventricle. (From AN DeMaria: *Am J Cardiol* 46:1097, 1980.)

valve regurgitation showed diastolic high-frequency flutter of the anterior mitral leaflet, 36 percent showed flutter of the interventricular septum, and 72 percent showed at least one or both. Hence, the sensitivity of this sign for aortic regurgitation was 72 percent and the specificity was found to be 83 percent [4].

Severe acute aortic regurgitation produces a characteristic and unique abnormality on the M-mode echocardiogram. The high regurgitant flow causes an early, profound rise in left ventricular end-diastolic pressure such that the left ventricular pressure exceeds the left atrial pressure. In this setting, the mitral valve

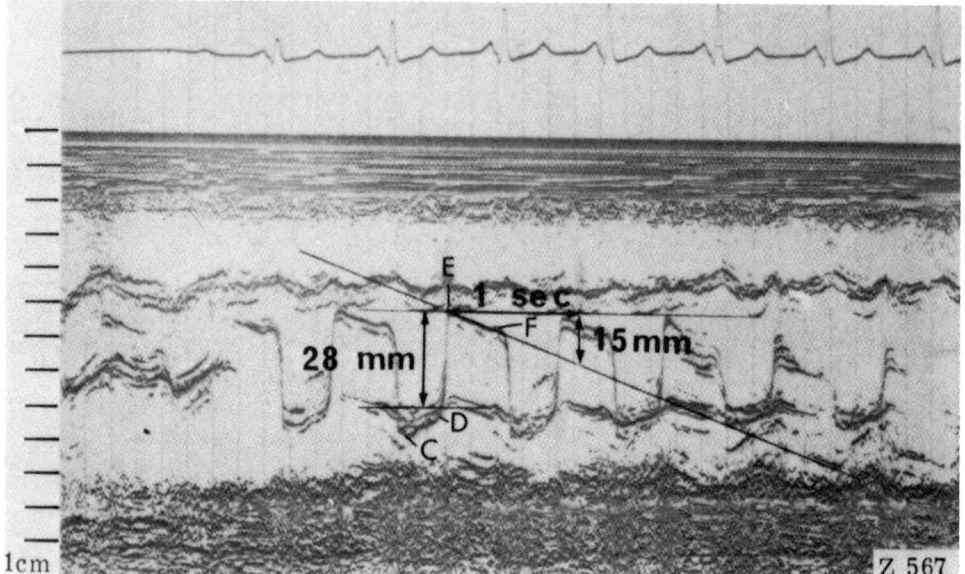

FIGURE 5-8. Echocardiogram in a patient with moderate mitral stenosis and a pliable mitral valve. Note how the diastolic closing velocity, or E–F slope, is measured and how one may measure the amplitude of opening of the mitral leaflet, or D–E amplitude. (From S Chang: *M-mode Echocardiographic Techniques and Pattern Recognition.* Philadelphia: Lea & Febiger, 1976.)

closes before the onset of systole; i.e., the C point occurs before the onset of the Q wave of the electrocardiogram (Fig. 5-11). This finding is seen only where the aortic regurgitation is severe and constitutes a cogent indication for consideration of emergency valve replacement.

Mitral Valve Prolapse

Prolapse of the mitral valve has been described in widely varying frequencies, and in one study was seen on echocardiography in 18 percent of 100 healthy young females [5]. This figure is substantially higher than most: Chandraratna et al found a prevalence of 7 percent by echo in newborn baby girls [6]. Procacci et al found the auscultatory signs in 6.3 percent of 1169 young Air Force wives; 80 percent of these had corroborating echo findings [7]. On auscultation of 107 male medical students and house officers, Darsee et al found four with mid-systolic clicks and seven with both click and murmur [8]. All seven of the latter had positive echocardiograms; none of the four subjects with click only or of the subjects with normal auscultation had mitral prolapse by echo. Thus, the incidence of mitral prolapse on echocardiography varies with the criteria utilized for diagnosis. Currently, although there is no consensus on echocardiographic criteria — nor, for that matter, on angiographic criteria — for its diagnosis, mitral prolapse consti-

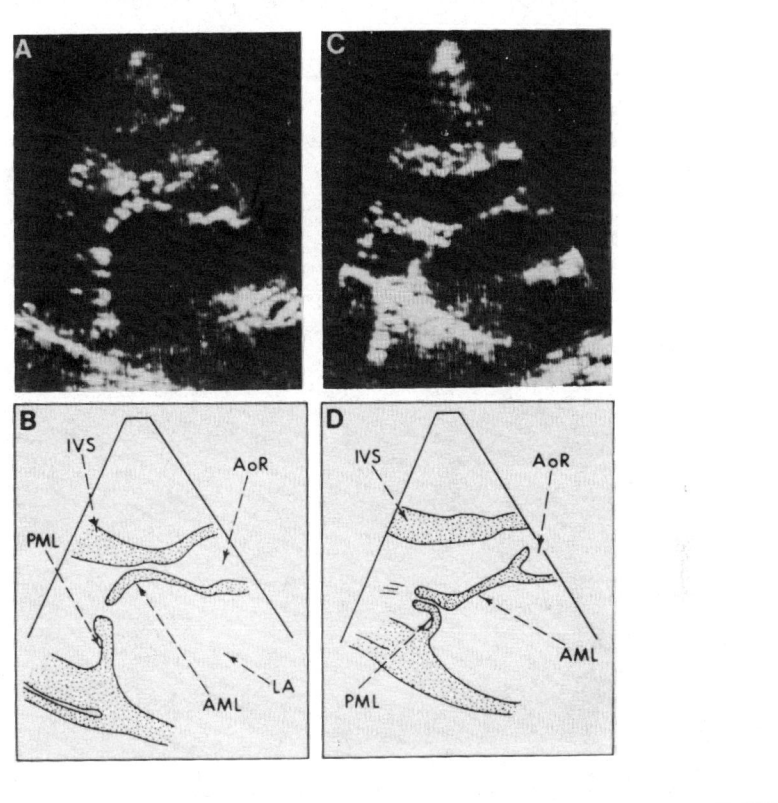

FIGURE 5-9. Sequential diastolic (panel *A*) and systolic (panel *C*) frames through the long axis of the mitral valve in a patient with mitral stenosis. In panel *A* note the thickening of the valve leaflets and arching of the mid-portion of the anterior mitral leaflet as the valve apparatus is open in diastole. In panel *C* note the superior arching of the posterior mitral leaflet as both mitral leaflets coapt in systole. *AML* = anterior mitral leaflet, *AoR* = aortic root, *IVS* = interventricular septum, *LA* = left atrium, *PML* = posterior mitral leaflet. (From J Kisslo: *Two-Dimensional Echocardiography.* New York: Churchill Livingstone, 1980, p 46.)

tutes one of the most frequent causes for referral of patients for echocardiography. The echocardiographic appearance in patients with unequivocal mitral valve prolapse consists of a bowing backward and upward into the left atrium of a portion of the mitral leaflets during systole. Prolapse may be seen to be holosystolic, initiating at the C point and terminating at the onset of diastole, or it may be confined to late systole, beginning some time after the C point. Late systolic prolapse is a much more specific echocardiographic diagnosis than holosystolic prolapse. The timing of prolapse on echocardiography usually correlates with the timing of click and/or murmur in the clinical examination. A trace amount of posterior deviation of the mitral leaflets during systole may be normal. One rather liberal criterion for concluding the diagnosis calls for at least 3 mm of mitral leaflet deviation below a line drawn between the C and D points. This criterion was utilized

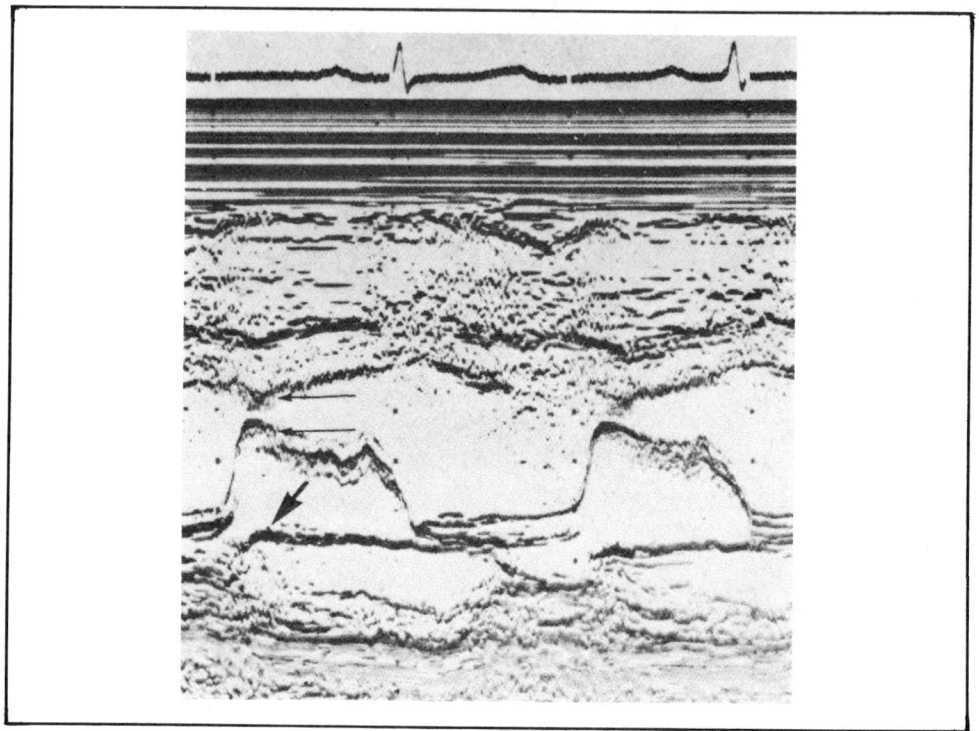

FIGURE 5-10. M-mode echocardiogram of diastolic flutter (*small arrows*) on the interventricular septum and anterior mitral leaflet in a patient with aortic regurgitation. The posterior mitral leaflet is not well seen; the large arrow indicates a portion of mitral apparatus. (From DJ Skorton: *Am J Med* 69:337, 1980.)

by Markiewicz et al in determining an 18 percent incidence of prolapse in healthy women [5].

Other abnormalities seen in the presence of mitral prolapse include (1) an increased anterior leaflet excursion, that is, a high D–E amplitude; and (2) a thickened or "smudgy" appearance of the redundant mitral leaflet tissue, which may be confused with bacterial vegetations on the leaflets (Fig. 5-12). Although M-mode echo cannot identify which of the two mitral leaflets is prolapsing, this question is readily resolved by two-dimensional echo. The M-mode appearance of mitral prolapse may be produced spuriously by (1) incorrect transducer location (e.g., directed caudad, rather than perpendicular to the chest or slightly cephalad), and (2) large pericardial effusion.

The two-dimensional echo appearance of mitral and, for that matter, tricuspid prolapse is a bowing toward the atrium of a portion of one or both leaflets, breaking the plane of the valve ring. This abnormality can be appreciated both in parasternal long axis and apical four-chamber views (Fig. 5-12).

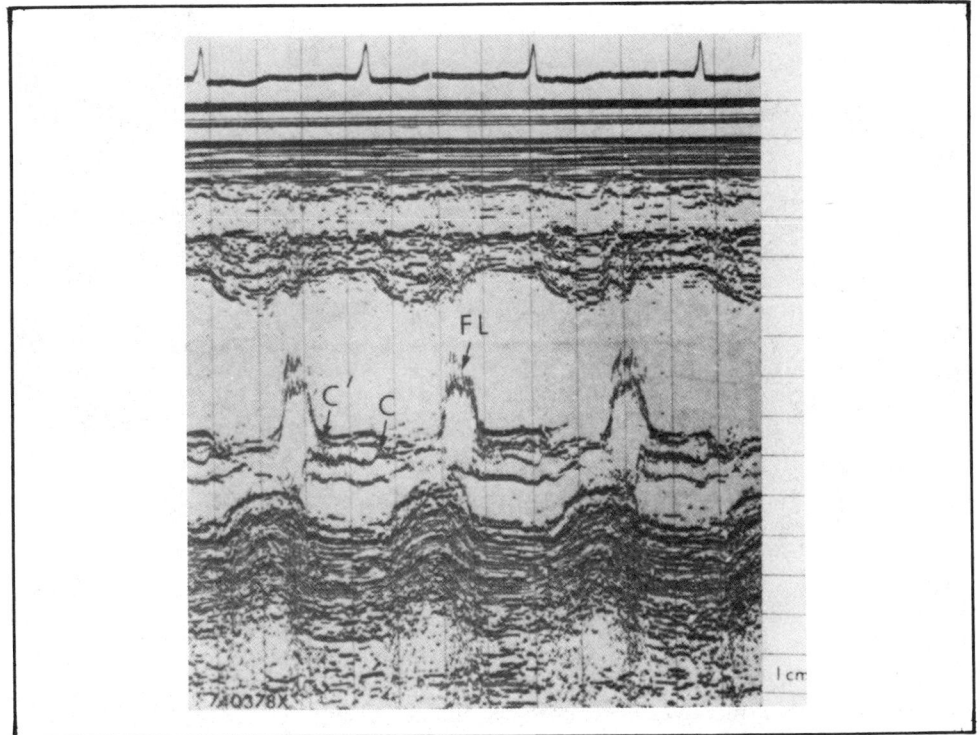

FIGURE 5-11. Mitral valve echocardiogram of a patient with acute severe aortic regurgitation. The valve is almost completely closed (C') before ventricular systole. The valve does not reopen with atrial systole and closes completely with ventricular systole (C). (From H Feigenbaum: *Echocardiography.* Philadelphia: Lea & Febiger, 1981, p 282.)

Mitral Regurgitation
Mitral regurgitation can only infrequently be identified directly on the echocardiogram. In the presence of a flail leaflet, due to ruptured chordae tendineae or papillary muscle, the unphysiologic motion of the affected leaflet, usually involving dramatic prolapse of a portion of the valve into the left atrium during systole and erratic movements into the left ventricle during diastole, is distinctive (Fig. 5-13). Most other forms of mitral regurgitation must be assessed indirectly via the effects of the regurgitation. The indirect signs of mitral regurgitation include an enlarged left ventricle (usually with well-preserved left ventricular function), a large left atrium, and prominent distension of the left atrium during systole. The degree of enlargement of both chambers is directly related to the magnitude of regurgitation. Other clues to the presence as well as cause of mitral regurgitation are the readily apparent thickening of the valve in rheumatic valve disease; the marked calcification of the annulus in regurgitation due to annular disease (Fig. 5-14); the akinesis or dyskinesis of portions of the left ventricle with papillary muscle

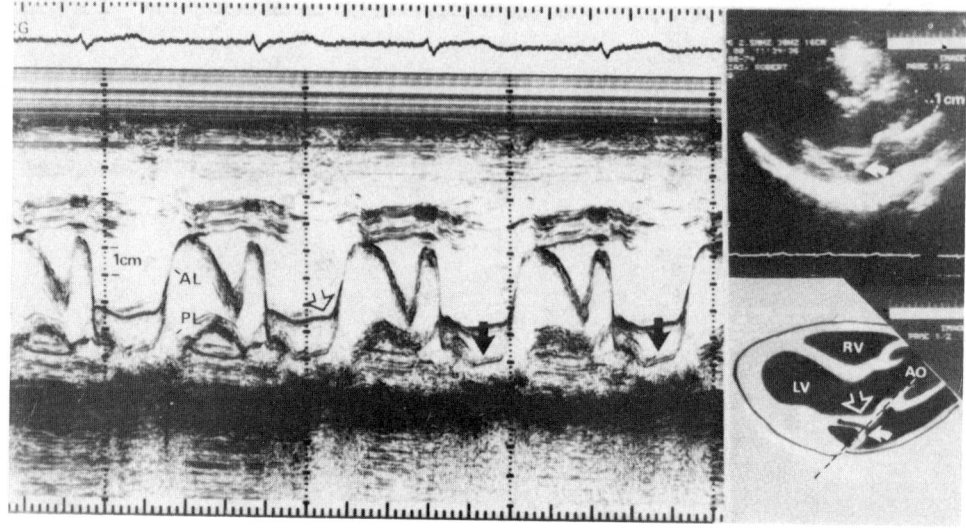

FIGURE 5-12. M-mode (*left*) and two-dimensional (2-D) (*upper right*) echocardiograms with a diagrammatic overlay (*lower right*) in a patient with the clinical click-murmur syndrome. Systolic posterior bowing (*solid black arrows*) is recorded after the mitral anterior leaflet (*AL*) and posterior leaflet (*PL*) echoes meet and before they separate in early diastole. Note the more anterior echo in systole (*open black arrow*). The 2-D images in late systole indicate marked displacement of the closed mitral valve (*solid white arrow*) beyond the atrioventricular junction toward the left atrium. A dashed line connecting the posterior atrioventricular junction and junction of the aorta with the mitral valve places the posterior leaflet on the atrial side of this line. Motion of the middle portion of the anterior mitral leaflet (*open white arrow*) corresponds to the motion indicated by the open black arrow on the M-mode record. AO = aorta, LV = left ventricle, RV = right ventricle. (From RL Popp: *Ann Intern Med* 93:844, 1980.)

dysfunction; and the presence of vegetations on the leaflets consistent with endocarditis.

Infective Endocarditis Involving the Mitral Valve

Vegetations on cardiac valves in clinically diagnosed infective endocarditis are seen in 40 to 80 percent of cases [9, 10]. Although vegetations visualized in patients with endocarditis clearly indicate more severe disease [11], this appearance cannot be utilized as an indication for cardiac surgery [12]. There is controversy regarding the relative sensitivities of M-mode and 2-D echo for identifying valvular vegetations. Martin et al [10] found definite vegetations by M-mode in only 14 percent but by 2-D echo in 81 percent of patients; similarly, Melvin et al [13] found an M-mode sensitivity of 49 percent compared with an 80 percent sensitivity of 2-D echo. In contrast, Mintz et al [9] found the two techniques to have similar sensitivities of 45 percent. However, 2-D echo is superior in demonstrating the complications of endocarditis; Mintz et al [9] found complications of endocarditis

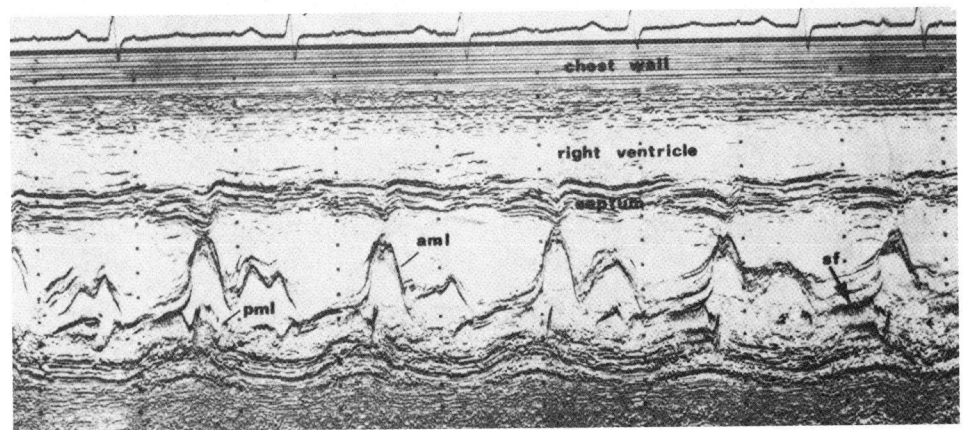

FIGURE 5-13. Representative M-mode echocardiogram of flail posterior mitral leaflet. The transducer angulation has been varied throughout this tracing. Thus, systolic flutter (*sf*) of the mitral closure line is more easily seen on the right side, whereas the diastolic motion abnormalities are more dramatic on the left. *aml* = anterior mitral leaflet, *pml* = posterior mitral leaflet. (From JS Child: *Am J Cardiol* 44:1383, 1979.)

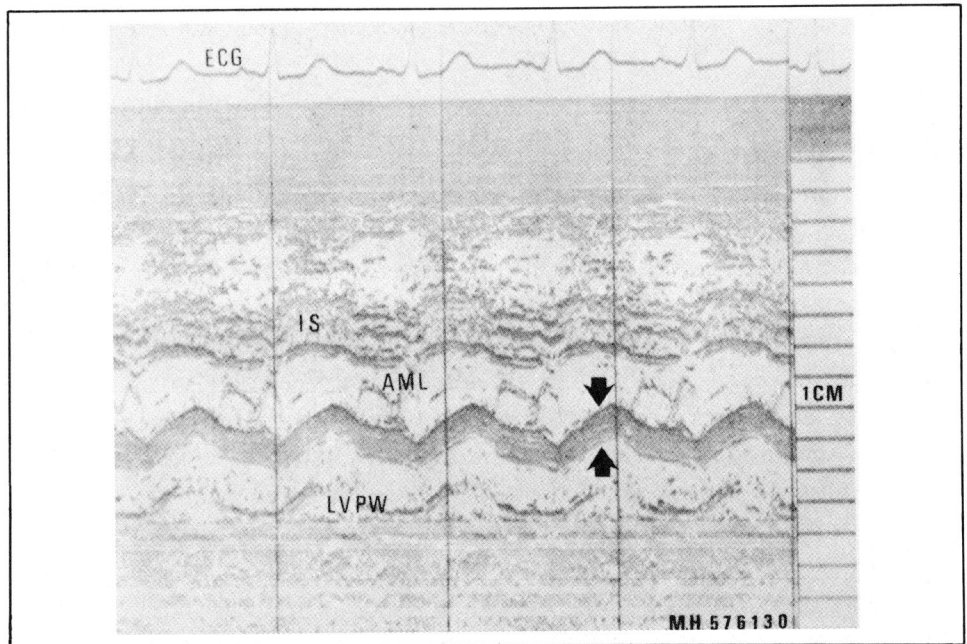

FIGURE 5-14. Echocardiogram in a patient with calcified mitral valve annulus. Note the dense echoes (*arrows*) emanating from the mitral valve annulus just posterior to the mitral valve leaflets and riding upon the endocardium of the left ventricular posterior wall (*LVPW*). *AML* = anterior mitral leaflet, *IS* = interventricular septum. (Reprinted with permission from AN DeMaria: The mitral echogram. In DT Mason [ed]: *Advances in Heart Disease*, Vol 2. New York: Grune & Stratton, 1978, p 32.)

in only 10 percent of subjects by M-mode but in 45 percent of the same subjects with 2-D echo. Such complications include flail cusps and leaflets, aortic root abscess, and sinus of Valsalva aneurysms. Furthermore, 2-D echo is superior to M-mode in determining the exact size, shape, and location of vegetations. The echocardiographic appearance of vegetations cannot be utilized as an index of response to therapy, since vegetations may persist without major change for months and years even after successful clinical cure [14].

The Prosthetic Mitral Valve

Prosthetic valves can be evaluated with both M-mode and 2-D echo techniques. The amplitude of motion of both the occluder and the valve housing can be assessed by echo. In addition, the timing of motion can be assessed; in the presence of a regular rhythm, a valve that opens with varying delay after S_2 suggests an intermittently "sticking" valve and often constitutes a surgical emergency. The presence of thrombus in the region of the valve can also be identified. Occasionally, tissue ingrowth to the valve can be detected. Paravalvular leak can be suspected on the basis on increased motion of the valve housing or by the usual criteria for the presence of mitral regurgitation. The leaflets in bioprosthetic (porcine) valves are normally thin and mobile but may become thickened or flail with degenerative changes.

Systolic Anterior Motion

Systolic anterior motion of the anterior mitral leaflet (SAM) is an abnormality associated most commonly with obstructive hypertrophic cardiomyopathy. By M-mode echo, the normal mitral valve executes a gradual anterior motion during systole, defining a relatively straight line between the C and D points (see Fig. 5-7A). This anterior motion is a consequence of the motion of the entire heart anteriorly rather than of the leaflets alone. In mitral prolapse, the leaflets bulge posteriorly during systole. In SAM, the anterior leaflet describes an arc anteriorly away from the posterior leaflet; the arc returns to baseline before the mitral valve opens, as shown in Figure 5-15. It is thought that the anterior leaflet is drawn into this anterior position as a consequence of the deformed geometry of the left ventricular outflow tract in hypertrophic cardiomyopathy. The presence of SAM correlates with the presence of obstruction, and the proximity of the anterior leaflet to the interventricular septum during systole correlates inversely with the pressure gradient measured at catheterization. Although the picture of SAM is most commonly associated with hypertrophic cardiomyopathy with obstruction, SAM is also seen in normal persons who are hypovolemic; SAM is abolished in this setting by the replenishment of normal intravascular volume. SAM can be appreciated on 2-D echo, but it is much more readily apparent with the M-mode technique.

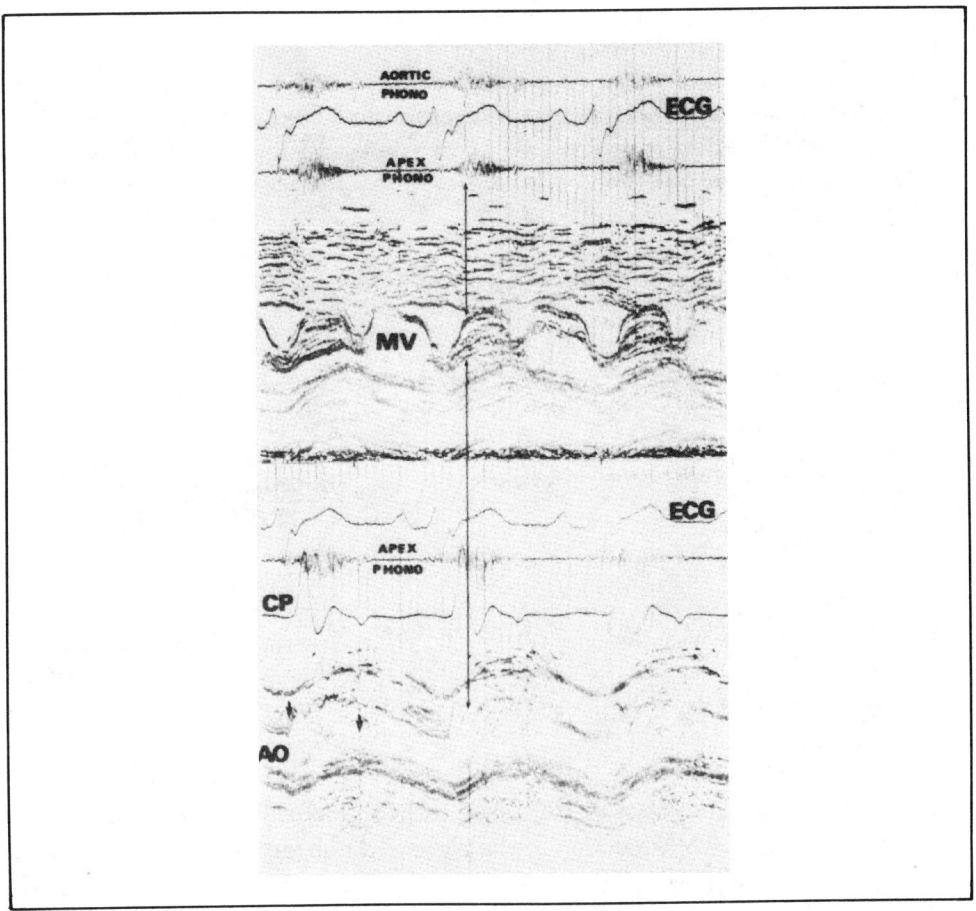

FIGURE 5-15. Mitral (*top*) and aortic valve (*bottom*) echoes in obstructive hypertrophic cardiomyopathy. The two panels were sequentially recorded and mounted to demonstrate valve motion and murmur timing at the same heart rate. The end-systolic crescendo murmur becomes most intense as the mitral valve (*MV*) maximally approaches the septum (*long vertical arrow*) and the aortic cusps move to a partially closed position. Two small arrows on the first aortic cycle denote the beginning and end of systole. There is a prominent mid-systolic carotid pulse (*CP*) trough coincident with maximal murmur intensity. *AO* = aorta. (From RL Popp: Echocardiographic assessment of cardiac disease. *Circulation* 54:538, 1970, by permission of the American Heart Association, Inc.)

THE AORTIC VALVE AND ROOT

Normal and Bicuspid Aortic Valve

The aortic valve is depicted by a distinctive M-mode pattern, shown in Figure 5-16. Two of the three aortic valve leaflets, the right and noncoronary cusps, are imaged. In diastole, the leaflets are seen as a single diastolic closure line, typically

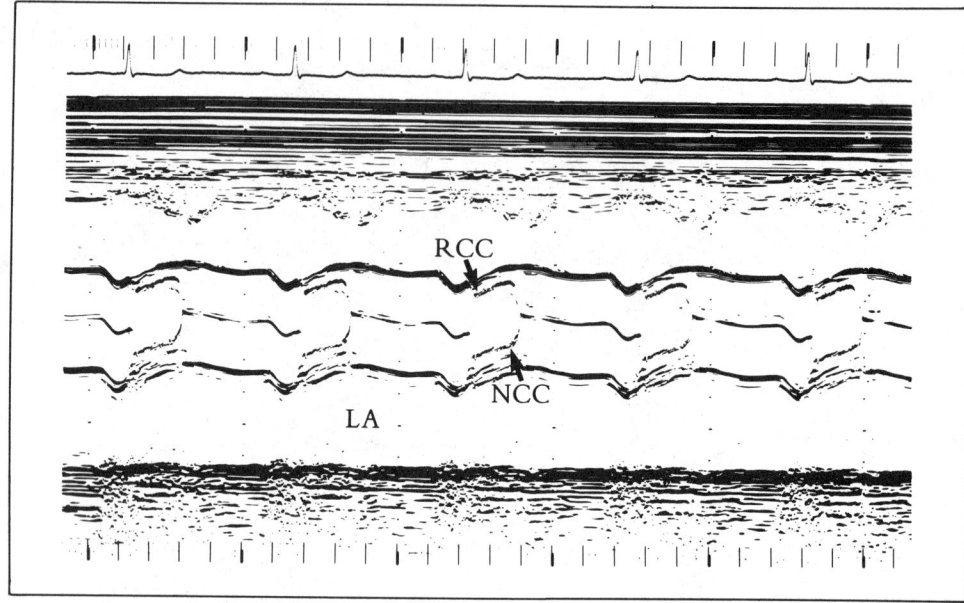

FIGURE 5-16. M-mode tracing of a normal aortic valve. The right (*RCC*) and noncoronary cusps (*NCC*) separate during systole and form a thin line of closure during diastole. *LA* = left atrium.

in the midline of the aortic root. Multiple parallel echo lines suggest valve thickening. The leaflets move away from each other in systole, forming a box-like shape. The amplitude of excursion of the right and noncoronary cusps away from the diastolic closure line should be equal. In congenitally bicuspid aortic valve, the diastolic closure line deviates from the middle of the aorta toward either the anterior or posterior aortic root wall, reflecting the asymmetric size of the two cusps in this disorder. This configuration can be defined by the so-called eccentricity index, which is the quotient of one-half the aortic root diameter divided by the distance from the diastolic closure line to the nearest aortic wall. The normal eccentricity index is less than or equal to 1.3. Using this criterion, the sensitivity for bicuspid aortic valve has been reported to be 75 to 100 percent and the specificity 100 percent [15, 16]; 2-D echo aids in the assessment of aortic valve disease (Fig. 5-17).

Valvular Aortic Stenosis

Valvular aortic stenosis is characterized on the M-mode echo as dense multiple echoes within the aortic root in both diastole and systole. Aortic leaflet excursion is either not apparent or diminished, as seen in Figure 5-18. A nonthickened aortic valve on M-mode excludes significant valvular aortic stenosis in middle-aged and elderly adults. However, the converse is not true — a valve may show

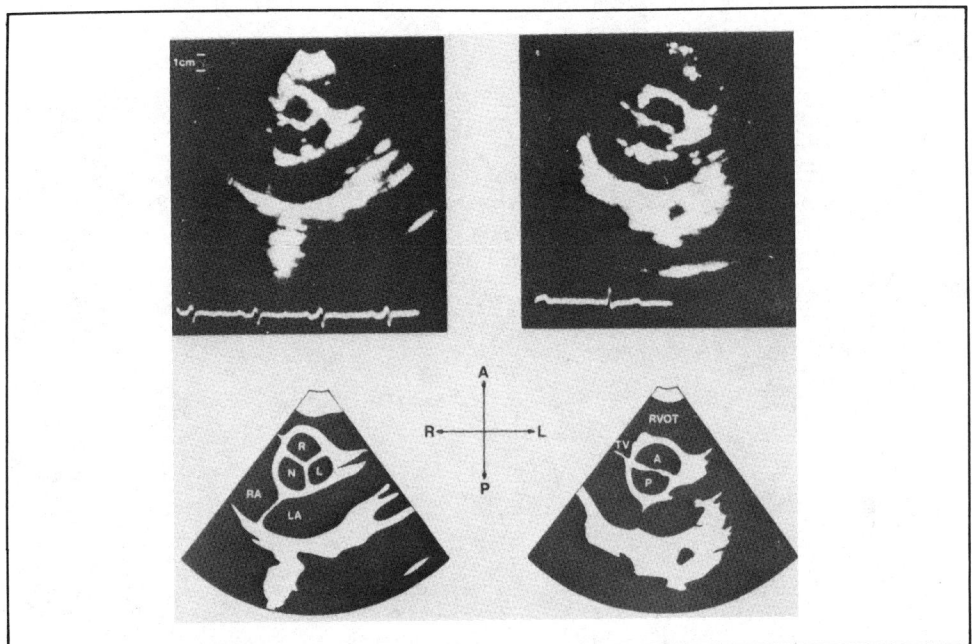

FIGURE 5-17. Two-dimensional echocardiogram, short-axis view in a normal patient (*left*) and in a patient with a bicuspid aortic valve (*right*). The trileaflet aortic valve is demonstrated in the left panel and the two cusps separated by a single commissure is demonstrated in the right panel. A = anterior cusp, L = left coronary cusp, LA = left atrium, N = noncoronary cusp, P = posterior cusp, R = right coronary cusp, RA = right atrium, $RVOT$ = right ventricular outflow tract, TV = tricuspid valve. (From MN Kotler et al: *Am J Cardiol* 45:1061, 1980.)

marked thickening and diminished or absent leaflet excursion on M-mode and yet have no significant gradient at catheterization. Furthermore, children and young adults with congenital valvular stenosis may demonstrate thin leaflets and a normal valve excursion on M-mode echo if the echo beam passes through the base or mid-portion of the leaflets; the stenotic portion of the valve may be cephalad to the echo beam, and severe stenosis may thus be entirely missed. Hence, M-mode echo cannot exclude valvular aortic stenosis in youthful patients, even with a normal-appearing aortic valve study.

On 2-D echo, stenotic aortic leaflets appear thickened, and motion is diminished. In contrast to mitral stenosis, the aortic valve orifice area measured by planimeter on the short-axis view correlates poorly with the aortic valve area calculated by the Gorlin equation from catheterization data. The distinction between a normal aortic valve and severe aortic stenosis usually can be made on the 2-D echocardiogram. Differentiating moderate from severe aortic stenosis may be more difficult, particularly if there is concomitant left ventricular dysfunction; cardiac catheterization is usually required to make this distinction. Finding left

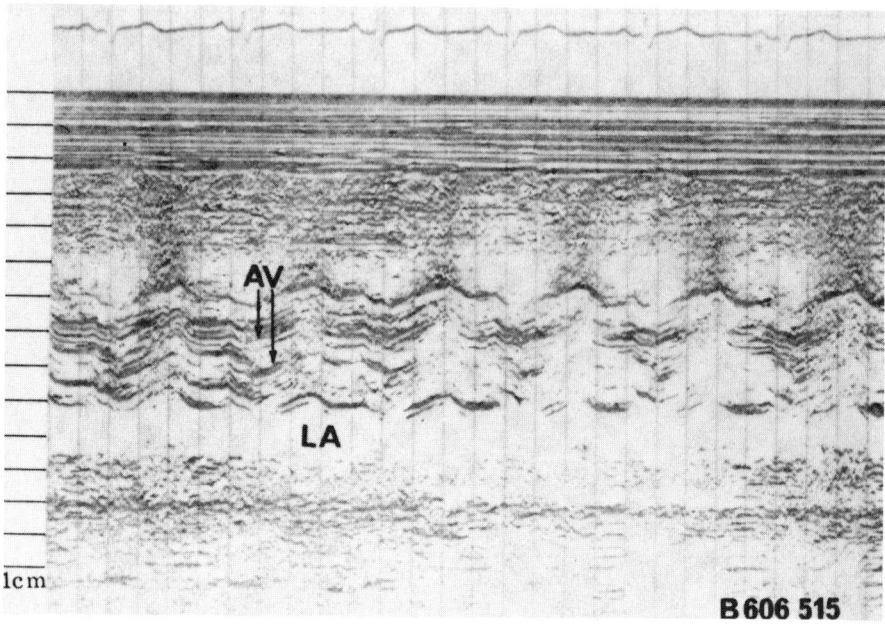

FIGURE 5-18. Fairly typical aortic valve echocardiogram of a patient with aortic stenosis. Thickened aortic leaflets are readily apparent, although the distance between the cusps is difficult to evaluate. AV = aortic valve leaflets, LA = left atrium. (From S Chang: *M-mode Echocardiographic Techniques and Pattern Recognition*. Philadelphia: Lea & Febiger, 1976.)

ventricular hypertrophy by either M-mode or 2-D examination increases the likelihood of significant aortic stenosis.

Subvalvular aortic stenosis due to either fixed (i.e., subvalvular ring or tunnel) or dynamic (i.e., hypertrophic cardiomyopathy) obstruction may cause characteristic abnormalities in the aortic valve echocardiogram, consisting of partial closure, or notching, of the aortic leaflet echoes in systole, as shown in Figure 5-15. Like systolic anterior motion of the mitral valve, this finding occurs only when outflow obstruction is present and is the physiologic correlate of the early systolic carotid pulse wave fall-off, the so-called spike and dome configuration, which is seen in obstructive hypertrophy cardiomyopathy. The notch coincides with approach of the anterior mitral leaflet to the interventricular septum and with the loudest phase of the murmur. Fixed subvalvular aortic stenosis can be diagnosed with the 2-D technique, either by direct imaging of the diaphragm or by the coarse aortic leaflet systolic fluttering that invariably occurs in this situation.

Aortic Regurgitation

Echocardiographic diagnosis of aortic regurgitation (AR) is more definitive than for mitral regurgitation. The characteristic echo feature of AR is high-frequency diastolic vibration of either the anterior mitral leaflet or of the interventricular septum (see Fig. 5-10); the reliability of this finding was discussed earlier (The Mitral Valve and Aortic Regurgitation). Fine fluttering of the aortic leaflets in systole is found in normal subjects. However, vibration of the aortic leaflets in diastole is distinctly abnormal and suggests aortic regurgitation. Furthermore, a flail aortic leaflet may be identified prolapsing into the left ventricle by both M-mode and 2-D techniques. Echocardiography can frequently determine the cause of aortic regurgitation, including vegetations in endocarditis; leaflet thickening in rheumatic and calcific disease; and enlargement of the root with normal cusps in aortic regurgitation due to hypertension, aortic aneurysm, or annuloaortic ectasia.

The echo picture pathognomonic for severe acute aortic regurgitation features a normal sized left ventricle; vibration of the anterior mitral leaflet or high interventricular septum; aortic valve vegetation; and premature closure of the mitral valve, i.e., C point before QRS onset (see Fig. 5-11). Because of the virulence of this condition, and in the face of its diagnostic echo findings, one can usually proceed directly to aortic valve replacement without further diagnostic studies.

As with mitral regurgitation, the extent of left ventricular enlargement is a rough index of severity of isolated aortic regurgitation.

Aortic Root Aneurysm
Saccular aneurysm of the aortic root can be readily diagnosed by M-mode echo on the basis of marked enlargement in diameter. However, dissection of the aortic root is a much more difficult echo diagnosis. Multiple longitudinal lines in the region of the anterior or posterior wall of the root, especially when asymmetric from the opposite side, have been suggested as a means of diagnosing aortic root dissection. This finding, however, is seen in normal subjects too often to be a reliable indicator of aortic root aneurysm. Should diastolic prolapse of an aortic leaflet into the left ventricular outflow tract be seen in the setting of multiple asymmetric aortic root wall echoes, on the other hand, dissection is more likely. Although efforts have been made to identify disease of the arch and of the descending aorta, this imaging is extremely demanding technically and cannot be reliably accomplished in most hospitals.

Two-dimensional echo can be diagnostic of root dissection, and occasionally even an intimal tear can be identified. However, false-positive examinations do occur, and the technique is not sufficiently sensitive to exclude the diagnosis.

Infective Endocarditis of the Aortic Valve
The same precepts that apply to the identification and interpretation of vegetations on the mitral valve apply to those on the aortic valve. The problem of previously

existing valve thickening obscuring the presence of vegetations is true of both valves. Fortunately, however, the confusion of vegetations with the "smudgy" appearance of the redundant leaflets in the mitral prolapse syndrome is not encountered with the aortic valve.

Prosthetic Aortic Valve

Prosthetic valves in the aortic position can be analyzed in precisely the same way as those placed in the mitral position. With regard to M-mode views, the transducer should be placed in a line parallel with the occluder motion. Accordingly, the mitral valve is best evaluated from the apical position and the aortic valve from the right supraclavicular fossa. Using 2-D echo, however, occluder motion can be evaluated in both positions from the parasternal position. The 2-D echo is particularly valuable in identifying abnormalities of the cusps of bioprostheses.

THE TRICUSPID VALVE

On M-mode echocardiography, the normal tricuspid valve bears a strong resemblance to the mitral valve (Fig. 5-19). However, the tricuspid valve appears as an anterior structure, lying anterior to the interventricular septum and projecting into the right ventricle in diastole. The valve is seldom visualized in its entirety by M-mode echo, although portions of the valve, especially in systole, can usually be imaged. On 2-D echo, the valve can be visualized in either the parasternal right ventricular inflow tract view, the subcostal view, or the apical four-chamber view, where it is seen alongside the mitral valve (see Fig. 5-6).

Tricuspid stenosis, a rare entity, can be diagnosed by echo, utilizing the same criteria as in mitral stenosis. Furthermore, clinically significant tricuspid stenosis virtually never occurs without associated rheumatic mitral stenosis.

Tricuspid regurgitation is suggested by the presence of right ventricular and right atrial enlargement on M-mode echo associated with paradoxical septal motion, as seen in any right ventricular volume overload state. Two-dimensional echo is fast becoming the diagnostic procedure of choice for tricuspid regurgitation. After intravenous injection of contrast material (most commonly 10 ml of forcefully injected normal saline), multiple echo signals can be seen to regurgitate into the inferior vena cava and hepatic veins during each systole.

Ebstein's anomaly of the tricuspid valve is readily appreciated from the four-chamber apical view, which shows the tricuspid valve ring to be located substantially lower in the right ventricle compared with the mitral valve ring in the left ventricle. On M-mode echo, the tricuspid valve is imaged in its entirety from many transducer positions, even during simultaneous imaging of the mitral echo; tricuspid closure may be quite delayed.

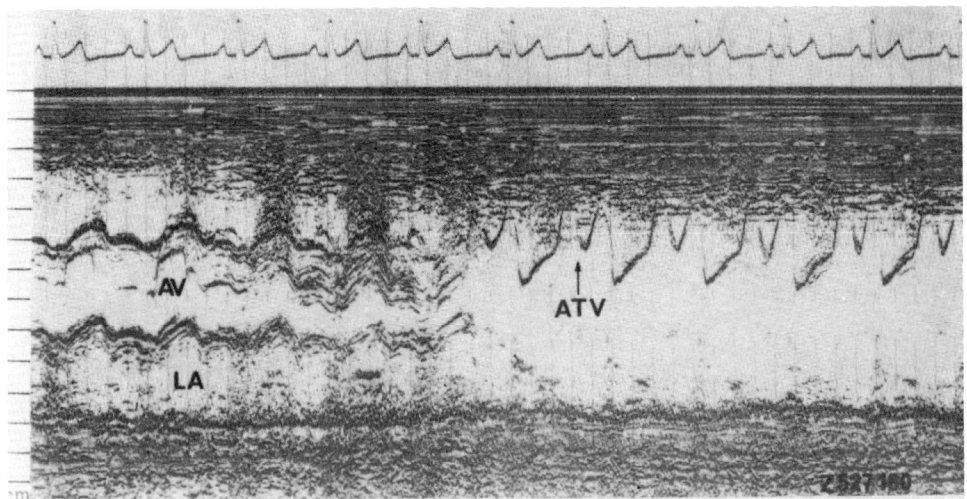

FIGURE 5-19. M-mode echocardiographic scan from the aortic valve to the anterior tricuspid valve leaflet (*ATV*). The echo resembles that of the anterior mitral valve leaflet. *AV* = aortic valve, *LA* = left atrium. (From H Feigenbaum: *Echocardiography.* Philadelphia: Lea & Febiger, 1981, p 65.)

THE PULMONIC VALVE

The pulmonic valve is the most difficult of the four valves to visualize by both M-mode and 2-D echo. If the entire pulmonic valve could be visualized by M-mode, the appearance would be similar to that of the aortic valve. However, it is uncommon to visualize the anterior leaflet during systole, and the pulmonary artery walls are virtually never imaged. Accordingly, only the leaflet closure line in diastole and the posterior leaflet in systole are seen (Fig. 5-20). A few diagnostic signs are present even with this limited imaging, however. A pronounced *a* wave suggests forceful right atrial contraction, often due to right ventricular hypertrophy, as seen in pulmonic valve stenosis. A diminished *a* wave suggests pulmonary arterial hypertension, with a mean pressure greater than 20 mm Hg. This is unfortunately an insensitive sign. Pulmonary hypertension is also associated with systolic notching of the valvular leaflets, reminiscent of the aortic valve appearance in obstructive hypertrophic cardiomyopathy. Unfortunately, in the case of the pulmonic valve, this is not a pathognomonic finding. In atrial fibrillation, the *a* wave is absent altogether.

The pulmonic valve, although difficult to image with either technique, proves less elusive on 2-D than on M-mode echo. The pulmonic valve is seen on the parasternal short-axis view of the aortic valve, wherein the pulmonic valve lies slightly anterior and lateral to the aortic valve. Because the outflow tracts are at

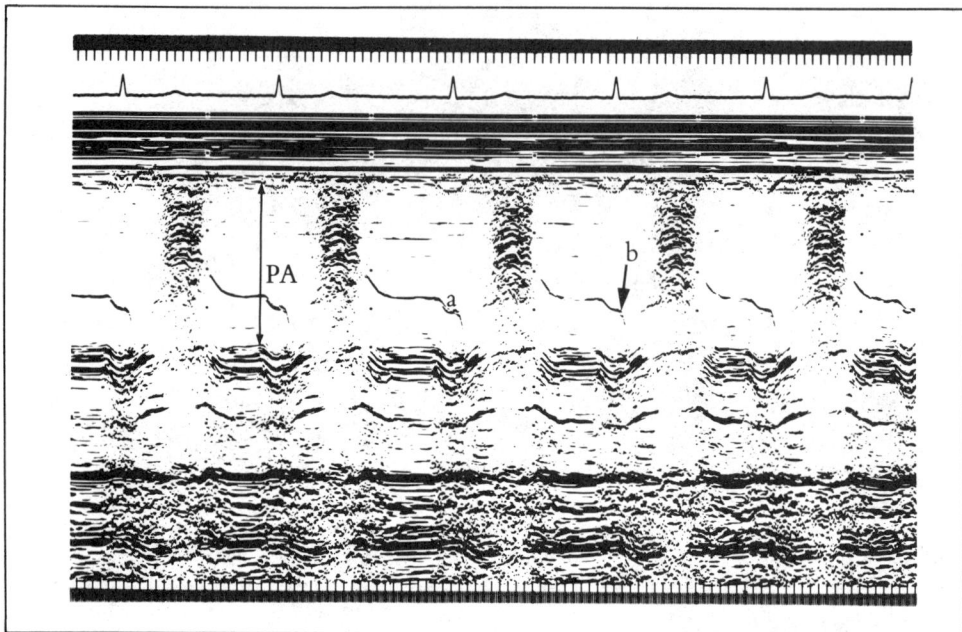

FIGURE 5-20. Normal pulmonary valve echocardiogram showing M-mode recording of the motion of the posterior pulmonary valve cusp. Posterior motion (a) of the cusp follows atrial systole prior to systolic opening of the valve (b). PA = pulmonary artery.

right angles to each other, the pulmonic valve is seen in long axis while the aortic valve is seen in short axis. Pulmonic stenosis, valvular vegetations, and flail leaflets can all be observed with this view, and the appearances are similar to those seen in the aortic valve. In the presence of normal valve thickness and motion, pulmonic stenosis can be excluded. However, hemodynamically significant pulmonic stenosis can usually not be diagnosed with certainty by echo techniques.

THE LEFT ATRIUM

The left atrium is seen on M-mode echo behind the aortic root, measured from the leading edge of the posterior aortic wall to the leading edge of the posterior left atrial wall. Ordinarily, the left atrium is roughly the same diameter as the aortic root, as shown in Figure 5-16. It is enlarged in the presence of mitral valve disease, both stenosis and regurgitation, and in the presence of left ventricular hypertrophy and left ventricular failure. The posterior left atrial wall is motionless in its mid and cephalad portions. The caudad end toward the mitral annulus moves well; comparison with the ECG demonstrates that this portion of the left atrial wall moves before the QRS complex, consistent with atrial systole (see Fig. 5-3). The left atrium can be examined for masses such as myxomas or, in the case of atrial fibrillation or mitral valve disease, thrombus.

THE LEFT VENTRICLE

Left ventricular dimensions on M-mode echo are measured by convention at the level of the chordae tendineae, that is, apical to the mitral valve leaflet tips but basal to the papillary muscles. Optimally, this measurement is made in the same left parasternal transducer position that allows imaging of the mitral valve leaflets with the transducer perpendicular to the chest wall. This standardization of transducer position minimizes oblique imaging of the cavity, allowing for more reproducible measurements. There is evidence, however, that measurements taken from the subxiphoid position are comparable to those from the standard left parasternal position [17].

Left ventricular performance measurements include maximum amplitude of motion of both interventricular septum and left ventricular posterior wall. These figures are only crude guides, however, since they reflect movement of the entire heart within the chest wall as well as individual wall motion proper. A more reliable measurement is the change in left ventricular dimension from end-diastole to end-systole. By American Society of Echocardiography recommendations, end-diastolic dimension is measured at the onset of the QRS complex and end-systolic dimension at the nadir of the interventricular septal motion [1]. The change in cavity dimension is independent of movement of the heart within the chest. This change in dimension can be manipulated in a number of ways to yield more clinically useful results. First, without correcting for heart size, the change in dimension would be higher for larger patients than for smaller ones. Hence, by dividing the change in dimension by the end-diastolic dimension, the figure is normalized for chamber size, yielding the so-called percent fractional shortening, or $\%\Delta D$

$$\%\Delta D = \frac{EDD - ESD}{EDD} \times 100\%$$

where EDD = end-diastolic dimension and ESD = end-systolic dimension. The percent fractional shortening can be further refined by dividing it by the ejection time (ET), as measured either by carotid pulse tracing or by the aortic valve echo, yielding the mean velocity of circumferential fiber shortening, or mean Vcf.

$$\text{mean Vcf} = \frac{EDD - ESD}{EDD \times ET} = \frac{\%\Delta D}{ET}$$

The dimension change can also be converted to ejection fraction (EF), a more familiar entity to most physicians. Several formulas are available. The best known is the so-called cube formula, based on the geometric assumption that the left ventricle is an ellipse of revolution in which the two short axes are equal, and the long axis is twice the length of the short axis.

$$EF_{cube} = \frac{EDD^3 - ESD^3}{EDD^3}$$

Ejection fractions computed with this formula correlate reasonably well with angiographic ejection fraction in the case of normal sized hearts. However, in either enlarged or unusually small hearts, the geometric assumptions are no longer applicable, and ejection fraction by the cube formula deviates widely from angiographic ejection fraction. A regression formula devised by Teichholz helps correct for this disproportion [18]:

$$EF_{Teichholz} = \frac{7.0}{2.4 + EDD} \times \frac{EDD^3 - ESD^3}{EDD^3} = \frac{7.0}{2.4 + EDD} \times EF_{cube}$$

It is important to remember that all left ventricular performance parameters (echo or otherwise) that measure dimension change are afterload-dependent. Hence, ejection fraction, percent fractional shortening, and mean Vcf cannot be sequentially compared in the same patient unless the blood pressure is roughly the same. Furthermore, because mean Vcf involves the ejection time, which varies with heart rate, mean Vcf cannot be compared sequentially in any given patient unless the heart rate (HR) is roughly the same or the mean Vcf is corrected for heart rate according to a regression equation, which then yields the so-called relative velocity of contraction (RVC) [19]:

$$RVC = \frac{Vcf}{0.14 + 0.014\ HR}$$

Volume measurements derived from M-mode studies correlate substantially less well with angiographic volumes than the functional parameters discussed above correlate with their angiographic equivalents. Techniques for determining left ventricular performance with 2-D echo have been appearing over the past several years. As with M-mode, 2-D echo determinations of volume are substantially less well-correlated with angiographic volumes than are the ejection fraction, the %ΔD, and the Vcf. Commercial systems for computer-assisted determination of these functional parameters from both M-mode and 2-D echoes are now generally available, and some of these systems are built into the echo machines themselves. Because of the continued need for geometric assumptions in deriving these global left ventricular function parameters, however, the echo determinations still deviate moderately from the "gold standards" of contrast angiography and radionuclide angiography. We anticipate considerable improvement in the reliability of these echo determinations in the next few years.

In addition to global left ventricular function, regional wall function can be assessed with increasing precision by 2-D echo. M-mode echo is restricted by convention to a single region of the interventricular septum and left ventricular posterior wall. Accordingly, M-mode left ventricular function parameters are valid only in hearts with symmetric wall motion throughout, as in valve disease and cardiomyopathy. In the case of regional wall motion abnormalities, however, as in coronary artery disease, M-mode determinations are unreliable when extrapolated to reflect global function. The two-dimensional technique examines much more wall area and is therefore less prone to error in the presence of regional wall motion abnormalities. Two-dimensional echo is generally considered not yet sufficiently refined to be a useful index of response of left ventricular function to therapy. Radionuclide angiography remains the most useful noninvasive technique for such purposes. However, 2-D echo may begin to yield comparably reliable results within this decade [20].

Regional wall motion is usually graded by echocardiography as hyperkinetic, normal, hypokinetic, akinetic, and dyskinetic (paradoxical). A number of schemes for dividing the left ventricle into regions for qualitative and quantitative assessment have been devised. One problem faced by echocardiography in the assessment of regional wall motion is the paucity of intraventricular landmarks for reproducibility of imaging plane. Landmarks typically used are the papillary muscles and the junctures of the right ventricular free wall with the left ventricular wall. All left ventricular imaging techniques, however, have their own special advantages and disadvantages [21].

A number of studies have demonstrated that two-dimensional echocardiographic assessments of myocardial infarct size based on wall motion abnormalities overestimate infarct size as determined by tissue examination. One reason for this finding is that uninfarcted tissue adjacent to infarcted tissue undergoes a "tethering effect," being pulled by adjacent infarcted tissue in an akinetic or dyskinetic fashion. Accordingly, analysis of endocardial motion has been shown to be less precise an echocardiographic index of myocardial viability than myocardial thickening [22]. Unfortunately, left ventricular wall thickening does not correlate linearly with the magnitude of infarction in any given region. Normal wall thickening averages about 40 percent. With transmural infarction of 1 to 20 percent of any given region, thickening continues to occur but is diminished in magnitude. When transmural infarction involves anywhere from 21 to 100 percent of left ventricular wall in any given segment, wall thickening is absent altogether, and thinning occurs [22]. Two-dimensional echo is qualitatively useful in detecting myocardial fibrosis or necrosis. In an autopsy study of 20 patients undergoing 2-D echocardiography shortly before death, 14 of 15 myocardial infarcts were detected on the basis of wall motion abnormality, ranging from hypokinesis to dyskinesis [23]. With regard to myocardial segments, 79 of 88 infarcted segments revealed some form of motion abnormality. Interestingly, 38 of 82 segments that were morphologically normal were also associated with wall motion abnormality, and most were adjacent to scar tissue. While 2-D echo is unreliable in determining the size of a myocardial infarct, it is nonetheless of value in predicting the presence of myocardial necrosis or fibrosis and is of great value in excluding transmural infarction. Studies in progress attempting to categorize tissue on the basis of echocardiographic signals as normal, ischemic, or infarcted hold great promise for the future; such tissue characterization may permit the determination of histopathology from echo images.

Left Ventricular Aneurysm

Left ventricular aneurysm can be diagnosed relatively easily with two-dimensional echo. Even more important, however, is the capability to diagnose false or pseudoaneurysm [24, 25]. False aneurysm is created by focal rupture of the left ventricular wall with formation of an extramyocardial cavity enclosed solely by thrombus and pericardium. The walls of such cavities are prone to rupture, resulting in sudden death due to pericardial tamponade. Diagnosis is made by comparing the ratio of the width of the neck of the aneurysm to the largest parallel internal diameter of the aneurysm: when this fraction is less than 0.5, a pseudoaneurysm is likely. Most true aneurysms bear a ratio of 0.9 to 1.1 Because of their penchant for rupture, all pseudoaneurysms should be excised surgically in appropriate candidates. The diagnosis can be life-saving and constitutes an important contribution of 2-D echo to the evaluation of patients with ischemic heart disease. The 2-D echo is also useful in identifying the intracavitary thrombus that is often found within a left ventricular aneurysm, although experience and caution are required in differentiation of thrombus from artifact.

Hypertrophic Cardiomyopathy

Hypertrophic cardiomyopathy (HCM) is defined as left ventricular hypertrophy without identifiable cause. More than 90 percent of cases show asymmetric involvement, with the septum being the hypertrophied portion in the great majority of cases. The criterion for asymmetric septal hypertrophy (ASH) is an interventricular septal thickness of greater than or equal to 1.3 times the left ventricular posterior wall thickness. Occasionally, the interventricular septum may be imaged tangentially by M-mode technique, resulting in a spurious diagnosis of ASH. Two-dimensional echo can rectify this problem easily. Where ASH is associated with left ventricular outflow tract obstruction, systolic anterior motion of the mitral valve and midsystolic notching of the aortic valve leaflets are also seen (see Fig. 5-15). Other echo findings in HCM include narrowed left ventricular outflow tract, reduced septal movement and thickening during systole, normal or increased posterior wall motion, small left ventricular cavity size, reduced mitral leaflet E–F slope, and mitral valve prolapse. Echocardiography has become the procedure of choice for evaluating patients with suspected hypertrophic cardiomyopathy.

Ventricular Septal Defect
Congenital ventricular septal defect (VSD) most commonly occurs in the membranous septum, near the base of the heart. When large, septal drop-out on slow sweep can be appreciated by M-mode technique. Two-dimensional echo allows this diagnosis to be made with much greater confidence. However, small VSDs are not easily seen by either technique. The rapid intravenous injection of saline permits contrast evaluation of the ventricles. In the presence of left-to-right shunting, as with a small VSD, a negative defect may be seen as blood without contrast mixes with contrast. In right-to-left shunt, however, contrast can be observed to pass readily from the right to the left ventricle and out the aorta. Routine echo contrast materials are defeated by the pulmonary capillaries. A new agent consisting of encapsulated microbubbles is presently being tested; this agent permits bubbles to pass through the pulmonary circulation and into the left heart after intravenous injection [26]. Such an agent will allow relatively easy identification of left-to-right shunt by the observation of bubbles traversing the left heart directly into the right heart.

A number of reports have described imaging of muscular ventricular septal defects arising post myocardial infarction [27]. Direct imaging of such defects is challenging at best, inasmuch as most such septal defects are porous and follow a serpiginous course through the muscle.

Interventricular Septal Motion
The interventricular septum normally moves posteriorly toward the posterior left ventricular wall. Several situations result in systolic movement of the interventricular septum toward the transducer and away from the left ventricular posterior wall, however. The conditions associated with so-called paradoxical septal motion can be organized, as shown in Figure 5-21, by the presence or absence of right ventricular enlargement and systolic septal thickening greater than 30 percent of its diastolic thickness. In the presence of right ventricular enlargement and abnormal septal thickening, septal paradox may be caused by cardiomyopathy and coronary artery disease with biventricular failure. Right ventricular enlargement with normal septal thickening is caused by right ventricular diastolic volume

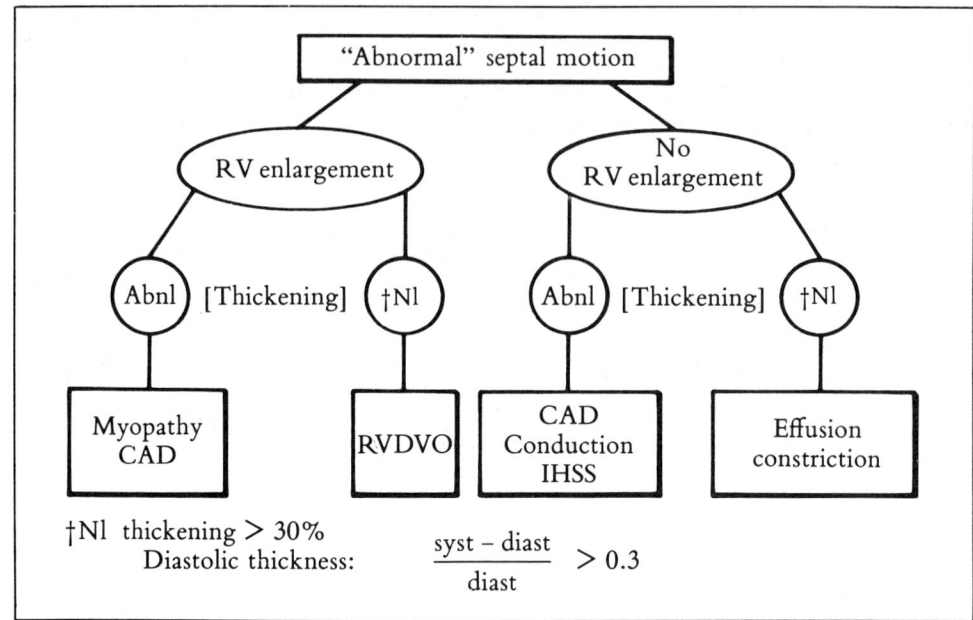

FIGURE 5-21. Schematic approach to elucidating the cause of abnormal septal motion on echocardiography. The presence or absence of right ventricular (*RV*) enlargement, and normal (*Nl*) or abnormal (*Abnl*) septal thickening allows the determination of the cause of septal abnormality. *CAD* = coronary artery disease, *IHSS* = hypertrophic cardiomyopathy, *RVDVO* = right ventricular diastolic volume overload (as in atrial septal defect). (From RL Popp: Echocardiographic assessment of cardiac disease. *Circulation* 54:538, 1970, by permission of the American Heart Association, Inc.)

overload secondary to atrial septal defect, tricuspid regurgitation, pulmonic regurgitation, or anomalous pulmonary venous drainage.

In the setting of normal right ventricular size but abnormal septal thickening, differential diagnosis includes coronary artery disease involving the left anterior descending branch; hypertrophic cardiomyopathy with septal involvement; or conduction disorders causing delayed activation of the septum, as in left bundle branch block. Finally, in the presence of normal right ventricular size and septal thickening, septal paradox is associated with the presence of pericardial effusion and constriction and with the post-cardiac surgery state. The explanation for paradoxical septal motion in the right ventricular volume overload, pericardial effusion, and postoperative settings is probably related to increased motion of the entire heart toward the anterior chest wall. A plot of instantaneous left ventricular dimension changes throughout the cardiac cycle, and therefore all calculated parameters of global left ventricular function, is within normal limits in these situations. Furthermore, the amplitude of the posterior wall motion increases proportionate to the magnitude of septal paradox. The septum moves normally with respect to the heart; the movement of the entire heart is what causes the abnormality seen on echo, which is spurious [28].

THE PERICARDIUM

Because of the major difference in acoustic impedance between the pericardium and air-filled lung, the posterior pericardium usually produces the echo of greatest amplitude seen by M-mode technique. The normal parietal pericardium is closely apposed to the visceral pericardium, with less than 15 ml of pericardial fluid in the entire sac. Hence, the normal pericardium moves in concert with the posterior epicardium. When a separation occurs between the epicardium and pericardium, a pericardial effusion is present (see Fig. 5-3).

M-mode echo can determine the quantity of pericardial fluid in semiquantitative terms. Effusions are usually classified as small, moderate, and large: small when only posterior systolic separation between epicardium and pericardium occurs; moderate if there is separation throughout both systole and diastole; and large when there is also an anterior echo-free space. When gross cardiac oscillation within this sac occurs, electrical alternans is often found on the electrocardiogram. Due to the problem of oscillation, one should not read mitral valve prolapse, systolic anterior motion, or paradoxical septal motion by M-mode in the presence of pericardial effusion.

The minimum effusion volume detectable is between 15 and 50 ml [29]. False-positive diagnosis of pericardial effusion by M-mode can occur with medial angulation of the transducer, by the presence of pericardial thickening, pericardial fat, juxtacardiac tumor, and by pleural effusion. The presence of echo-free space anteriorly raises the likelihood of pericardial effusion. Where effusion is suspected, a continuous M-mode scan from the left ventricle to the aortic root should be performed. In most cases, pericardial effusion is seen to terminate at the level of the atrioventricular groove, since the pericardium adheres to the pulmonary veins where they enter the posterior left atrium. However, the pericardial oblique sinus continues between the pulmonary veins up the posterior left atrium and can fill with fluid with large pericardial effusions. In this case, the depth of effusion at the atrial level is always smaller than at the ventricular level [29] (see Fig. 5-3).

Two-dimensional echo can often provide additional useful information in the evaluation of a patient with a suspected pericardial effusion. In the absence of loculation, the effusion can be seen to move to the most dependent portion of the sac as the patient's posture is changed. When present, fibrin strands can be identified in the effusion, usually stretching from the visceral to the parietal pericardium. In the case of large effusions, cardiac oscillation is even more apparent than with M-mode.

When the distinction between pericardial and pleural fluid is not clear on 2-D echo, the location of the descending aorta on the parasternal long-axis view may be diagnostic; this structure is seen in cross-section as a circle at the level of the atrioventricular ring. The descending aorta remains apposed to the parietal pericardium regardless of effusion. If the descending aorta is seen to be removed from the heart itself, pericardial effusion is present. If the descending aorta continues to be apposed to the region of the posterior left atrium, the effusion is pleural.

The echo identification of pericardial thickening is less reliable than for effusion; the presence of multiple dense parallel echoes in the region of the posterior myocardium moving concordantly is suggestive of pericardial thickening.

ATRIAL SEPTAL DEFECT

Atrial septal defect (ASD) can be diagnosed echocardiographically either by direct imaging of the defect or, more commonly, by identifying its consequences. M-mode echo can reliably image only a portion of the interatrial septum via its view through the tricuspid valve. Two-dimensional technique, however, can scan the septum from a number of views: short axis at the aortic level; four-chamber at the apical level; and long axis at the subcostal level. The last of these views is the most reliable for imaging ASDs; however, some degree of atrial septal dropout in the region of the foramen ovale is normal, so one must be careful in diagnosing secundum defects without seeing a reproducible defect through multiple sweeps.

Indirect signs of ASD include right ventricular enlargement, paradoxical septal motion, and contrast study abnormalities. Right ventricular enlargement is quite constant in the presence of significant shunt; septal paradox may be absent.

Even in ASDs with predominant left-to-right shunting, a mild degree of right-to-left shunt may be present. Accordingly, saline injected forcefully through a peripheral vein may demonstrate a few signals crossing into the left atrium from the right heart. A negative contrast effect in the right atrium may be seen, but this is a subjective and equivocally reliable finding. Right-to-left shunting of a major degree, as found in Eisenmenger's syndrome, usually is easily demonstrated with contrast with either M-mode or 2-D echo technique.

References

1. Sahn DJ, DeMaria A, Kisslo J, Weyman A: The Committee on M-mode Standardization of the American Society of Echocardiography. *Circulation* 58:1072, 1978
2. Tajik AJ, Seward J, Hagler DJ, Mair D, Lie JT: Two-dimensional real-time ultrasonic imaging of the heart and great vessels. Technique, image orientation, structure identification, and validation. *Mayo Clin Proc* 53:271, 1978
3. Henry WL, DeMaria A, Gramiak R, King DL, Kisslo JA, Popp RL, Sahn DJ,

Schiller NB, Tajik A, Teichholz LE, Weyman AE: Report of the American Society of Echocardiography on Nomenclature and Standards in Two-Dimensional Echocardiography. *Circulation* 62:212, 1980
4. Skorton DJ, Child JS, Perloff JK: Accuracy of the echocardiographic diagnosis of aortic regurgitation. *Am J Med* 69:377, 1980
5. Markiewicz W, Stoner J, Londen E, Hunt SA, Popp RL: Mitral valve prolapse in one hundred presumably healthy young females. *Circulation* 53:464, 1976
6. Chandraratna P, Vlahovich G, Kong Y, Wilson D: Incidence of mitral valve prolapse in one hundred clinically stable newborn baby girls: An echocardiographic study. *Am Heart J* 98:312, 1979
7. Procacci PM, Sauran SV, Schreiter SL, Bryson AL: Prevalence of clinical mitral valve prolapse in 1169 young women. *N Engl J Med* 294:1086, 1976
8. Darsee JR, Mikolich RJ, Nicoloff NB, Lesser LE: Prevalence of mitral valve prolapse in presumably healthy young men. *Circulation* 59:619, 1979
9. Mintz GS, Kotler MN, Segal BL, Parry WR: Comparison of two-dimensional and M-mode echocardiography in the evaluation of patients with infective endocarditis. *Am J Cardiol* 43:738, 1979
10. Martin RP, Meltzer RS, Chia BL, Stinson EB, Rakowski H, Popp RL: Clinical utility of two dimensional echocardiography with infective endocarditis. *Am J Cardiol* 46:379, 1980
11. Davis RS, Strom JA, Frishman W, Becker R, Matsumoto M, Le Jemtel, Thierry L, Sonnenblick EH, Frater RWM: The demonstration of vegetations by echocardiography in bacterial endocarditis—an indication for early surgical intervention. *Am J Med* 69:57, 1980
12. Stewart JA, Silimperi D, Harris P, Wise NK, Fraker TD, Kisslo J: Echocardiographic documentation of vegetative lesions in infective endocarditis: Clinical implications. *Circulation* 61:374, 1980
13. Melvin ET, Berger M, Lutzker LG, Goldberg E, Mildvan D: Noninvasive methods for detection of valve vegetations in infective endocarditis. *Am J Cardiol* 47:271, 1981
14. Stafford A, Wann LS, Dillon JC, Weyman AE, Feigenbaum H: Serial echocardiographic appearance of healing bacterial vegetations. *Am J Cardiol* 44:754, 1979
15. Radford DJ, Bloom KR, Izukawa T, Moes CAF, Rowe RD: Echocardiographic assessment of bicuspid aortic valves. *Circulation* 53:80, 1976
16. Nanda NC, Gramiak R, Manning J, Mahoney EB, Lipchik EO, De Weese JA: Echocardiographic recognition of the congenital bicuspid aortic valve. *Circulation* 49:870, 1974
17. Starling MR, Crawford MH, O'Rourke RA, Graves BN, Amon KW: Accuracy of subxiphoid echocardiography for assessing left ventricular size and performance. *Circulation* 61:367, 1980
18. Teichholz LE, Kreulen T, Herman MV, Gorlin R: Problems in echocardiographic volume determinations: Echocardiographic-angiographic correlations in the presence of asynergy. *Am J Cardiol* 37:7, 1976

19. Knapp W: Relationship between mean VCF and heart rate — the diagnostic value of normalization of VCF to heart rate. *J Clin Ultrasound* 6:10-15, 1978
20. Crawford MH: Value and limitations of echocardiography for determining left ventricular size and performance. Council on Clinical Cardiology Newsletter, American Heart Association 6:1-6, 1981
21. Falsetti HL, Marcus ML, Kerber RE, Skorton DJ: Quantification of myocardial ischemia and infarction by left ventricular imaging (Editorial). *Circulation* 63:747, 1981
22. Lieberman AN, Weiss JL, Jugdutt BI, Becker LC, Bulkley BH, Garrison JG, Hutchins GM, Kallman CA, Weisfeldt ML: Two-dimensional echocardiography and infarct size: Relationship of regional wall motion and thickening to the extent of myocardial infarction in the dog. *Circulation* 63:739, 1981
23. Weiss JL, Bulkley BH, Hutchins GM, Mason SJ: Two-dimensional echocardiographic recognition of myocardial injury in man: Comparison with postmortem studies. *Circulation* 63:401, 1981
24. Gatewood RP, Nanda NC: Differentiation of left ventricular pseudoaneurysm from true aneurysm with two-dimensional echocardiography. *Am J Cardiol* 46:869, 1980
25. Catherwood E, Mintz GS, Kutler MN, Parry WR, Segal BL: Two dimensional echocardiographic recognition of left ventricular pseudoaneurysm. *Circulation* 62:294, 1980
26. Bommer WJ, Tickner EG, Rasor J, Grehl T, Mason DT, DeMaria AN: Development of a new echocardiographic contrast agent capable of pulmonary transmission and left heart opacification following peripheral venous injection (Abstract). *Circulation* 62(Suppl III):34, 1980
27. Farcot JC, Boisante L, Rigaud M, Bardet J, Bourdarias JP: Two-dimensional echocardiographic visualization of ventricular septal rupture after acute myocardial infarction. *Am J Cardiol* 45:370, 1980
28. Waggoner AD, Shah AA, Schuessler JS, Crawford ES, Miller RR, Quinones MA: Effect of cardiac surgery on echocardiographic septal motion: Assessment by intraoperative and post-operative echocardiography (Abstract). *Circulation* 62(Suppl III):20, 1980
29. Teichholz LE: Echocardiographic evaluation of pericardial diseases. *Prog Cardiovasc Dis* 21:133, 1978

Chapter 6

External Pulse Recordings, Systolic Time Intervals, Apexcardiography, and Phonocardiography

Kenneth M. Borow and Joshua Wynne

The advent of high-quality echocardiographic and radionuclide imaging techniques in the 1970s marked a major advance toward the goal of accurate and reproducible noninvasive assessment of cardiac disease. These newer techniques, however, commonly provide anatomic rather than physiologic information. In order to produce a comprehensive, integrated noninvasive assessment of cardiac pathophysiology, our practice for the past 10 years has been to complement these techniques with the physiologic information available from the phonocardiogram, carotid arterial, jugular venous, and apical pulse tracings, systolic time intervals, and clinical history. We recently reported the accuracy of this approach in 108 consecutive patients (60 percent of whom had predominant single-valve disease, 11 percent double-valve disease, 1 percent triple-valve disease, 9 percent coronary artery disease, 7 percent cardiomyopathy, and 12 percent congenital heart disease) prospectively evaluated prior to cardiac catheterization [1]. Diagnostic predictions employing combined clinical and noninvasive cardiac evaluation were completely correct in 86 percent of patients and management strategy formulations were correct in 97 percent of individuals. Subsequently, we reported on 35 patients who underwent valve surgery at our institution based solely on the findings of our integrated noninvasive evaluation without preoperative cardiac catheterization [2]. Patients with clinical evidence of coronary artery disease were excluded from the study. Eighty-three percent of the patients were New York Heart Association functional class III or IV preoperatively. In all cases, the noninvasive diagnosis was corroborated at the time of surgery; there were no unexpected findings. There were no deaths related to incomplete or incorrect diagnosis. Thus, a careful and comprehensive noninvasive assessment of patients with heart disease can give accurate information regarding cardiac anatomy *and* pathophysiology.

The first five sections of this chapter present an overview of the clinical utility and interpretation of standard pulse tracings and systolic time intervals. The final section of the chapter combines this information with echocardiographic data to present an integrated noninvasive method of assessing and evaluating specific cardiovascular disease states.

The Arterial Pulse

Normal Carotid Pulse Morphology

The morphology of the carotid pulse tracing (CPT) closely resembles that of the aortic pressure tracing recorded just above the aortic valve [3, 4] (Fig. 6-1). The externally recorded carotid pulse is delayed by the 10 to 50 msec required for the pulse wave to travel from the heart to the cervical area. The major factor determining this delay in adults is the velocity of the pulse wave [5]. The external carotid pulse tracing recorded from either the right or left carotid artery reflects fluctuations in pulse pressure and volume. In the normal subject, the ascending or anacrotic limb of the tracing is characterized by a rapid upstroke terminating in an initial peak or percussion wave. The percussion wave is followed by a less prominent, somewhat more rounded systolic or tidal wave. Freis et al have suggested that the percussion wave corresponds to peak aortic flow rate and the tidal wave corresponds to peak aortic pressure [6]. In patients with fixed left ventricular (LV) outflow tract obstruction, such as valvular aortic stenosis, the percussion wave is diminished in amplitude, resulting in an anacrotic notch or shoulder. Patients given isoproterenol or dobutamine infusions have prominent percussion waves due to increased early systolic flow velocity [6, 7]. The prominence of the tidal wave frequently increases with infusion of a peripheral vasoconstrictor such as methoxamine or phenylephrine, with systemic hypertension, and with the diminished aortic distensibility noted in elderly patients. The tidal wave becomes relatively low after administration of a peripheral vasodilator such as amyl nitrite or nitroprusside.

The descending limb of the CPT, which is normally less steep than the ascending limb, is interrupted by the incisura or dicrotic notch. The dicrotic notch of the aortic pressure tracing recorded from within the ascending aorta occurs essentially simultaneously with aortic valve closure. The notch of the CPT, however, follows the aortic closure sound (A_2) by an interval equal to the pulse transmission time. Aortic closure thus never follows the dicrotic notch of the CPT. However, the pulmonary closure sound (P_2) may occur prior to, synchronous with, or after the CPT dicrotic notch. Following the dicrotic notch, the pulse wave rises slightly and then falls until the next ventricular systole occurs. Occasionally, a small rise will precede the steep ascending limb of the carotid pulse, reflecting LV isovolumic contraction.

The morphology of the arterial pressure wave changes as the waveform is transmitted from the central aorta to the peripheral arteries [8]. The systolic upstroke

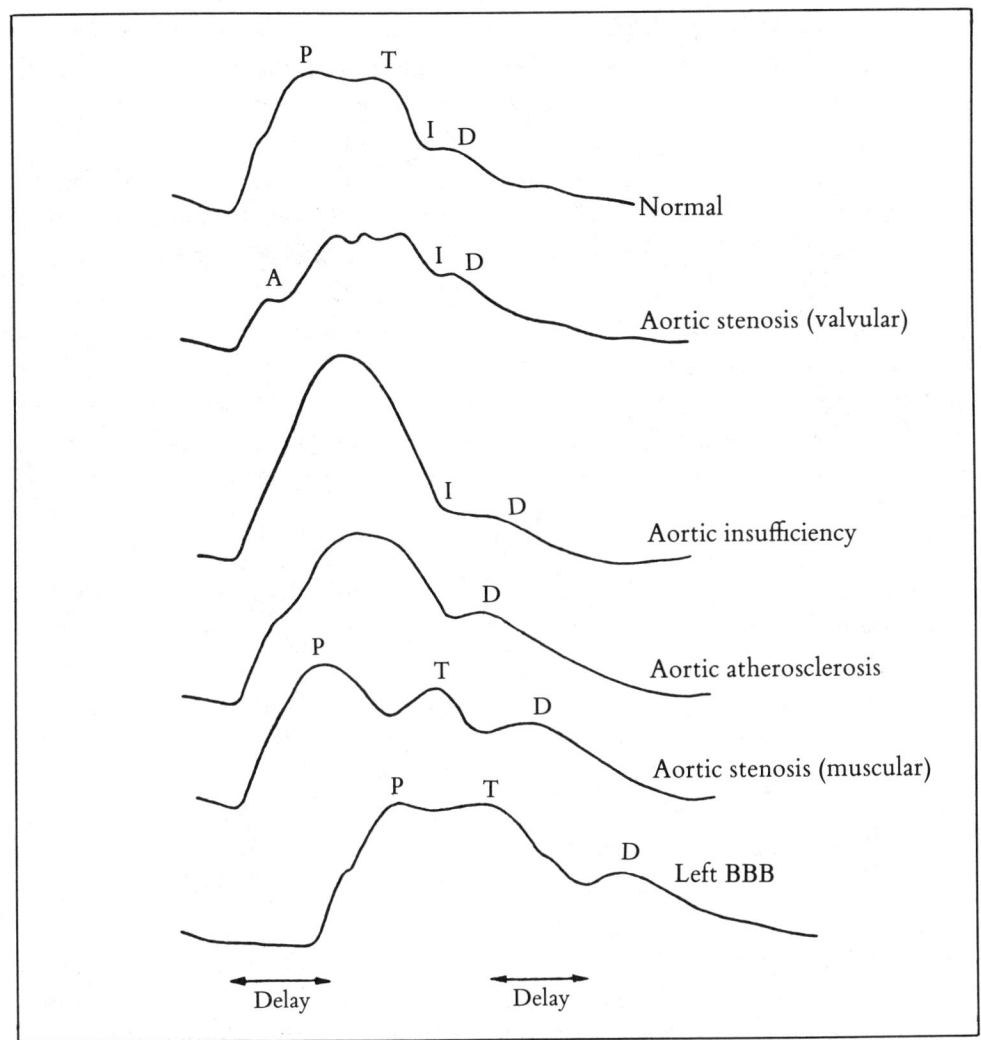

FIGURE 6-1. Carotid pulse tracing in health and disease. A = anacrotic shoulder, BBB = bundle branch block, D = dicrotic wave, I = incisura, P = percussion wave, T = tidal wave. (Adapted from AA Luisada: *Med Clin N Am* 64:24, 1980.)

time shortens, reflecting the steeper initial pulse upstroke; the anacrotic shoulder is blunted or disappears; and the systolic ejection time increases in duration [9]. The dicrotic wave after the dicrotic notch becomes more prominent. Distortion and damping of the pulse wave, amplification of parts of the pulse wave by reflected or standing wave effect, differential transmission rates of various components of the pulse wave, and differences in elastic behavior of the periphery compared with central arteries all contribute to modification of the morphology of the pulse wave.

Abnormal Carotid Pulse Morphology: Pathophysiologic Correlation

In the absence of local arterial disease, arterial pulse abnormalities can be generally categorized as those resulting in either hyperkinetic (bounding) or hypokinetic (weak) pulses [8, 10]. A *hyperkinetic* pulse can result from a high cardiac output state (such as found with anxiety, fever, exercise, pregnancy, hyperthyroidism, anemia, and the idiopathic hyperkinetic heart syndrome), or high LV preload with normal forward cardiac output (i.e., complete heart block with bradycardia, ventricular septal defect, mitral regurgitation). Other causes of hyperkinetic pulses include abnormal runoff of blood from the systemic arterial tree resulting in widened pulse pressure (i.e., aortic regurgitation, persistent ductus arteriosus, aorticopulmonary window, peripheral arteriovenous shunt, Paget's disease of the bone, cirrhosis of the liver) and decreased arterial distensibility. This latter finding is most frequently found in the elderly population, where systolic hypertension is associated with normal or low aortic diastolic pressure resulting in widening of the arterial pulse pressure. The *hypokinetic* pulse can be found in patients with fixed LV outflow tract (LVOT) obstruction (i.e., valvular aortic stenosis, discrete subaortic stenosis), low forward stroke volume states (i.e., myocardial infarction with LV dysfunction, cardiomyopathy, severe mitral, pulmonary, or tricuspid valve disease), conditions resulting in a narrow arterial pulse pressure (cardiac tamponade, constrictive pericarditis), and conditions marked by high systemic vascular resistance.

Several indexes derived from the CPT have been developed in an attempt to quantify the magnitude of fixed LV outflow tract obstruction. The *upstroke time* (U-time) is the interval from initial rapid ascent of the carotid pulse to the peak of the pulse. This index is usually of limited value since either the peak of the percussion or tidal wave may be more prominent depending upon aortic pressure and LV flow velocity. A significant variation in U-time with only slight variation in pulse contour is not uncommon. There is considerable overlap of U-time values between patients with and without valvular aortic stenosis (AS) [9, 11]. The *T-time* ($T_{1/2}$ time) is the interval required for the externally recorded pulse to reach one-half of its maximal amplitude. The $T_{1/2}$ time is relatively insensitive to minor changes in pulse height and usually is less than 50 msec. The *maximal rate of carotid rise* is an index of the rate of pressure development in the carotid artery. It is obtained by fitting a line to the steepest portion of the carotid upstroke. This line is then extrapolated to the peak of the CPT. The time required to reach maximal pulse pressure along this line is measured and divided into the pulse pressure determined using sphygmomanometric measurement of the brachial artery blood pressure. Several authors have found this measurement to be useful in assessing the severity of aortic stenosis [12, 13].

Certain carotid pulse contours are characteristic of specific disease states.

Pulsus Parvus et Tardus
"Small, slow pulse" is found in moderate to severe fixed left ventricular outflow tract obstruction (valvular or subvalvular) and is characterized by a small hypokinetic pulse with a delayed systolic peak [8, 14]. An anacrotic shoulder occurring in the early to mid portion of the ascending limb of the CPT reflects decreased aortic flow velocity secondary to obstruction to LV emptying and intracardiac blood turbulence [15]. A carotid "shudder" (i.e., vibrations on the ascending limb of the CPT) reflects the turbulent blood flow across the stenotic LVOT but may also be seen in aortic regurgitation (AR), where it is probably due to increased initial flow velocity [16]. In mild to moderate aortic stenosis, the anacrotic shoulder may be relatively high and may even disappear as one palpates the more peripheral pulses. In supravalvular aortic stenosis, there is frequently an hourglass narrowing of the aorta just above the aortic valve that preferentially directs a high-velocity stream of blood to the right innominate artery. This results in a higher blood pressure, stronger pulse, and more rapid upstroke in the right carotid as compared with the left carotid and brachial arteries (termed the Coanda effect) [17]. In coarctation of the aorta, the pulses proximal to the coarctation (including both carotid and right brachial arteries) are full and bounding. This in part reflects the systolic hypertension and wide pulse pressure present in these vessels. In contrast, the pulse pressure in vessels distal to the coarctation is diminished owing to the decreased rate of arterial filling through the coarctation site and collateral channels. The lower extremity pulses characteristically have a slow rate of rise with a late systolic peak. This latter finding is due to loss of the initial percussion wave resulting in palpation of only the tidal wave. The percussion wave is retained in arterial pulses proximal to the coarctation site. This in part explains the physical sign of brachial-femoral delay noted on simultaneous palpation or pulse recordings of these vessels.

Pulsus Bisferiens
Characterized by a double systolic impulse separated by a mid-systolic trough, a bisferiens pulse is typically seen in combined aortic stenosis/regurgitation with regurgitation the predominant lesion, in hypertrophic obstructive cardiomyopathy (HOCM), and occasionally in isolated AR [8]. In chronic AR, the prominent percussion wave reflects large initial LV flow into the aorta followed by rapid runoff into the peripheral vessels with a normally timed tidal wave. In HOCM, the percussion wave has a large amplitude with a rapid upstroke rate [18]. As the LV volume decreases with ventricular ejection, the subaortic geometry is altered sufficiently to allow dynamic LVOT obstruction to occur as the anterior leaflet of the mitral valve moves toward the septum and narrows the LVOT. This results in a sudden decrease in the carotid pulse amplitude reflecting

a sudden fall in LV ejection rate. Following this dip, LV ejection continues, although at a slower rate. The secondary systolic wave summates with the reflected wave from the periphery resulting in a rounded tidal wave. The net result is the "spike and dome" pulse wave configuration that is characteristic of HOCM.

Dicrotic Pulse

Like the bisferiens pulse, the dicrotic pulse is characterized by two positive impulses; however, its second pulse wave occurs after aortic valve closure, is associated with a low dicrotic notch, and reflects an accentuation of the dicrotic wave during early diastole [19]. It is most frequently found in low cardiac output states associated with high systemic vascular resistance such as primary or hypertensive cardiomyopathy, myocardial infarction, and after open heart surgery. Normalization of the pulse contour may occur on the beat following a premature ventricular contraction or with administration of a peripheral vasodilator.

Pulsus Alternans

This abnormality, characterized by a beat-to-beat alteration of the carotid pulse amplitude that is independent of respiratory variation, occurs despite a regular cardiac rhythm. Thought to be due to variations in LV contractile state and stroke volume, pulsus alternans may be seen in patients with severe LV dysfunction, following an episode of supraventricular tachycardia, or after a premature atrial or ventricular depolarization [20]. It is frequently associated with a third heart sound and may be more prominent in peripheral rather than central pulses owing to accentuation by reflected waveforms.

Bigeminal Pulse

Unlike pulsus alternans, which occurs with a regular cardiac rhythm, the bigeminal pulse occurs in patients with premature beats in which the ectopic beat occurs relatively close to the preceding beat. This results in a small preload and stroke volume for the premature beat followed by a compensatory increase in preload with augmented stroke volume and pulse amplitude in the beat following the premature depolarization.

Pulsus Paradoxus

An inspiratory fall in arterial pulse amplitude and a greater than 10 mm Hg decline in systolic blood pressure in a patient with a regular cardiac rhythm are characteristic of pulsus paradoxus. It is most frequently found in patients with cardiac tamponade or conditions associated with wide fluctuations in intrathoracic pressure, such as chronic obstructive pulmonary disease or asthma. In patients with cardiac tamponade, the major factor resulting in pulsus paradoxus appears to be preservation of right ventricular (RV) preload augmentation during inspiration with subsequent rise in intrapericardial pressure within the taut pericardial sac. This results in compromised LV filling, a fall in LV stroke volume, and a large decline in LV systolic pressure during inspiration [21].

The Jugular Venous Pulse

Although the jugular venous pulse (JVP) tracing records only volume displacement in the internal jugular vein, it generally gives a reliable noninvasive approximation of the right atrial (RA) pressure curve contour (Fig. 6-2). The JVP contour is altered on occasion by contamination with carotid pulse waves. Jugular venous pulsations can usually be distinguished from the carotid pulse since the JVP may be ablated by digital compression. Estimation of central venous pressure from visual inspection of the jugular veins can give worthwhile information about right heart hemodynamics.

NORMAL JUGULAR VENOUS PULSE MORPHOLOGY

The normal JVP recording consists of two major peaks (*a* and *v*) and two major descents (*x* and *y*) [10, 22]. Although the JVP recording cannot be calibrated to measure RA pressure directly, the relative timing and amplitude of its major components may provide useful diagnostic information. The *a* wave of the JVP tracing is a positive deflection beginning after the P wave of the electrocardiogram and after the *a* wave of the right atrial pressure tracing. It is due to volume displacement into the jugular veins following right atrial systole. The pulse transmission time between RA and detection over the jugular vein is dependent on the volume and compliance of the systemic venous system. The relative amplitude of the *a* wave reflects the vigor of RA contraction, the effective tricuspid valve orifice size, and RV compliance. The peak of the *a* wave occurs synchronous with or slightly later than a right ventricular fourth heart sound. The atrial relaxation phase following atrial systole is characterized by the *x* descent, which is frequently interrupted by the *c* wave. The *c* wave is caused by the upward bulging of the tricuspid valve toward the RA during RV isovolumic contraction, possibly with a small contribution from transmitted carotid arterial pulsations [23]. Following the *c* wave, the *x* descent resumes. This latter portion of the *x* descent is thought to be due to the downward displacement of the tricuspid valve ring and lower portion of the RA during ventricular systole. The *x* descent ends when the rate of RA filling from the inferior and superior vena cavae becomes greater than the downward displacement rate of the RA. This results in the positive *v* wave, which begins 0.06 to 0.08 second before and terminates 0.10 to 0.12 second after pulmonary valve closure (P_2) [24]. The normal *v* wave reflects passive rather than active accumulation of blood in the RA, which occurs while the tricuspid valve is

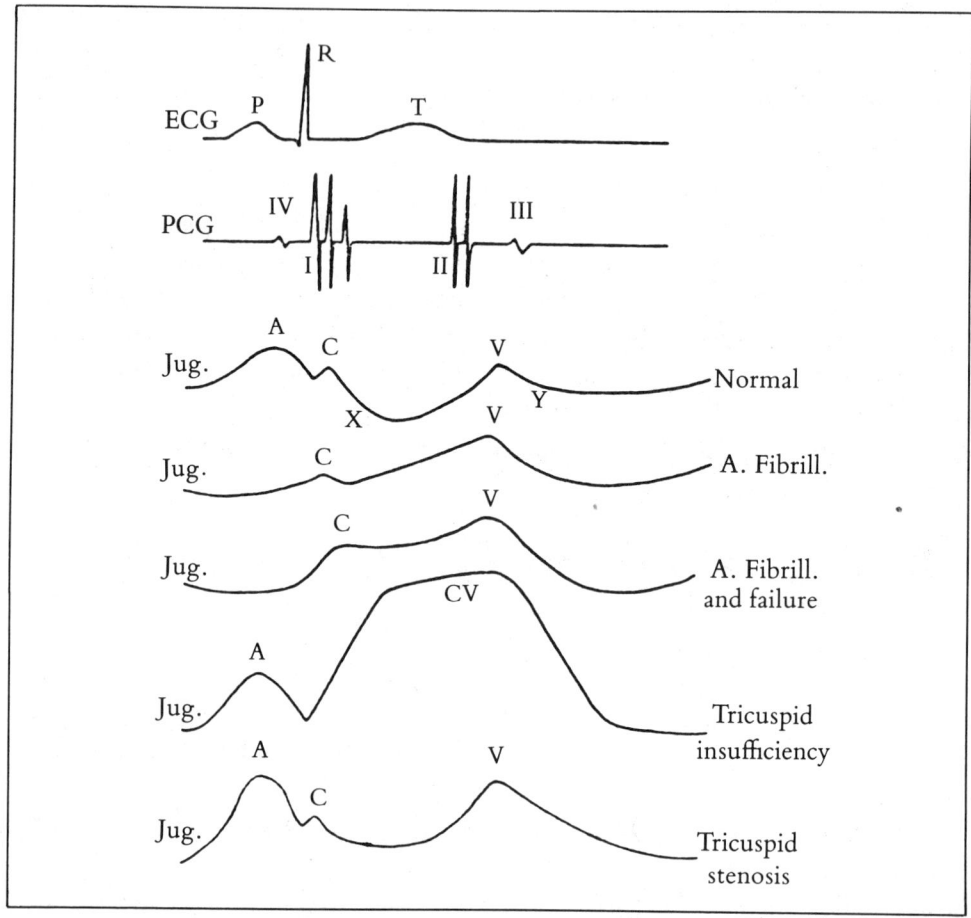

FIGURE 6-2. Jugular venous tracing (*Jug*) in health and disease. *A. Fibrill* = atrial fibrillation, *I, II, III, IV* = heart sounds, *PCG* = phonocardiogram. (Adapted from AA Luisada: *Med Clin N Am* 64:25, 1980.)

closed. Its amplitude reflects the volume of caval blood returning to the RA, as well as the size and distensibility of the RA. The *y* descent occurs when the tricuspid valve opens in early diastole and terminates with rapid emptying of the RA. Hemodynamically, the *y* descent reflects the abrupt decompression of the RA during the RV rapid filling period and is altered by events retarding RA emptying. A final small positive deflection, the *h* wave, may be evident during late diastole in the patient with bradycardia. This wave reflects RV slow filling and ends when filling is completed.

The normal RA pressure or JVP recording is characterized by an *a* wave that is more prominent than its *v* wave, in contrast to the left atrium, where the *v* wave predominates. Normally, the *x* descent is lower than the *y* descent. At rapid heart rates, summation of various components of the JVP tracing can occur, decreasing somewhat the clinical utility of this tracing. Recording of the hepatic venous pulse tracing is difficult in normal subjects; however, when hepatic congestion occurs, as seen in tricuspid regurgitation or right ventricular failure, valuable information can be acquired.

ABNORMAL JVP MORPHOLOGY: PATHOPHYSIOLOGIC CORRELATION

The clinical utility of the JVP tracing depends on identifying abnormalities in timing, contour, and amplitude of various component parts.

Abnormalities of the a Wave

A prominent *a* wave reflects impediment to RA emptying in the patient in normal sinus rhythm. This may be due to obstruction at the valvular level (tricuspid stenosis, RA myxoma), alteration in RV compliance (RV infarction, chronic obstructive pulmonary disease), and pulmonary artery hypertension secondary to mitral valve disease or acute RV pressure overload (massive pulmonary embolism)[25, 26]. Interestingly, the patient with tetralogy of Fallot does not usually have a prominent *a* wave, since the RV diastolic pressure is decompressed through the ventricular septal defect. Patients in atrial fibrillation do not have *a* waves on their JVP recording [27]. In patients with atrioventricular dissociation such as in ventricular tachycardia, junctional rhythm, complete heart block, or occasionally premature ventricular contractions, prominent *a* waves ("cannon waves") may be present when the RA contracts against a completely closed tricuspid valve. In atrial flutter, or paroxysmal atrial tachycardia with block, small *a* waves occur at a regular rate, reflecting the underlying atrial tachycardia. These waves become more prominent when atrial systole occurs during ventricular systole.

Abnormalities of the x Descent

The *x* descent frequently becomes diminutive in the presence of atrial fibrillation. It is shallow or even obliterated in moderate to severe tricuspid regurgitation and restrictive cardiomyopathy. In contrast, it is typically prominent in cardiac tamponade and occasionally exaggerated in constrictive pericarditis, especially in the presence of effusoconstrictive disease [28].

Abnormalities of the v Wave

The *v* wave is more prominent than the *a* wave in patients with atrial septal defects, probably reflecting left rather than right atrial events [29]. In tricuspid regurgitation, a systolic wave may interrupt the *x* descent and is characterized by increasing amplitude and earlier onset as the hemodynamic significance of the lesion increases [30]. Eventually the *c* and *v* waves seem to merge into a single positive deflection, the so-called *c-v*, systolic, or regurgitant wave, which reflects both passive RA filling from the cavae and active RA filling due to tricuspid regurgitation. This is in contrast to the normal *v* wave, which is produced solely by passive RA filling. In patients with atrial fibrillation, the *c-v* wave may be the only deflection visible on the JVP tracing. Since the *c-v* wave in tricuspid regurgitation is still a reflection of relatively low pressure venous events, it can be obliterated by digital compression over the base of the neck. The morphology of the hepatic pulse tracing in tricuspid regurgitation closely resembles that of the jugular venous recording (Fig. 6-3).

Abnormalities of the y Descent

In constrictive pericarditis the *y* descent is quite rapid and brief, interrupts a relatively high venous plateau, and ends in early RV diastasis [31]. This reflects the small RV end-diastolic volume and restriction to RV filling, resulting in the so-called square root sign. A deep and sharp *y* descent may also be evident in RV failure. In this case, it probably reflects an elevated RA pressure, reduced RV compliance, and diminished systemic venous blood return. In cardiac tamponade, a prominent *y* descent is generally not present.

In the normal individual, jugular venous pressure falls and neck veins collapse during inspiration owing to the negative intrathoracic pressure drawing blood from peripheral veins into the central venous system. This inspiratory decline in venous pressure is diminished or obliterated when the RV is unable to accommodate the increased systemic venous return. Thus, in cases of RV failure (i.e., RV infarction, massive pulmonary embolism, severe cor pulmonale) or constrictive pericarditis, an inspiratory rise (Kussmaul's sign) of jugular venous pressure is frequently noted. Although this physical finding may not be evident in patients with congestive heart failure vigorously treated with diuretics, it is usually preserved in patients with constrictive pericarditis. In contrast, a normal or only slightly diminished inspiratory fall of jugular venous pressure may be evident in cardiac tamponade.

The Apexcardiogram

The apexcardiogram (ACG) gives a graphic representation of the low-frequency vibrations generated by pressure and volume fluxes within the left ventricle [32, 33] (Fig. 6-4).

Normal Apexcardiographic Morphology

During ventricular systole, the LV myocardial fibers contract in a spiral fashion about the long axis of the ventricle. This results in a brief period of contact between the anterior wall of the LV and the inner surface of the chest wall. The impulse transmitted to the left precordial surface is a gentle outward motion occurring during early systole followed by a palpable retraction in mid to late systole.

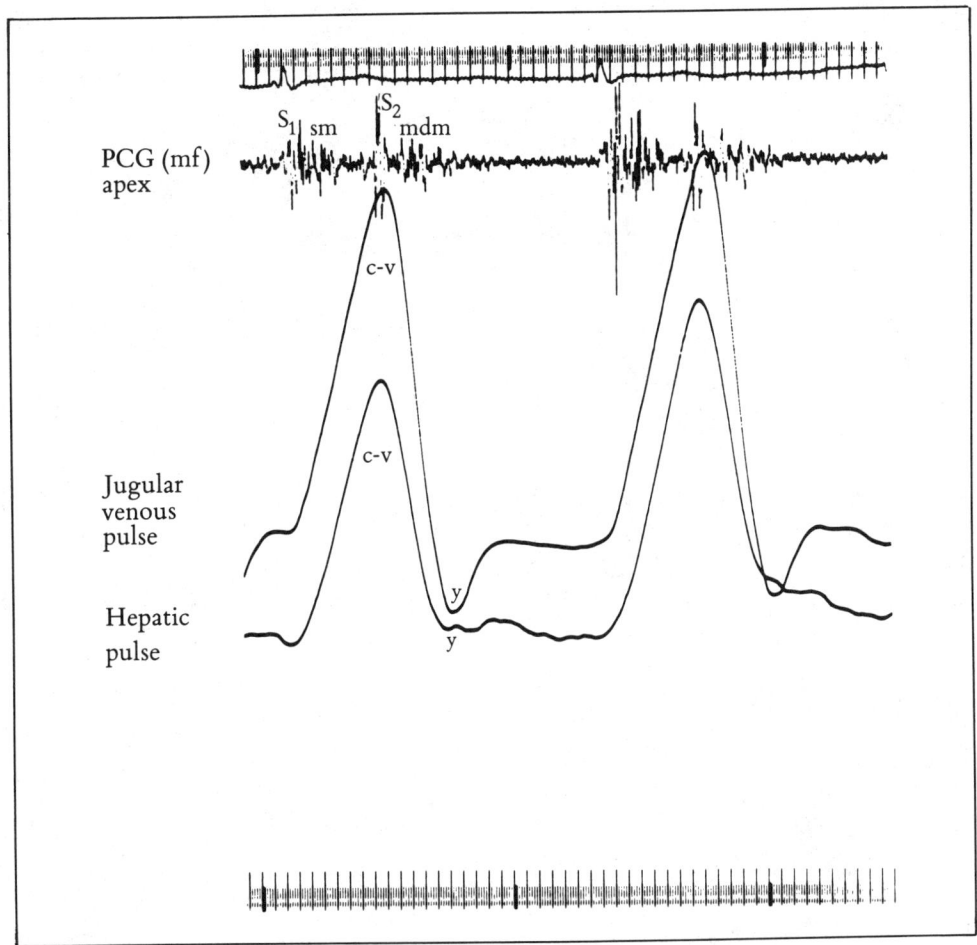

FIGURE 6-3. Jugular venous and hepatic pulse tracings in a patient with Ebstein's anomaly and tricuspid regurgitation. The JVP recording demonstrates a giant *c-v* systolic wave followed by rapid diastolic runoff producing an abrupt *y* descent. The hepatic pulse recording is similar to the jugular pulse and synchronous with it. *mdm* = mid-diastolic murmur, *mf* = mid frequency, *PCG* = phonocardiogram, *sm* = systolic murmur.

The rapid upstroke of the ACG begins with LV isovolumic systole (C point). The period from the onset of the QRS complex on the electrocardiogram to the C point approximates the electromechanical association interval. During isovolumic systole, the LV changes shape but maintains a constant volume despite rising LV pressure [32]. The upstroke of the ACG terminates at the E point, which seems to coincide approximately with the onset of LV ejection [34, 35]. During the second half of LV systole, the curve usually undergoes a gentle decline. At approximately the time of aortic valve closure, the curve begins a sharp decline correlating with the onset of the ventricular isovolumic relaxation period [36].

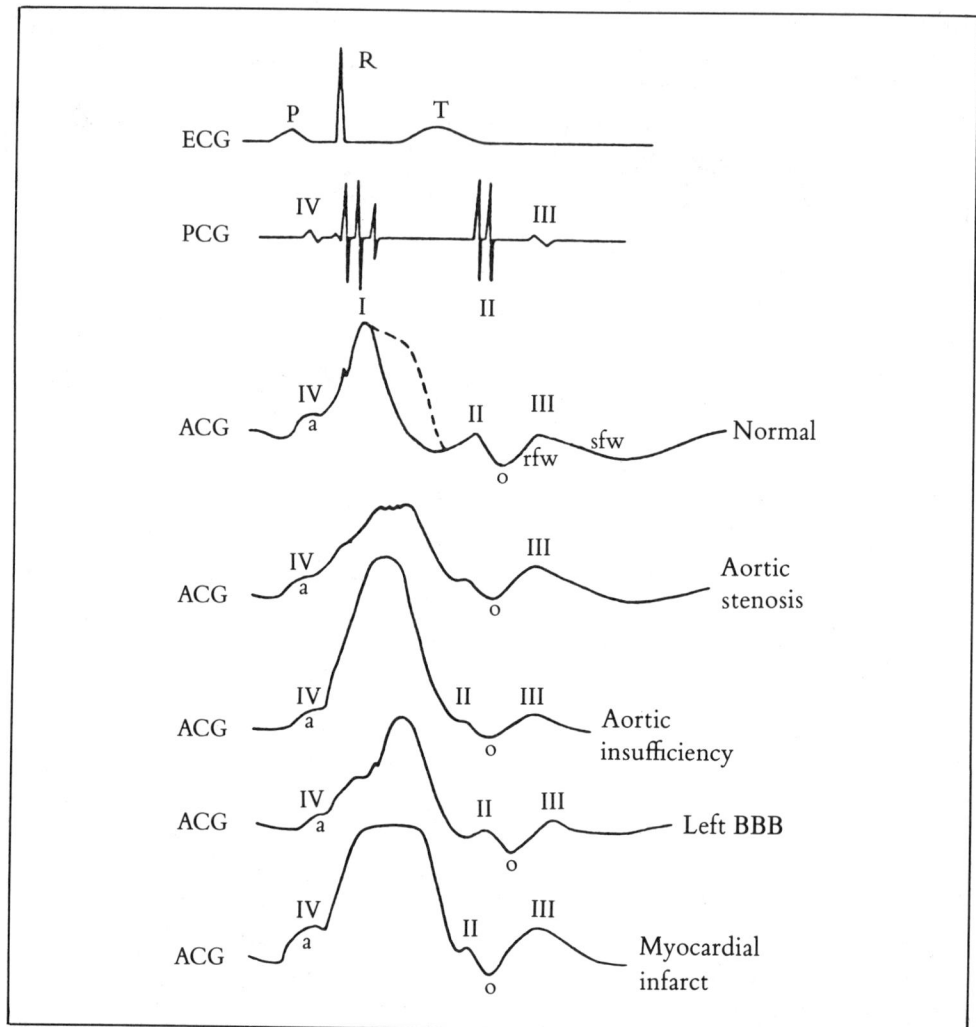

FIGURE 6-4. The apexcardiogram (ACG) in health and disease. BBB = bundle branch block, PCG = phonocardiogram, rfw = rapid filling wave, sfw = slow filling wave. (Adapted from A A Luisada: *Med Clin N Am* 64:23, 1980.)

This downward deflection terminates near the end of mitral valve opening (end of isovolumic relaxation period), an event that is variably approximated by the O point on the ACG tracing. The curve next undergoes a relatively steep rise, the rapid filling wave (RFW), which terminates in the F point. A much slower phase of ventricular filling, the slow filling period (SFP), follows the F point. The *a* wave is the final diastolic wave and corresponds to the distension of the LV caused by left atrial contraction. The *a* wave is absent in patients with atrial fibrillation and prominent in patients with diminished left ventricular compliance. In several studies, the contour and timing of these diastolic events correlated closely with LV pressure recordings [34, 37].

Abnormal ACG Morphology: Pathophysiologic Correlation

Systolic Events

Several patterns of systolic movement on ACG have been shown to correlate with physiologic alteration of LV size, wall thickness and/or function [32, 38, 39]. These systolic motion patterns can be categorized as (1) hyperdynamic, (2) sustained, and (3) bifid.

HYPERDYNAMIC MOTION. The hyperdynamic apical impulse is characterized on precordial palpation by an exaggerated apical movement of brief duration that ends within the first half of ventricular systole. Despite an increased systolic amplitude on ACG, the morphology of the tracing is normal. This pattern is found in patients with large LV stroke volumes and compensated ventricular function (aortic regurgitation, mitral regurgitation, ventricular septal defect, persistent ductus arteriosus), hyperkinetic circulatory states (thyrotoxicosis, marked anxiety), thin chest walls, or pectus excavatum.

SUSTAINED MOTION. On precordial palpation, an apical impulse is sustained, heaving, or thrusting if it can be felt past mid-systole. The ACG tracing shows a prolonged systolic plateau that is horizontal or rising during ventricular ejection in contrast to the gentle systolic decline noted with the normal and hyperdynamic tracings. This pattern is seen in patients with LV pressure overload (aortic stenosis, chronic systemic hypertension), chronic LV volume overload with ventricular dysfunction, primary myocardial disease, and coronary artery disease (CAD). In a study of 41 patients with CAD and altered LV contraction patterns on ventriculography, the following correlations were noted [40]:

1. Early sustained systolic bulge on ACG correlated with a large ventricular aneurysm with large end-diastolic volume
2. Mid to late systolic bulge on ACG correlated with ventricular asynergy
3. Prominent rapid filling wave during diastolic filling correlated with large zones of ventricular asynergy

BIFID MOTION. On precordial palpation, there is a double systolic impulse. This pattern is most frequently seen on ACG in HOCM [35, 41]. It may also be noted in patients with mitral valve prolapse (where the trough may coincide with the systolic click) and in some patients with left atrial myxoma [42].

Early to Mid-Diastolic Events

Numerous studies have shown that the O point of the ACG coincides with the nadir of the LV pressure tracing and only indirectly with mitral valve opening. In addition, the O point appears to correlate well with the time of peak rate of LV outward movement on a simultaneously recorded M-mode echocardiogram of the LV [43]. The ACG can be helpful in distinguishing an opening sound (O.S.) of the mitral valve from a third heart sound (S_3) since the O.S. always precedes the peak of the rapid filling wave, while the S_3 occurs synchronously with the peak of the RFW [33, 44].

Abnormalities of the RFW can provide diagnostic information. A prominent RFW with a sharp peak and steep slope is frequently seen in patients with augmented early diastolic filling due to an LV volume overload (i.e., mitral regurgitation, ventricular septal defect, persistent ductus arteriosus) [32]. Diminished LV compliance, as seen in valvular aortic stenosis, may cause reduction or absence of the RFW by interfering with the left ventricle's ability to expand in early diastole. In mitral stenosis (MS), the RFW is frequently blunted and shortened in duration (<0.08 second) [45]. The presence of normal RFW morphology and duration suggests that a patient with isolated mitral valve disease does not have high-grade or dominant mitral stenosis. The duration of the slow filling period in mitral stenosis is increased, reflecting the time required for decompression of the left atrium and completion of LV filling. In severe MS, a period of diastasis is not attained even when bradycardia is present. In contrast, the patient with mild to moderate mitral stenosis will generally attain diastasis on the ACG recording, provided the heart rate is less than 80 beats/min [45].

Late Diastolic Events

The left atrium responds to LV hypertrophy or dilatation by increasing its volume and the vigor of its contraction. This is frequently reflected in the relative size of the *a* wave during late diastole. A standard method of assessing *a* wave amplitude is the *a*/OE ratio, where the height of the *a* wave is divided by the vertical excursion of the ACG tracing from the O point to the following E point. Usually less than 0.11 to 0.15, the *a*/OE ratio frequently is increased when alterations in LV end-diastolic pressure, volume, or compliance occur [46]. This alteration in the *a*/OE ratio is usually associated with a fourth heart sound on auscultation or phonocardiography. Voight and Freisinger [47], using simultaneous LV pressure measurements and ACG to study these relationships, found that patients with an *a*/OE ratio of greater than 0.15 consistently had elevations in LV end-diastolic pressure (LVEDP). Patients with increased LVEDP and *a*/OE ratio less than 0.15 uniformly had elevated early LV diastolic pressure, which often rose further before atrial systole. The small *a* wave size in these cases was suggestive of impaired left atrial function with diminished delivery of blood to the LV with atrial contraction. Thus, a normal *a* wave on ACG does not necessarily rule out an elevation in LVEDP.

In patients over 40 years of age with physical findings suggestive of valvular aortic stenosis, an a/OE ratio greater than 0.15 is frequently associated with aortic valve areas less than 0.75 cm² and/or peak LV-to-aorta systolic pressure gradients over 75 mm Hg [48]. The absence of an enlarged a wave, however, does not exclude severe LV outflow tract obstruction [49]. Prominent a waves may also be found in patients with chronic systemic hypertension or longstanding aortic regurgitation. In the latter patients, the degree of regurgitation is usually severe and is associated with elevation of the LVEDP.

Patients with coronary artery disease will frequently demonstrate increased a/OE ratios during myocardial ischemia or after an LV infarction. In these cases, the large a wave correlates with diminished LV compliance to the ischemic or fibrotic myocardium [50]. Benchimol and Dimond, in a study using ACG in arteriosclerotic heart disease, found that 55 percent of their patients had abnormally large a waves at rest [51]. With exercise, an additional 40 percent developed large a waves. Thus, over 90 percent of patients with ischemic heart disease had resting or exercise-induced abnormalities in the a wave of the ACG.

Absent or diminished a waves are seen in conditions that limit blood flow from the left atrium to left ventricle such as mitral stenosis and constrictive pericarditis [52]. The presence of an a wave in a patient with rheumatic heart disease with multivalvular involvement essentially excludes mitral stenosis as a predominant lesion. In acute severe AR, the LV pressure may exceed left atrial pressure prior to ventricular systole, resulting in early closure of the mitral valve. In this case, the ACG shows prominent continued filling throughout diastole with a high C point. Since the mitral valve is already closed when atrial systole occurs, the a wave on the ACG is absent.

Systolic Time Intervals

Systolic time intervals (STI), when used in conjunction with pulse tracings and echocardiography, can provide a measure of LV performance and compensation in patients with suspected or known heart disease. Because STI utilize totally noninvasive techniques, they can provide serial assessment of the natural history of cardiac disorders prior to, during, or after therapy.

In adults, the most common method of determining STI utilizes simultaneous recordings of the electrocardiogram (ECG), carotid pulse tracing (CPT), and phonocardiogram (PCG) (Fig. 6-5) [53, 54]. The following specific landmarks are required for accurate and reproducible measurement of STI:

1. The surface ECG lead utilized must have a distinct initial deflection that accurately reflects the onset of electrical depolarization of the ventricles. Traditionally, an inferior or lateral limb lead with a well-demarcated Q wave has

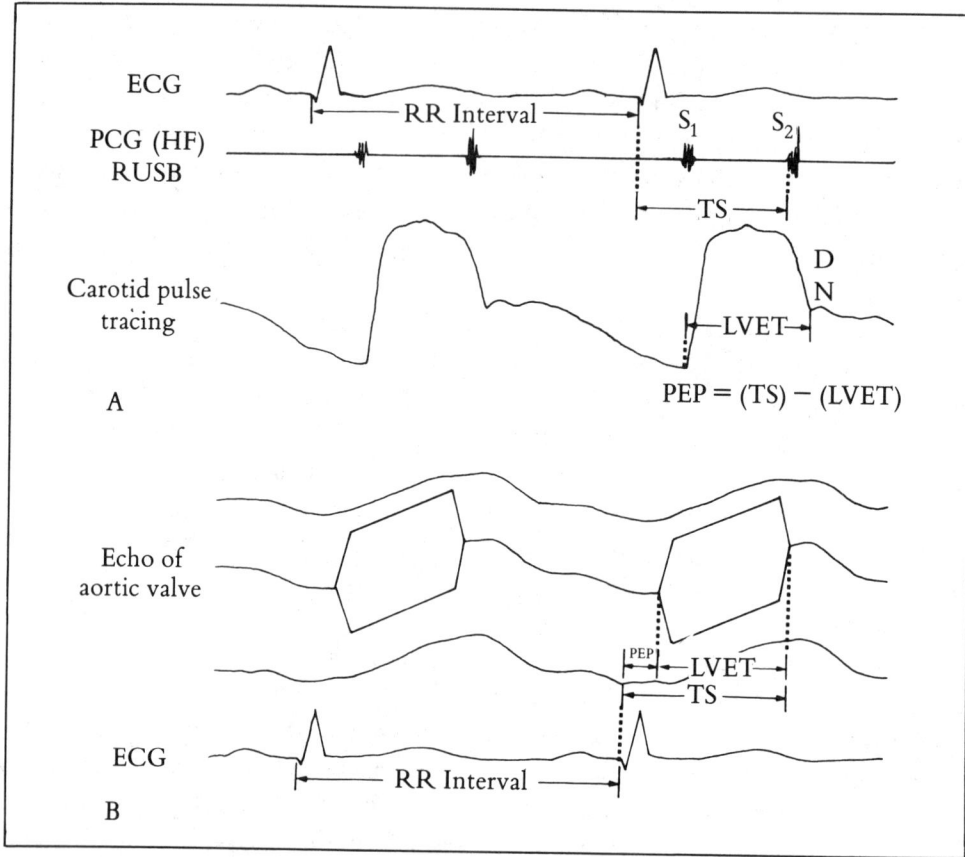

FIGURE 6-5. Left ventricular systolic time intervals. Schematic drawings indicating major intervals derived from (A) simultaneous phonocardiogram (PCG), indirect carotid pulse tracing and electrocardiogram (ECG), (B) echocardiogram of the aortic valve and electrocardiogram. DN = dicrotic notch, HF = high frequency, LVET = left ventricular ejection time, PEP = left ventricular preejection period, RR = beat cycle length, RUSB = right upper sternal border, TS = total systole.

been used to define the onset of electrical systole. Recently, the onset of the QRS complex in a right precordial lead (V1 or V2) has been shown to precede the onset of the limb lead QRS complex (specifically lead II) in over one-third of 319 subjects studied [55]. This suggests that leads V1 or V2 rather than limb leads should be used in the measurement of STI.

2. A well-defined first high-frequency vibration of the aortic component of the second heart sound (A_2) on PCG.
3. A clearly demarcated rapid upstroke of the CPT with care taken to exclude the gentle upstroke often seen during isovolumic systole
4. A discrete dicrotic notch on the CPT.

The three intervals most commonly used in clinical practice are the total electromechanical systole ($Q-A_2$), the LV ejection time (LVET), and the preejection period (PEP). The $Q-A_2$ is measured from the onset of ventricular depolarization (earliest portion of QRS complex) to the first high-frequency component of A_2. The LVET is determined as the interval from the beginning of the CPT upstroke to the dicrotic notch. The PEP is obtained by subtracting the LVET from $Q-A_2$ and equals the electromechanical association time plus the isovolumic contraction time. This value is a derived rather than measured value, since the pulse transmission time (15–40 msec) from the central aorta to the carotid artery must be excluded. Several studies in humans have demonstrated very close agreement of STI values determined with high-fidelity catheter-tip micromanometers placed in the LV or proximal aorta and values calculated externally from the carotid pulse [56, 57].

An alternative method of measuring STI utilizes simultaneous recording of the ECG, PCG, and M-mode echocardiogram of the aortic valve [58]. By this method, $Q-A_2$ is calculated from the onset of ventricular depolarization to either A_2 on PCG or, since they occur essentially simultaneously, aortic valve closure on echocardiography. The PEP is measured directly as the time from the onset of the QRS to aortic valve opening. The LVET is the interval from opening of the aortic valve to either aortic valve closure on the echocardiogram or onset of A_2 on the PCG. This method has the advantage that all values are measured directly from the graphic recordings. Unfortunately, aortic valve opening and closure points are not always well defined, especially in patients with some degree of aortic valve disease. In addition, the CPT should still be recorded to assess pulse contour and measure T-time or maximal carotid pulse upstroke time. In studies comparing STI values derived from the traditional CPT and echocardiographic methods, the correlation has been excellent, especially in younger patients [58]. Right ventricular STI can be calculated using the echocardiographic technique with total electromechanical systole measured as the interval from the onset of the QRS to closure of the pulmonary valve on the M-mode echocardiogram or onset of pulmonary valve closure sound (P_2) on a PCG recorded from the left upper sternal border area [58, 59]. The RV preejection period is the time between onset of the QRS to pulmonary valve opening on the echocardiogram. The RVET is the interval from pulmonary valve opening to closure on the echocardiogram or pulmonary valve opening on the echocardiogram to onset of P_2 on the phonocardiogram.

Factors Affecting the LV Preejection Period

In most instances, the major physiologic parameters influencing the PEP affect the isovolumic contraction time rather than the electromechanical association time (Tables 6-1 and 6-2). These factors include the LV contractile state as reflected

TABLE 6-1. Factors Influencing Systolic Time Intervals

	Increase	Decrease
PEP	Decreased LV contractile state Intrinsic LV dysfunction Negative inotropic drugs Hypothyroidism Decreased LV preload Systemic hypertension with high aortic diastolic pressure Left bundle branch block Bradycardia	Increased LV contractile state Anxiety, exercise Positive inotropic drugs Hyperthyroidism Increased LV preload Afterload reduction therapy with low aortic diastolic pressure Aortic valve disease with normal LV function Tachycardia
LVET	Increased LV stroke volume Aortic valve disease with normal LV function Increased LV afterload (systolic wall stress)	Decreased LV stroke volume LV dysfunction Positive inotropic drugs Negative inotropic drugs
PEP/LVET	LV dysfunction Decreased LV stroke volume Decreased LV preload Mitral regurgitation Negative inotropic drugs Left bundle branch block	Aortic valve disease Increased LV stroke volume Positive inotropic drugs

PEP = preejection period, LV = left ventricular, LVET = left ventricular ejection time.

by the rate of LV isovolumic pressure development (dp/dt), the LV end-diastolic pressure (LVEDP) and volume, and the aortic diastolic pressure [53, 60, 61]. Interventions that increase LV contractility shorten the isovolumic interval while those that decrease contractility lengthen this interval. Similarly, increased LV preload or end-diastolic wall stress acting through the Starling mechanism will augment the rate of LV pressure rise and thus decrease PEP. Conditions with diminished pulmonary venous return to the left atrium as seen in hypovolemia, assumption of the standing position and chronic obstructive pulmonary disease lengthen the PEP by decreasing LV preload [62–64]. The magnitude of the pressure rise required to open the aortic valve (aortic diastolic minus LV end-diastolic pressure) will also directly influence the PEP. This is illustrated in the patient with chronic aortic regurgitation where aortic diastolic pressure is low and LVEDP is somewhat

TABLE 6-2. Typical Alterations in Systolic Time Intervals in a Variety of Disease States

	PEP	LVETc	PEP/LVET	$T_{1/2}$ time
Left ventricular dysfunction	↑	↓	↑	±N
Aortic valve disease				
Aortic stenosis	↓	↑	↓	↑↑
AS + LV dysfunction	±N	±N	±N	↑↑
Aortic regurgitation	↓	↑	↓	N/sl↑
AR + LV dysfunction	±N	±N	±N	N/sl↑
Mitral valve disease				
Mitral regurgitation	↑	↓	↑	N
MR + LV dysfunction	↑	↓	↑↑	N
Mitral stenosis	↑	↓	↑	N
COPD or hypovolemia	↑	↓	↑	N

PEP = preejection period, LVETc = rate-normalized LV ejection time, LVET = left ventricular ejection time, ↑ = increase, ↓ = decrease, ± = more or less, N = normal, ↑↑ = great increase, AS = aortic stenosis, LV = left ventricular, AR = aortic regurgitation, sl = slight, MR = mitral regurgitation, COPD = chronic obstructive pulmonary disease.

elevated. The small magnitude of isovolumic pressure rise required to open the aortic valve in conjunction with the increased preload results in a shortened PEP. Afterload reduction therapy with increase in aortic diastolic runoff and decrease in systemic vascular resistance will also shorten the PEP if LV preload is maintained relatively constant. Right bundle branch block in the absence of LV dysfunction does not alter the left ventricular PEP. Complete left bundle branch block, on the other hand, prolongs the PEP, probably through delay in the electromechanical association time [65]. Whether isolated left anterior hemiblock significantly alters the LV preejection period remains controversial.

Over the physiologic range of heart rates, the normal values for PEP are fairly constant. At heart rates below 60 beats/min and above 100 beats/min, the PEP tends to increase and decrease, respectively. In our laboratory, we consider any PEP value within the range of 0.08 to 0.11 second to be within normal limits. Weissler and associates, in an attempt to further define the normal PEP range, have proposed the following regression equations suitable for various heart rates (HR) [60]:

Males: PEP = (−0.4) (HR) + 131; SD = 13

Females: PEP = (−0.4) (HR) + 133; SD = 11

Factors Affecting the LVET

The major physiologic parameters influencing the LVET are the LV stroke volume, the condition of the aortic valve, LV contractile state, LV afterload (or systolic wall stress), and heart rate (see Tables 6-1 and 6-2) [53, 60]. Augmentation of LV stroke volume prolongs the LVET since the aortic valve must stay open for a longer period to allow egress of blood from the LV. When left ventricular preload is decreased, as in hypovolemia, or when LV stroke volume is small relative to end-diastolic volume, as in cardiomyopathy, the LVET is short [60]. When a therapeutic intervention results in improvement of LV stroke volume, the LVET frequently returns to the normal range. In valvular and fixed subvalvular aortic stenosis with normal LV function, LV outflow tract obstruction results in prolongation of mechanical systole and ejection time [66]. Elevation of LV afterload or systolic wall stress as in systemic hypertension also prolongs LVET [67]. Positive inotropic drugs such as digitalis or calcium generally shorten LVET in patients with normal LV function by increasing LV velocity of fiber shortening and ejection rate [68, 69]. In patients with LV dysfunction, positive inotropic interventions may increase LVET if sufficient improvement in stroke volume occurs. Negative inotropic agents shorten LVET by diminishing stroke volume and decreasing LV contractile state [53, 70]. Left ventricular conduction abnormalities have little direct effect on LVET, although they are often found in association with myocardial diseases that may impair contractility.

Left ventricular ejection time varies inversely with heart rate. Many centers normalize LVET for a heart rate of 60 beats/min using the formula

$$LVET_c = \frac{LVET}{\sqrt{RR}}$$

where $LVET_c$ = rate-normalized ejection time in msec, LVET = measured ejection time in msec, and RR = the cycle length of the preceding beat in sec. In this instance, the normal range for $LVET_c$ is 290 to 340 msec. Weissler et al have proposed the following regression equations relating LVET to heart rate [60]:

Males: LVET = (−1.7) (HR) + 413; SD = 10

Females: LVET = (−1.6) (HR) + 418; SD = 10

In patients with atrial fibrillation without mitral stenosis, gross variations in RR intervals can occur. Selection of cycles with RR intervals greater than 800 msec gives the best correlation between pre- and post-cardioversion values for rate corrected LVET and PEP [53, 71].

FACTORS AFFECTING THE PEP/LVET RATIO

The ratio of PEP to measured LVET as an index of intrinsic LV muscle performance has several advantages over the use of either the PEP or LVET alone. First, the PEP/LVET is not significantly influenced by heart rate over a large physiologic range (40–110 beats/min) [65]. Second, the PEP/LVET may reflect intrinsic LV dysfunction when either the PEP and/or LVET are still within the normal range. Finally, the PEP/LVET correlates better with the angiographic LV ejection fraction (r = −0.90) than does either of its component parts [72]. The PEP/LVET correlates fairly well with LV stroke volume but less well with cardiac index, since the latter parameter may remain normal in patients with LV dysfunction due to compensatory tachycardia.

In normal subjects, the average value for PEP/LVET is 0.34 ± 0.036 (SD); thus, 95 percent of the values should fall between 0.27 and 0.41 [73]. Left ventricular dysfunction, decreased LV stroke volume or preload, mitral regurgitation, negative inotropic drugs, severe pulmonary disease with diminished pulmonary venous blood return to the left atrium, acute increases in LV afterload due to vasopressor drugs, and complete left bundle branch block may all result in increases in the PEP/LVET above the normal range [53, 73, 74]. A PEP/LVET ratio greater than 0.50 in a patient with mitral regurgitation suggests the presence of associated LV dysfunction [75, 76]. Diminution of the PEP/LVET ratio is seen in patients with aortic valve disease, high LV stroke volume states such as persistent ductus arteriosus or hyperthyroidism, and receiving positive inotropic drugs including digitalis. When LV dysfunction complicates aortic valve disease, the PEP/LVET ratio frequently returns to the normal range. The PEP/LVET ratio in patients with atrial fibrillation correlates best with postcardioversion values when beats with preceding RR intervals longer than 800 msec are analyzed [71].

RIGHT VENTRICULAR SYSTOLIC TIME INTERVALS

In the normal subject, the pulmonary artery diastolic pressure (PADP) is much lower than the aortic diastolic pressure. Therefore, RV isovolumic systole terminates earlier and at a lower pressure than does its left ventricular counterpart. The right ventricular PEP thus is shorter than the left ventricular PEP. In contrast, the RVET is longer than the LVET owing to a greater delay of pulmonary compared with aortic valve closure following the fall in ventricular pressure at the end of systole. The duration of this delay, called the hangout interval, is related to the impedance of the vascular bed into which blood is being injected. The more compliant the bed, the longer is the hangout interval and the more delayed is semilunar valve closure [77].

Values for RVPEP and RVET vary inversely with heart rate. The net result is an RVPEP/RVET ratio that is both relatively independent of heart rate and lower than the LVPEP/LVET ratio [58]. In patients with congenital heart disease, the RVPEP/RVET has been shown to accurately predict changes in the pulmonary vascular bed either after surgical therapy or during the natural history of the disease [59, 78]. Patients who have normal pulmonary artery diastolic pressure (PADP) at cardiac catheterization without complete right bundle branch block on ECG usually have a RVPEP/RVET less than 0.30. In contrast, patients with ratios over 0.35 virtually always demonstrate a PADP >20 mm Hg and usually >30 mm Hg [58]. Unfortunately, the RVPEP/RVET does not correlate well with PADP when other causes of an increased ratio exist, such as complete right bundle branch block (where the onset of RV systole is delayed, resulting in a prolonged PEP) and global cardiomyopathy. Several centers are currently utilizing right ventricular systolic time intervals to noninvasively assess the hemodynamic effects of pulmonary vasodilator therapy for such problems as primary pulmonary hypertension.

The Phonocardiogram

Throughout the course of this chapter we have noted the value of the phonocardiogram in timing various events recorded with other graphic techniques. In addition, phonocardiography is useful in documenting cardiac murmurs. The following (last) section of this chapter specifically integrates phonocardiographic findings with data from other graphic techniques. For detailed information on phonocardiographic recording principles, devices, and so forth, the reader is referred to Tavel's text [24].

An Integrated Noninvasive Approach to Specific Cardiovascular Disease States

This last section combines the previously discussed procedures with echocardiography to present an integrated approach for evaluating specific disease states.

VALVULAR AORTIC STENOSIS
Phonocardiography

The murmur is systolic ejection in timing. A systolic ejection click frequently initiates the murmur in patients with congenital aortic stenosis but is absent in calcific aortic stenosis. In severe valvular aortic stenosis (VAS), the aortic component of S_2 is reduced in intensity or absent. The loudness of the murmur is dependent on the volume of blood flowing across the stenotic valve. Thus, a patient with low cardiac output may have severe VAS but only a relatively soft murmur. When the interval from onset of the QRS complex on ECG to the peak of the systolic murmur is greater than 190 msec, severe VAS is usually present.

Jugular Venous Pulse Tracing
A prominent *a* wave may be present, reflecting altered RV filling (Bernheim's syndrome).

Carotid Pulse Tracing
In severe VAS, the CPT typically shows pulsus parvus et tardus with an early anacrotic shoulder and mid-systolic shudder (Fig. 6-6). Over 90 percent of individuals with peak systolic ejection gradients (PSEG) greater than 50 mm Hg will have maximal rate of carotid rise less than 450 mm Hg/sec. Most patients with rate-corrected $T_{1/2}$ times over 55 msec will have at least 45 mm Hg PSEG across the aortic valve. A normal $T_{1/2}$ time does not, however, exclude severe VAS and may be found in elderly patients with inelastic arteries.

Apexcardiography
VAS is characterized by a heaving precordial impulse with dome-shaped configuration in systole. The *a* wave may be exaggerated, especially in severe VAS (Fig. 6-7).

Systolic Time Intervals
The PEP is usually shortened due to rapid rise of the LV pressure during isovolumic systole and a relatively small isovolumic pressure gradient. The LVETc is increased (if LV function is adequate to maintain a relatively normal stroke volume) owing to prolonged time in ejection of blood across the stenotic valve and delay in inscription of the incisural notch (perhaps related to increased hangout as a consequence of aortic root dilatation). The PEP/LVET is decreased owing to diminished PEP and prolonged LVET. When LV decompensation occurs, the LVET shortens and PEP is prolonged, resulting in "normalization" of the STI. With medical therapy, the LVET may once again lengthen as the PEP decreases. The prolonged LVETc usually returns to normal with aortic valve replacement and may even become abnormally short if underlying LV dysfunction is present.

Echocardiography
In severe VAS, M-mode echocardiography shows multiple dense echoes without discernible motion of the cusps. Two-dimensional (2-D) echo helps identify doming of the valve in bicuspid aortic valve disease. The 2-D echo can usually identify patients without significant VAS by demonstrating normal excursion of the valve cusps. Severe calcific aortic stenosis produces markedly reduced excursion and can usually be identified. Separating patients with moderate and severe VAS by 2-D echo is more difficult, particularly when there is concomitant LV dysfunction.

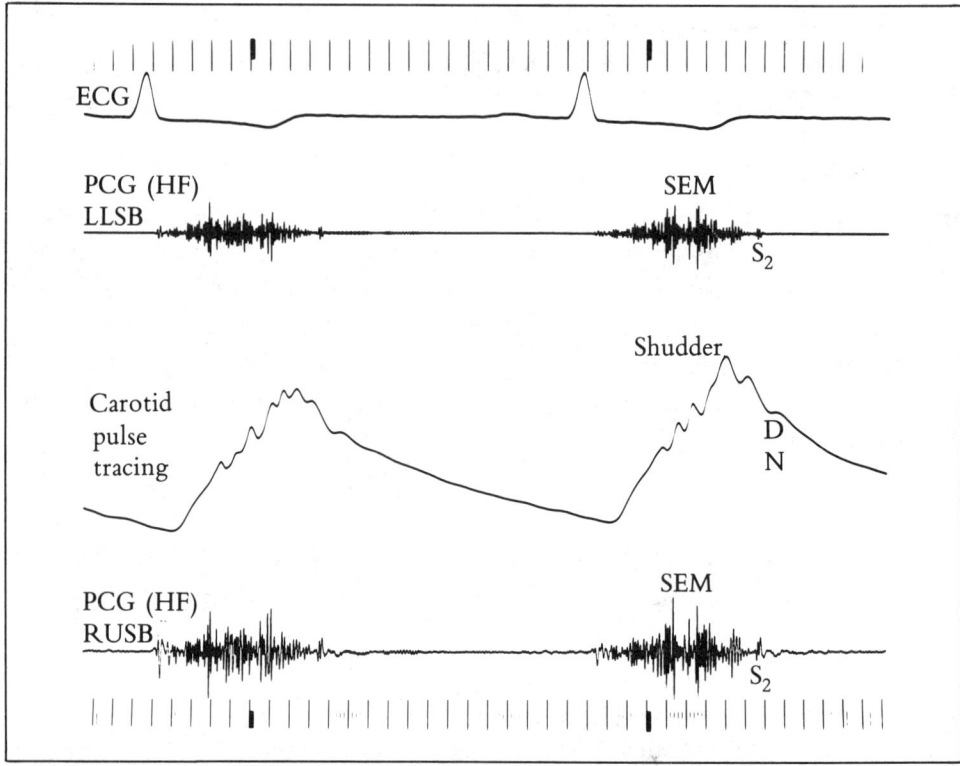

FIGURE 6-6. Carotid pulse tracing in a patient with severe valvular aortic stenosis showing a low anacrotic shoulder and systolic shudder. The phonocardiogram (*PCG*) demonstrates a mid to late peaking systolic ejection murmur (*SEM*) with soft aortic component of the second heart sound (S_2). *DN* = dicrotic notch, *HF* = high frequency, *LLSB* = left lower sternal border, *RUSB* = right upper sternal border.

Integration

In a patient with echocardiographic studies suggestive of severe aortic stenosis in association with a late peaking systolic murmur, prolonged corrected ejection time and $T_{1/2}$ time, and a reduced peak rate of carotid rise, moderate to severe VAS is usually present. One can distinguish the prolonged ejection time of aortic regurgitation from that of stenosis since only stenosis will markedly prolong the $T_{1/2}$ time. In a moribund patient with low forward cardiac output and congestive heart failure, the presence of echocardiographic findings of aortic stenosis, increased $T_{1/2}$ time and normal STI strongly suggest severe LV outflow tract obstruction. Conversely, a short LVETc suggests that VAS is not the cause of the heart failure. In patients with carotid bruits, analysis of suprasternal notch or subclavian artery pulse recordings may be helpful in distinguishing local carotid disease from fixed LV outflow tract obstruction.

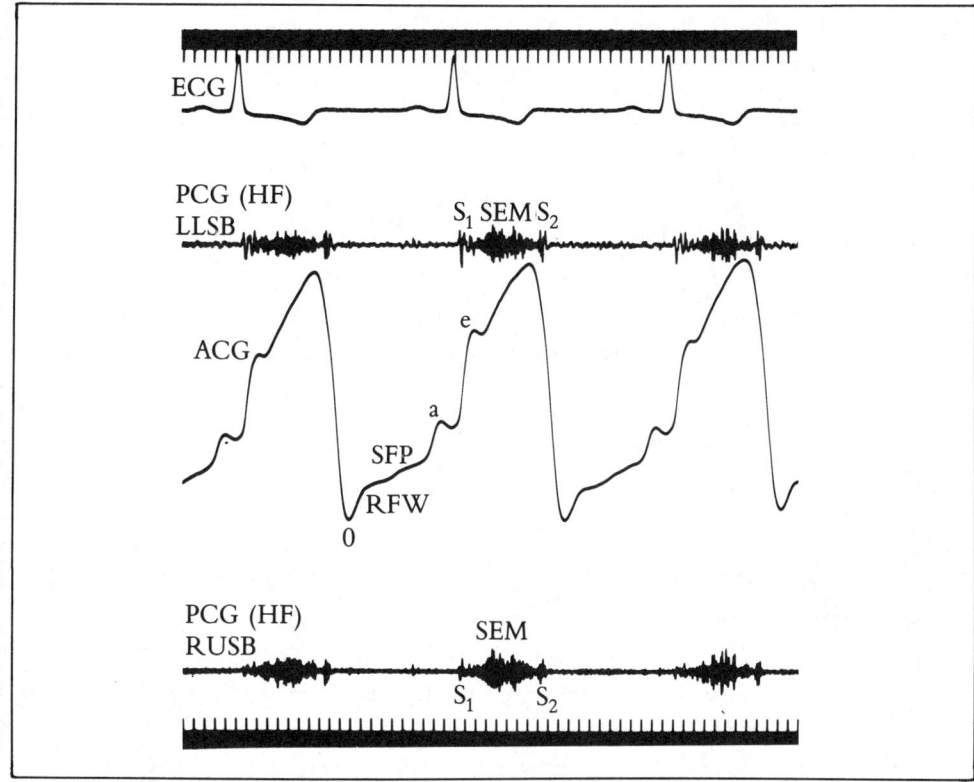

FIGURE 6-7. Apexcardiogram (ACG) in a patient with severe valvular aortic stenosis. The systolic wave is sustained with a continued rise throughout ventricular ejection. The *a* wave is exaggerated (*a*/OE ratio = 0.21). HF = high frequency, LLSB = left lower sternal border, PCG = phonocardiogram, RFW = rapid filling wave, SEM = systolic ejection murmur, SFP = slow filling phase (wave).

HYPERTROPHIC OBSTRUCTIVE CARDIOMYOPATHY
Phonocardiography

The aortic second heart sound is usually of normal intensity. Unlike VAS, an ejection click is uncommon, even in young patients. A fourth heart sound is often heard. When dynamic obstruction is present, a systolic ejection murmur occurs, which is loudest in the left mid-sternal border area with poor radiation to the cervical region. This murmur increases in intensity with maneuvers that decrease LV preload (standing, peak Valsalva maneuver), decrease LV afterload (amyl nitrite), or increase LV contractility (isoproterenol, digitalis). The murmur decreases upon prompt squatting, isometric hand grip, or use of vasoconstrictor medications. A murmur of mitral regurgitation is often associated with hypertrophic obstructive cardiomyopathy (HOCM).

Jugular Venous Pulse Tracing

The JVP occasionally shows a large *a* wave when RV filling characteristics are altered.

Carotid Pulse Tracing

The initial carotid upstroke is usually brisk with a subsequent dome-shaped curve during systole (Fig. 6-8). This spike and dome configuration, which is characteristic of dynamic HOCM, may not be present under resting conditions. However, typical carotid morphology may be provoked with amyl nitrite, isoproterenol, Valsalva maneuver, or following a premature atrial or ventricular beat (Fig. 6-9).

Apexcardiography

There is usually a large *a* wave due to altered LV compliance. A bifid systolic appearance is a common finding.

Systolic Time Intervals

Unlike VAS, the PEP in HOCM is usually normal. The LVETc is normal when resting obstruction is absent. When dynamic or resting obstruction occurs, the LVETc is prolonged. The degree of LVETc prolongation correlates with the magnitude of LV-to-aorta systolic pressure gradient. Maneuvers that increase outflow gradient, such as the Valsalva maneuver, will increase LVETc. This is in contrast to the normal decline in LVETc that occurs during the straining phase of the Valsalva maneuver (Table 6-3). In HOCM, the PEP/LVET is generally normal or low. If the PEP/LVET is less than 0.30, LV outflow obstruction is usually severe. Ratios greater than 0.35 are usually associated with little or no obstruction.

Echocardiography

M-mode and 2-D studies are characterized by asymmetric septal hypertrophy, systolic anterior motion of the anterior leaflet of the mitral valve, narrowed LV outflow tract, small LV chamber size, and diminished septal thickening during systole. The aortic valve cusps may show partial closure at the time of onset of the murmur.

Integration

Combined echophonocardiographic studies with simultaneous carotid pulse recording can demonstrate the onset of dynamic LV outflow tract obstruction with provocative maneuvers. Similarly, recordings made after a premature beat will demonstrate precipitation of a spike and dome configuration on carotid pulse tracing and echocardiographic findings of dynamic obstruction in many patients with HOCM. Patients with VAS will have a stronger pulse with pulsus parvus et tardus in the beat following a premature contraction. Other features which may be used to differentiate VAS from HOCM are listed in Table 6-4.

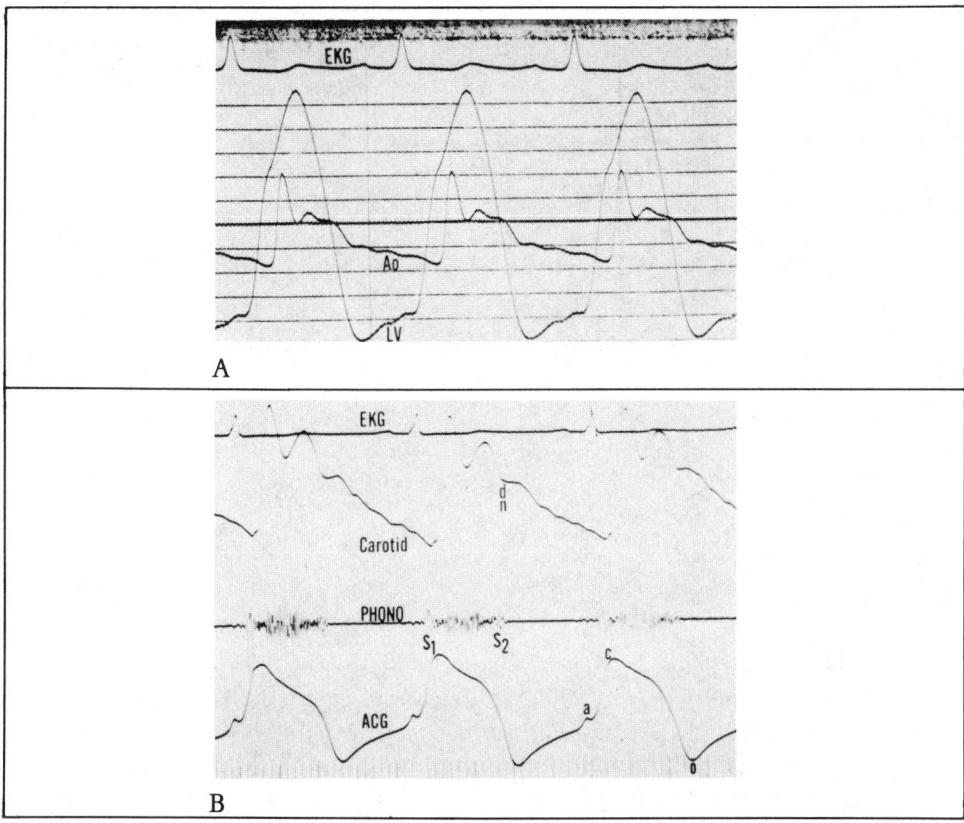

FIGURE 6-8. Recordings in a patient with hypertrophic obstructive cardiomyopathy (HOCM) and resting left ventricular (LV) outflow tract obstruction. (A) Simultaneous direct pressure tracings recorded with catheters in the LV and aortic root (Ao). The typical spike and dome configuration characteristic of dynamic LV outflow tract obstruction is demonstrated in the Ao. (B) Simultaneous indirect carotid pulse tracing and apexcardiogram (ACG) in the same patient. Note the similarity of pulse configuration between the recordings made using noninvasive and invasive techniques. dn = dicrotic notch.

AORTIC REGURGITATION

Phonocardiography

The typical murmur of aortic regurgitation (AR) is a decrescendo, high frequency, early diastolic murmur beginning with A_2 and continuing throughout most of diastole. A_2 is decreased in intensity or absent. If AR is due to cusp abnormality, the murmur is usually loudest in the lower left sternal border area. If it is due to aortic root dilation, maximal intensity is usually to the right of the sternum. An apical mid to late diastolic rumble (Austin Flint) may be present in pure AR. Acute AR may result in an absent mitral closure sound (M_1) due to premature closure of the mitral valve. Since it is the pressure gradient between the aorta and

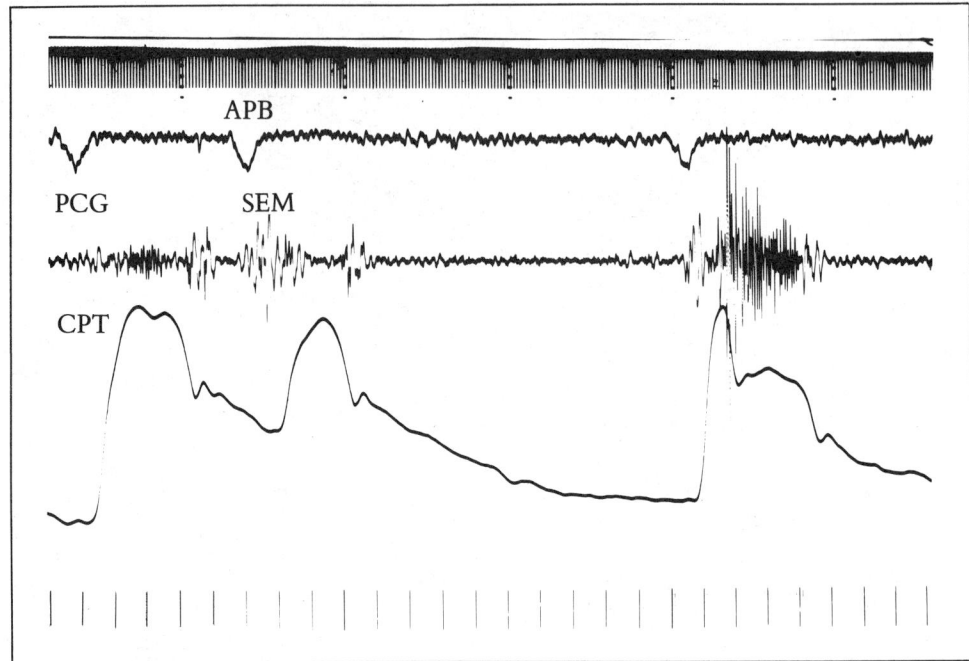

FIGURE 6-9. Carotid pulse tracing (*CPT*), phonocardiogram (*PCG*) recorded at the left lower sternal border, and electrocardiogram in a patient with HOCM without resting obstruction. Recordings made after an atrial premature beat (*APB*) demonstrate precipitation of a spike and dome configuration on CPT and accentuation of the systolic ejection murmur (*SEM*), indicating that dynamic obstruction was provoked.

LV that produces the retrograde flow and thus the murmur, acute severe AR often produces a short diastolic murmur, since there is virtual equilibration of aortic and LV pressures by mid-diastole. A short, early peaking systolic ejection murmur is frequently present in chronic AR due to high flow across the aortic valve. A third heart sound is frequently present. The murmur of AR increases with isometric exercise.

Carotid Pulse Tracing

A bisferiens pulse may be present in mixed AS/AR or occasionally in pure AR. In chronic AR, the dicrotic notch is frequently low or indistinct. In acute AR, the peripheral pulse contour and pulse pressure may remain relatively normal due to low cardiac output in association with a high systemic vascular resistance. The $T_{1/2}$ time is usually normal or slightly prolonged.

Apexcardiography

In uncomplicated AR of moderate or greater severity, the ACG is of a hyper-

TABLE 6-3. Alterations in Systolic Time Intervals in LVOT Obstruction with the Valsalva Maneuver

	Early Strain	Peak Strain	Recovery
Functional murmur or valvular aortic stenosis			
RR	↑	↓	Baseline or ↑
LVETc	↓	↓	Baseline or ↑
PEP	↑	↑	Baseline or ↓
PEP/LVET	↑	↑	Baseline or ↓
Murmur	↓	↓	Baseline or ↑
HOCM			
RR	↑	↓	Baseline or ↑
LVETc	↑ or N	↑ or N	Baseline or ↓
PEP	N or ↓	N or ↓	Baseline or ↑
PEP/LVET	N or ↓	N or ↓	Baseline or ↑
Murmur	↑	↑↑	Baseline or ↓

LVOT = left ventricular outflow tract, RR = beat cycle length, ↑ = increase, ↓ = decrease, LVETc = rate-normalized left ventricular ejection time, PEP = preejection period, LVET = left ventricular ejection time, HOCM = hypertrophic obstructive cardiomyopathy, N = normal.

TABLE 6-4. Findings in Valvular Aortic Stenosis and Hypertrophic Obstructive Cardiomyopathy

	VAS	HOCM
Location of murmur	RUSB	LMSB
Radiation of murmur	Well to neck	Poorly to neck
Ejection click	Frequent	Infrequent
Aortic regurgitation	Frequent	Infrequent
Carotid upstroke	Diminished	Rapid

VAS = valvular aortic stenosis, HOCM = hypertrophic obstructive cardiomyopathy, RUSB = right upper sternal border, LMSB = left mid-sternal border.

dynamic variety with accentuated rapid filling wave. In severe chronic AR with LV dilatation and decreased ejection fraction, the ACG becomes sustained in quality with a prominent *a* wave reflecting diminished LV compliance.

Systolic Time Intervals
The PEP is usually diminished, occasionally strikingly so, due to high LV end-diastolic pressure and low aortic diastolic pressure resulting in a small isovolumic pulse pressure. Furthermore, the increased LV preload shortens PEP. The LV cor-

rected ejection time is increased, since the LV ejects an increased stroke volume across the aortic valve. In addition, the aortic valve opens early (low aortic diastolic pressure) and closes late (delayed incisura). If LV function is preserved, the more severe the AR, the longer the LVETc. The PEP/LVET is shortened. As in aortic stenosis, LV decompensation tends to "normalize" the STI. Aortic valve replacement normalizes the STI if irreversible LV dysfunction is not present.

Echocardiography

In chronic AR, the LV is dilated and hyperkinetic. Although there is often high frequency diastolic vibration of the anterior leaflet of the mitral valve, its absence does not exclude AR. In acute aortic regurgitation, there may be early closure of the mitral valve due to early crossover of the LVEDP-LA pressure curves.

Integration

The physiologic significance of clinical, phonocardiographic, and echocardiographic findings of AR can be assessed by analyzing the STI. Normal STI in the presence of AR and preserved LV fractional shortening suggests that the regurgitation is of mild severity. In a patient with mixed AS/AR on physical examination in association with a prolonged LVETc and normal LV shortening on echocardiogram, the $T_{1/2}$ time becomes important since it will be significantly prolonged in predominant AS and relatively normal in duration if AR predominates. The dilated, poorly contracting heart of chronic AR with LV dysfunction can be distinguished from idiopathic cardiomyopathy by the LVETc, which is "normal" in the former and shortened in the latter.

MITRAL STENOSIS

Phonocardiography

The first heart sound is increased in intensity in the absence of significant mitral valve calcification. The $Q-M_1$ interval is often prolonged while the A_2-opening snap interval is decreased (normal A_2-mitral valve opening interval is >0.120 seconds). The more positive the difference between $Q-M_1$ and A_2-OS intervals, the more severe the mitral stenosis (MS). The P_2 is increased in intensity when pulmonary hypertension is present. The duration of the mid-diastolic rumble (due to turbulent blood flow across the stenotic valve) is greater the more severe the MS. This is due to persistence of a transvalvular gradient throughout much of diastole in moderate to severe MS. Presystolic accentuation of the murmur is common in patients in sinus rhythm but occasionally can also be heard when atrial fibrillation is present. The murmur of MS gets louder with exercise owing to increased cardiac output and decreased diastolic filling period.

Jugular Venous Pulse Tracing

The *a* wave may have increased amplitude due to diminished RV compliance in the presence of long-standing pulmonary hypertension.

Carotid Pulse Tracing

In severe MS with low cardiac output, there may be normal ascent of the CPT followed by early smoothing of the curve with a late systolic peak.

Apexcardiography

In mild to moderate MS, the ACG may have a normal systolic configuration and amplitude; however, the rapid filling wave will be somewhat blunted and the *a* wave amplitude diminished. In severe MS, there is slurring of the rapid and slow diastolic filling periods with failure to attain diastasis even on long cardiac cycles.

Systolic Time Intervals

Abnormalities, including increased PEP, decreased LVET, and increased PEP/LVET, occur only in severe MS with diminished LV preload. These findings are nonspecific, however.

Echocardiography

The severity of the mitral stenosis can be reliably determined by planimetry of the mitral valve orifice on 2-D echo study. The mitral valve appears thickened and shortened with diminished leaflet movement. There is often tethering of the anterior leaflet. The magnitude of associated mitral regurgitation cannot be directly determined by echo.

Integration

Use of integrated noninvasive studies can be particularly helpful when some degree of mitral or aortic regurgitation is present. The presence of a large LV end-diastolic dimension in association with a normal or increased *a* wave on ACG and increased PEP/LVET on STI suggests significant concomitant or predominant mitral regurgitation (Figs. 6-10 and 6-11).

MITRAL REGURGITATION

Phonocardiography

The first heart sound is frequently diminished in intensity. Chronic mitral regurgitation (MR) is characterized by a high-frequency holosystolic murmur that is best recorded from the cardiac apex. In moderate to severe MR, a third heart sound and mid-diastolic rumble may be present due to high transmitral flow. The murmur of acute MR frequently tapers off in mid to late systole. This abbrevia-

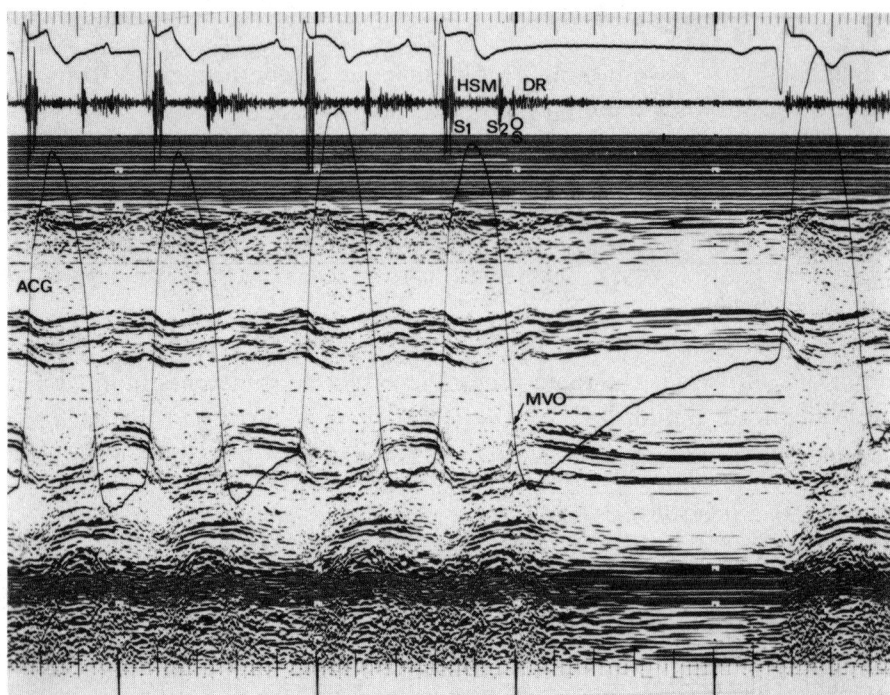

FIGURE 6-10. Echocardiogram of the mitral valve, apexcardiogram (*ACG*), phonocardiogram (*PCG*) recorded from the left ventricular (*LV*) apical area, and electrocardiogram in a patient with moderately severe mitral stenosis. Continued LV filling is noted on the echocardiogram and ACG throughout diastole even on the long diastolic cycle. There is slurring of the rapid and slow filling waves of the ACG. *DR* = diastolic rumble, *HSM* = holosystolic murmur, *MVO* = mitral valve opening, *OS* = opening snap of the mitral valve.

tion of the murmur is due to rapid rise in left atrial pressure as blood regurgitates into the relatively noncompliant LA, resulting in equalization of LV and LA pressures during systole. The murmur of MR gets louder with increases in LV afterload (sudden squatting, isometric handgrip); the converse is true with inhalation of amyl nitrite.

Carotid Pulse Tracing

The carotid pulse contour may be hyperkinetic although the peripheral pulse pressure is normal. This is due to a large volume of blood being ejected through two orifices during systole. The CPT has a brisk upstroke and rapid falloff.

Apexcardiography

The ACG is hyperkinetic due to an increased LV stroke volume. The pulse contour is normal in shape but exaggerated in magnitude. A prominent rapid filling

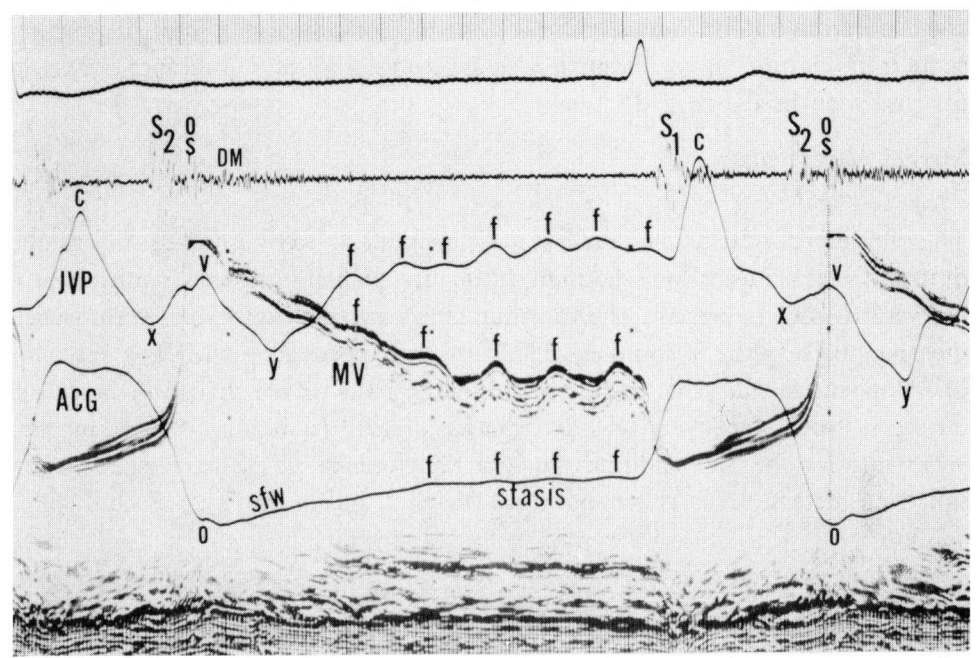

FIGURE 6-11. Simultaneous echocardiogram of the mitral valve (*MV*), jugular venous pulse (*JVP*), apexcardiogram (*ACG*), phonocardiogram and electrocardiogram in a patient with mild mitral stenosis. Fibrillatory waves (*f*) due to atrial fibrillation are demonstrated on the JVP, MV echocardiogram, and ACG. DM = diastolic murmur, OS = opening snap, *sfw* = slow filling wave.

wave is often present. Acute MR, unlike the chronic form, is frequently associated with a large *a* wave on ACG and a prominent fourth heart sound on PCG.

Systolic Time Intervals
Prolongation of the PEP, diminished LVETc, and increased PEP/LVET are characteristic findings of MR. The presence of a normal PEP/LVET suggests that LV contractile performance is compensated; a PEP/LVET greater than or equal to 0.50 correlates with coexistent LV dysfunction.

Echocardiography
The etiology of MR can often be ascertained by 2-D echocardiographic study. The degree of LV diastolic enlargement is often a reasonable guide to the severity of isolated MR. Prominent LA systolic expansion, when present, suggests severe MR.

Integration
The STI are helpful in assessing LV muscle performance in patients with clinical

and echocardiographic findings of MR. The ACG can be useful in distinguishing acute from chronic regurgitation as well as ascertaining the significance of MR in patients with mixed MS/MR.

MITRAL VALVE PROLAPSE

Phonocardiography

The typical presentation includes a systolic click followed by a mid to late systolic murmur, often musical or whooping in quality. When holosystolic mitral valve prolapse (MVP) is present, the murmur is holosystolic with the ejection click incorporated into the S_1 complex. The pathologic correlate for MVP is excessive or redundant mitral valve tissue with respect to the orifice that must be closed during systole. Maneuvers that decrease LV preload (standing, Valsalva maneuver) will cause the click and murmur to move closer to S_1. Passive leg raising and squatting increase LV preload and move the click and murmur closer to S_2 (Fig. 6-12).

Apexcardiography

A systolic notch may occur at the time of the click, resulting in a bisferiens configuration.

Systolic Time Intervals

If hemodynamically significant mitral regurgitation is present, the PEP lengthens, LVETc shortens, and the PEP/LVET is increased.

Echocardiography

Large, redundant mitral valve leaflets billow posteriorly into the LA during systole.

Integration

Echophonocardiography can demonstrate a systolic murmur associated with typical ultrasound findings of MVP. STI can be useful in assessing the physiologic significance of associated MR.

PERICARDIAL DISEASE

Phonocardiography

In constrictive pericarditis, the second heart sound may be widely split during inspiration due to early occurrence of A_2. A "pericardial knock" may occur approximately 100 to 120 msec after A_2. Generally, no characteristic murmurs are present.

Jugular Venous Pulse Tracing

In constrictive pericarditis, the JVP shows a rapid and brief y descent interrupting

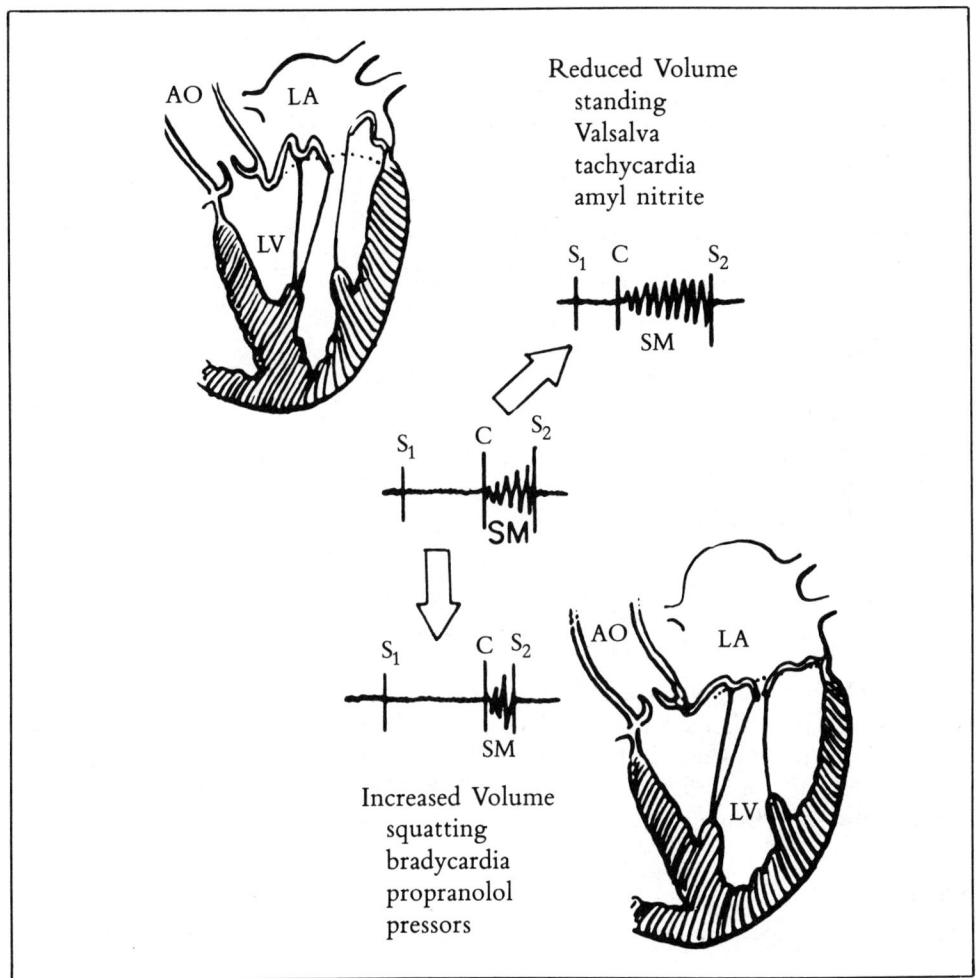

FIGURE 6-12. The effect of interventions on the timing of auscultatory events in mitral valve prolapse. Maneuvers that reduce left ventricular (*LV*) volume enhance leaflet redundancy, hasten prolapse, and move click (*C*) and murmur (*SM*) earlier in systole. An increase in left ventricular dimensions has the opposite effect. The loudness of auscultatory events is governed independently by LV systolic pressure. *AO* = aorta, *LA* = left atrium. (From RB Devereux et al: Mitral valve prolapse. *Circulation* 54:8, 1976, by permission of the American Heart Association, Inc.)

a relatively high venous plateau and ending in early diastasis. In many cases, the *v* wave peaks early. The JVP in cardiac tamponade does not characteristically show a prominent *y* descent.

Carotid Pulse Tracing

In hemodynamically compromising constrictive pericarditis or cardiac tampon-

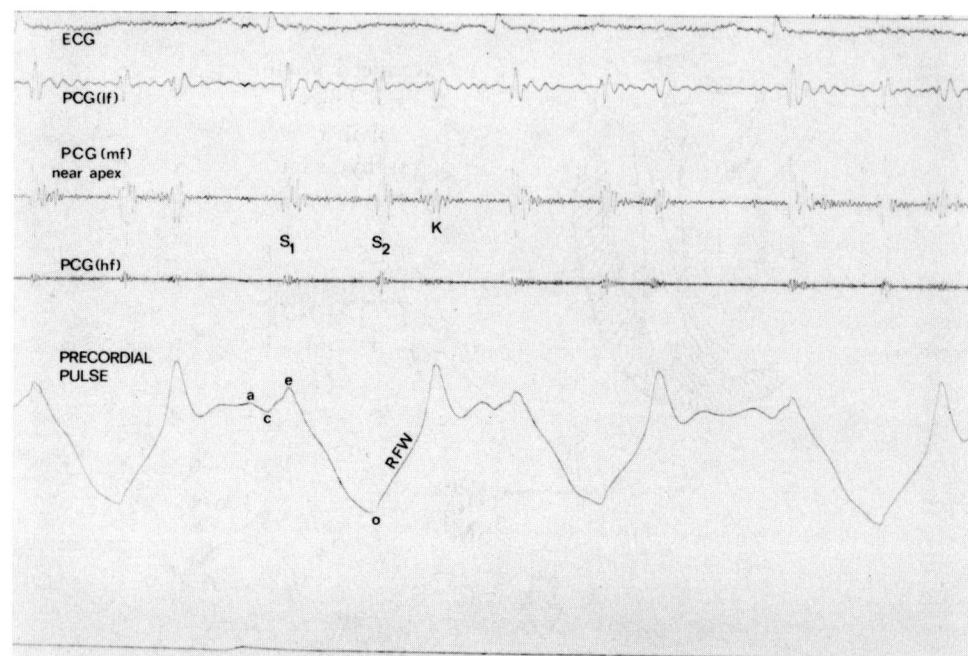

FIGURE 6-13. Precordial pulse recording in a patient with constrictive pericardial disease shows systolic retraction and abrupt cessation of the rapid filling wave (*RFW*) resulting in an early diastolic plateau. The phonocardiogram, recorded near the left ventricular apex, demonstrates a loud "pericardial knock" (*K*). hf = high frequency, lf = low frequency, mf = mid frequency.

ade, the pulse pressure may be narrow, resulting in a hypokinetic carotid pulse. In tamponade, pulsus paradoxus may be evident.

Apexcardiography
In constriction, the ACG, which is often difficult to record, shows systolic retractions that resemble a mirror image of the normal tracing. In early diastole, the rapid filling wave is suddenly halted resulting in an early diastolic plateau. The configuration of the ACG during diastole resembles the intraventricular pressure tracings seen in pericardial constriction (Fig. 6-13).

Systolic Time Intervals
In cardiac tamponade, the LVETc is shortened during inspiration by more than 20 msec. This is probably due to gross variations in LV filling and stroke volume with respiration. Chronic pericardial constriction is characterized by normal or slightly shortened PEP and LVETc with normal PEP/LVET.

Echocardiography
The echocardiogram is not diagnostic for constriction or tamponade. Findings of

a large pericardial effusion, thickened pericardium, phasic variation in RV and LV dimensions, and gross cardiac oscillations are all circumstantial evidence for hemodynamically significant pericardial disease.

Integration

The ACG can be helpful in assessing the significance of echo findings suggestive of pericardial constriction. Since the ventricle cannot continue to fill in mid to late diastole in constriction, the finding of a normal slow filling wave with normal to large *a* wave precludes the presence of hemodynamically significant constrictive pericarditis. The STI help distinguish circulatory congestion due to cardiomyopathy from that of pericardial disease, since the former will have an increased PEP/LVET, whereas the latter will have a normal ratio.

Acknowledgment

We note with pleasure and gratitude the support and assistance of our colleague, Laurence J. Sloss, M.D.

References

1. Alpert JS, Sloss LJ, Cohn PF, Grossman W: The diagnostic accuracy of combined clinical and noninvasive cardiac evaluation: Comparison with findings at cardiac catheterization. *Cath Cardiovasc Diag* 6:359, 1980
2. Borow KM, Wynne J, Sloss LJ, Cohn LH, Collins JJ: Definitive noninvasive assessment of valvular heart disease: Surgery without catheterization. *Am J Cardiol* 45:402, 1980
3. Martin CE, Shaver JA, Thompson ME, Reddy PS, Leonard JJ: Direct correlation of external systolic time intervals with internal indices of left ventricular function in man. *Circulation* 44:419, 1973
4. Van der Werf F, Piessens J, Kesteloot H, De Geest H: A comparison of systolic time intervals derived from the central aortic pressure and from the external carotid pulse tracing. *Circulation* 51:310, 1975
5. Jordan H: Investigations on the relationship between central pulse velocity and so-called delay-time. *Cardiologia* 35:228, 1959
6. Freis ED, Heath WC, Luchsinger PC, Snell RE: Changes in the carotid pulse that occur with age and hypertension. *Am Heart J* 71:757, 1966
7. Nathan D, Ongley PA, Rahimtoola SH: The dynamics of left ventricular ejection in "normal" man with infusion of isoproterenol. *Chest* 71:746, 1977
8. O'Rourke MF: The arterial pulse in health and disease. *Am Heart J* 82:687, 1971
9. Robinson B: The carotid pulse. II. Relation of external recordings to carotid, aortic and brachial pulses. *Br Heart J* 25:61, 1963
10. Fowler NO, Marshall WJ: Cardiac diagnosis from examination of arteries and veins. *Circulation* 30:272, 1964

11. Cousins AL, Eddleman EE, Reeves TJ: Prediction of aortic valvular area and gradient by noninvasive techniques. *Am Heart J* 95:308, 1978
12. Lyle DP, Bancroft WH, Tucker M, Eddleman EE: Slopes of the carotid pulse wave in normal subjects, aortic valvular disease and hypertrophic subaortic stenosis. *Circulation* 43:374, 1971
13. Bonner AJ, Sacks HN, Tavel ME: Assessing the severity of aortic stenosis by phonocardiography and external carotid pulse recordings. *Circulation* 48:247, 1973
14. Epstein EJ, Coulshed N: Assessment of aortic stenosis from the external carotid pulse wave. *Br Heart J* 26:84, 1964
15. Sabbah HN, Blick EF, Anbe DT, Stein PD: Effect of turbulent blood flow on systolic pressure contour in the ventricles and great vessels: Significance related to anacrotic and bisferious pulses. *Am J Cardiol* 45:1139, 1980
16. Starr I, Ambrosi C, Manchester JH, Shelburne JC: Disturbed blood flow in the carotid artery: Its physiological and clinical significance. *Am Heart J* 86:644, 1973
17. Logan WF, Jones EW, Walker E, Coulshed N, Epstein EJ: Familial supravalvular aortic stenosis. *Br Heart J* 27:547, 1965
18. Mason DT, Braunwald E, Ross J, Morrow AG: Diagnostic value of the first and second derivatives of the arterial pulse in aortic valve disease and in hypertrophic subaortic stenosis. *Circulation* 30:90, 1964
19. Ewy GA, Rios JA, Marcus FI: The dicrotic arterial pulse. *Circulation* 39:655, 1969
20. Mitchell JH, Sarnoff SJ, Sonnenblick EH: The dynamics of pulsus alternans: Alternating end-diastolic fiber length as a causative factor. *J Clin Invest* 42:55, 1963
21. Fowler NO: Physiology of cardiac tamponade and pulsus paradoxus. *Mod Concepts Cardiovasc Dis* 47:109, 1978
22. Hartman H: The jugular venous tracing. *Am Heart J* 59:698, 1960
23. Rich LL, Tavel ME: The origin of the jugular C wave. *N Engl J Med* 284:1309, 1970
24. Tavel ME: *Clinical Phonocardiography and External Pulse Recording.* 3rd ed. Chicago: Year Book Publishers, 1978, p 54
25. Gibson R, Wood P: The diagnosis of tricuspid stenosis. *Br Heart J* 17:552, 1955
26. Perloff JK, Harvey WP: Clinical recognition of tricuspid stenosis. *Circulation* 22:346, 1960
27. Borow KM, Henschke C, Sloss LJ, Wynne J: Tricuspid stenosis masquerading as right ventricular failure in a patient with a prosthetic mitral valve. *Cath Cardiovasc Diag* 7:409, 1981
28. Kesteloot H, Denef B: Value of reference tracings in diagnosis and assessment of constrictive epi- and pericarditis. *Br Heart J* 32:675, 1970
29. Nagel MR, Ronan JA, Roberts WC: Left-to-right shunt at atrial level after rupture of papillary muscle from acute myocardial infarction. *Am Heart J* 86:112, 1973
30. Constant J: *Bedside Cardiology.* 2nd ed. Boston: Little Brown, 1976, p 93
31. Lisa CP, Hood G, Tavel ME: The jugular pulse in pericardial constriction: Its differentiation from that of cardiomyopathy. *Am Heart J* 84:409, 1972

32. Abrams J: Precordial motion in health and disease. *Mod Concepts Cardiovasc Dis* 49:55, 1980
33. Benchimol A, Dimond EG, Carson JC: The value of the apexcardiogram as a reference tracing in phonocardiography. *Am Heart J* 61:485, 1961
34. Manolas J, Rutishauser W, Wirz P, Arbenz U: Time relation between apexcardiogram and left ventricular events using simultaneous high fidelity tracings in man. *Br Heart J* 37:1263, 1975
35. Tafur E, Cohen LS, Levine HD: The normal apexcardiogram, its temporal relationship to electrical, acoustic, and mechanical cardiac events. *Circulation* 30:381, 1964
36. Manolas J, Rutishauser W: Relation between apexcardiographic and internal indices of left ventricular relaxation in man. *Br Heart J* 39:1324, 1977
37. Willems J, De Geest H, Kesteloot H: On the value of apexcardiography for timing intracardiac events. *Am J Cardiol* 28:59, 1971
38. Craige E: Apexcardiography. In Weissler AM (ed): *Noninvasive Cardiology.* New York: Grune & Stratton, 1972, p 14
39. Sutton GC, Prewitt TA, Craige E: Relationship between quantitated precordial movement and left ventricular function. *Circulation* 41:179, 1970
40. Lane FJ, Carroll JM, Levine HD, Gorlin R: The apexcardiogram in myocardial asynergy. *Circulation* 37:890, 1968
41. Braunwald E, Lambrew CT, Rockoff SD, Ross J, Morrow AG: Idiopathic hypertrophic subaortic stenosis. I. A description of the disease based upon an analysis of 64 patients. *Circulation* 30(Suppl IV):3–119, 1964
42. Algary WP, Craige E: Left atrial myxoma. Diagnosis with the help of the phonocardiogram and apexcardiogram. *Arch Intern Med* 129:470, 1972
43. Prewitt T, Gibson D, Brown D, Sutton G: The rapid filling wave of the apexcardiogram — Its relation to echocardiographic and cineangiographic measurements of ventricular filling. *Br Heart J* 37:1256, 1975
44. Benchimol A, Dimond EG: Normal and abnormal apexcardiogram. *Am J Cardiol* 11:368, 1963
45. Nixon PGF, Wooler GH: Phases of diastole in various syndromes of mitral valvular disease. *Br Heart J* 25:393, 1963
46. Gibson TC, Madry R, Grossman W, McLaurin LP, Craige E: The A wave of the apexcardiogram and left ventricular diastolic stiffness. *Circulation* 49:441, 1974
47. Voigt G, Friesinger GC: The use of apexcardiography in the assessment of left ventricular diastolic pressure. *Circulation* 41:1015, 1970
48. Kavalier MA, Stewart J, Tavel ME: The apical A wave versus the fourth heart sound in assessing the severity of aortic stenosis. *Circulation* 51:324, 1975
49. Fleming JS: The assessment of failure in aortic stenosis from the diastolic movement of the left ventricle. *Am Heart J* 76:235, 1968
50. Ginn WM, Sherwin RW, Harrison KW, Baker BM: Apexcardiography: Use in coronary heart disease and reproducibility. *Am Heart J* 73:168, 1967

51. Benchimol A, Dimond EG: The apexcardiogram in normal older subjects and in patients with arteriosclerotic heart disease: Effect of exercise on the "A" wave. *Am Heart J* 65:789, 1963
52. El-Sherif A, El-Said G: Jugular, hepatic and praecordial pulsations in constrictive pericarditis. *Br Heart J* 33:305, 1971
53. Lewis RP, Rittgers SE, Forester WF, Boudoulas H: A critical review of the systolic time intervals. *Circulation* 56:146, 1977
54. Weissler AM: Current concepts in cardiology: Systolic time intervals. *N Engl J Med* 296:321, 1977
55. Wanderman KL, Loutaty G, Ovsyshcher I, Cantor A, Gussarsky Y, Gueron M: Choice of electrocardiographic leads for recording the earliest QRS onset in noninvasive measurements. *Circulation* 63:933, 1981
56. Martin CE, Shaver JA, Thompson ME, Reddy PS, Leonard JJ: Direct correlation of external systolic time intervals with internal indices of left ventricular function in man. *Circulation* 44:419, 1971
57. Van der Werf F, Piessens J, Kesteloot H, De Geest H: A comparison of systolic time intervals derived from the central aortic pressure and from the external carotid pulse tracing. *Circulation* 51:310, 1975
58. Hirschfeld S, Meyer R, Schwartz DC, Korfhagen J, Kaplan S: Measurement of right and left ventricular systolic time intervals by echocardiography. *Circulation* 51:304, 1975
59. Riggs T, Hirschfeld S, Borkat G, Knoke J, Liebman J: Assessment of the pulmonary vascular bed by echocardiographic right ventricular systolic time intervals. *Circulation* 57:939, 1978
60. Weissler AM, Harris WS, Schoenfeld CD: Systolic time intervals in heart failure in man. *Circulation* 37:149, 1968
61. Metzger CC, Chough CB, Kroetz FW, Leonard JJ: True isovolumic contraction time: Its correlation with two external indexes of ventricular performance. *Am J Cardiol* 25:434, 1970
62. Stafford RW, Harris WS, Weissler AM: Left ventricular systolic time intervals as indices of postural circulatory stress in man. *Circulation* 41:485, 1970
63. Alpert JS, Rickman FD, Howe JP, Dexter L, Dalen JE: Alteration of systolic time intervals in right ventricular failure. *Circulation* 50:317, 1974
64. Hooper RG, Whitcomb ME: Systolic time intervals in chronic obstructive pulmonary disease. *Circulation* 50:1205, 1974
65. Lewis RP, Leighton RF, Forester WF, Weissler AM: Systolic time intervals. In Weissler AM (ed): *Noninvasive Cardiology*. New York: Grune & Stratton, 1974, p 301
66. Bonner AJ, Tavel ME: Use in congestive heart failure due to aortic stenosis. *Arch Intern Med* 132:816, 1973
67. Shaver JA, Kroetz FW, Leonard JJ, Paley HW: The effect of steady state increases in systemic arterial pressure on the duration of left ventricular ejection time. *J Clin Invest* 47:217, 1968

68. Weissler AM, Snyder JR, Schoenfeld CD, Cohen S: Assay of digitalis glycosides in man. *Am J Cardiol* 17:768, 1966
69. Shiner PT, Harris WS, Weissler AM: Effects of acute changes in serum calcium levels on the systolic time intervals in man. *Am J Cardiol* 24:42, 1967
70. Hunt D, Sloman G, Clark RM, Hoffman G: Effects of beta-adrenergic blockade on systolic time intervals. *Am J Med Sci* 259:97, 1970
71. Tavel ME, Baugh DO, Feigenbaum H, Nasser WK: Left ventricular ejection time in atrial fibrillation. *Circulation* 46:744, 1972
72. Garrard CL, Weissler AM, Dodge HT: The relationship of alterations in systolic time intervals to ejection fraction in patients with cardiac disease. *Circulation* 42:455, 1970
73. Weissler AM, Harris WS, Schoenfeld CD: Bedside technics for the evaluation of ventricular function in man. *Am J Cardiol* 23:577, 1969
74. Stack RS, Sohn YH, Weissler AM: Accuracy of systolic time intervals in detecting abnormal left ventricular performance in coronary artery disease. *Am J Cardiol* 47:603, 1981
75. Boudoulas H, Lewis RP, Dervenagas S, Fontana ME, Vasko JS: Abbreviation of systolic time interval in acute mitral regurgitation: Effect of prosthetic mitral valve replacement. *Am J Cardiol* 44:595, 1979
76. Wanderman KL, Goldberg MJ, Stack RS, Weissler AM: Left ventricular performance in mitral regurgitation assessed with systolic time intervals and echocardiography. *Am J Cardiol* 38:831, 1976
77. Shaver JA, O'Toole JD: The second heart sound: Newer concepts. *Mod Concepts Cardiovasc Dis* 46:7, 1977
78. Spooner EW, Perry BL, Stern AM, Sigmann JM: Estimation of pulmonary/systemic resistance ratios from echocardiographic systolic time intervals in young patients with congenital or acquired heart disease. *Am J Cardiol* 42:810, 1978

Part III

Radioisotopic Examination of the Heart

Chapter 7

Radionuclide Ventriculography

Marvin A. Konstam and Joshua Wynne

Radionuclide ventriculography provides dynamic visualization of the cardiac chambers by detection of gamma radiation emanating from the blood pool. Some authors prefer the broader term blood pool scanning or radionuclide cineangiography, since the technique permits visualization of the atria and great vessels as well as the left and right ventricles. It is conceptually similar to routine contrast angiography in that an intravascular indicator, in this case a radioactive one, is used to identify the interior of the heart in a manner analogous to the use of an iodinated contrast agent for radiographic angiography. Radionuclide ventriculography became possible as a result of several technologic advances in the late 1960s and early 1970s. These include development of (1) the gamma (Anger) scintillation camera, permitting rapid formation of high-resolution images from emitted gamma radiation [1]; (2) imaging agents such as technetium-99m–human serum albumin, and in vivo labeled technetium-99m–red blood cells, permitting adequate visualization of the blood pool [2]; and (3) electrocardiographic gating and computer systems with which formation of the nuclear image could be linked to the cardiac cycle and the resulting data manipulated and analyzed.

The applications of radionuclide ventriculography continue to be defined, and presently include the following:

1. Assessment of resting global and regional left ventricular systolic function
2. Assessment of the capacity for augmentation of global and regional left ventricular systolic function with exercise
3. Assessment of resting right ventricular systolic function
4. Assessment of the capacity for augmentation of right ventricular systolic function with exercise
5. Measurement of left ventricular volumes
6. Identification of configurational abnormalities of the left ventricle, particularly ventricular aneurysms
7. Evaluation of aortic and mitral regurgitation

Radionuclide ventriculography offers several advantages over other imaging modalities. Compared to ventriculography using radiographic contrast medium, it is relatively noninvasive, involving only an intravenous injection; whereas contrast ventriculography entails the risks of arterial and left ventricular catheterization. Radionuclide ventriculography carries only the risk resulting from minimal radiation exposure, estimated at 0.15 to 0.30 rads to the whole body for equilibrium-gated scanning using technetium-99m–labeled human serum albumin, compared with up to 3.9 rads for cardiac catheterization and contrast angiography [3, 4]. The administration of contrast medium into the left ventricle is a stimulus to ventricular ectopy and depresses systolic function. It exposes the patient to a high osmotic volume load, the risk of adverse effects on renal function, and potential idiosyncratic reactions.

A single radionuclide ventriculographic study permits evaluation of biventricular function. In addition, if equilibrium-gated scanning is performed, multiple views and repeated images over several hours may be obtained without additional radiation exposure, whereas each additional contrast ventriculogram entails the risks of additional radiation and contrast medium.

Evaluation of global ventricular function by contrast angiography or by two-dimensional echocardiography requires a geometric analysis, which may become invalid with alterations in ventricular configuration. Each contrast angiogram yields only a two-dimensional perspective, and the two-dimensional echocardiogram is limited to examining a single cross-sectional "slice" of the ventricle at any one moment. The radionuclide ventriculogram permits evaluation of global function with a single view, largely free of geometric assumptions.

Disadvantages of the radionuclide ventriculogram are that present imaging techniques do not permit the spatial resolution possible with contrast angiography, and that nuclear studies are not as truly noninvasive as is echocardiography, since there is a small radiation exposure involved.

Techniques

Imaging Instruments

Development of the gamma scintillation camera represented a major breakthrough in the practice of clinical nuclear medicine [1]. At present, the vast majority of nuclear studies are performed using the gamma camera. Previously, nuclear imaging required the use of a rectilinear scanner, a moving device that forms images from multiple "points" on the subject, each point being examined individually by the scanner in a sequential manner. The rectilinear scanner quantifies activity arising from a series of points, line by line, and creates its image by integrating all of the points scanned. The images have relatively poor resolution and require many minutes to acquire, resulting in potential motion artifact and precluding dynamic studies that entail rapidly acquiring a series of images. The gamma camera (Fig. 7-1), a stationary device that detects radiation from the entire organ being studied simultaneously, forms its image by continuous spatial sorting of individual photons. Resolution with the gamma camera is considerably better than with the rectilinear scanner and, depending on the amount of radioactivity present, images may be formed rapidly (e.g., within 10–25 msec), permitting the performance of dynamic studies.

In devices employed for imaging gamma radiation, a sodium iodide scintillation crystal converts the energy from a gamma photon into a scintillation of light. A collimator, situated between the patient and the scintillation crystal, permits imaging with adequate resolution by preventing a gamma photon from reaching any region of the crystal if the photon did not arise from a corresponding region in the patient. The collimator most often used for cardiac imaging is made from a lead plate containing an array of parallel holes that absorb any photon that does not travel in a course approximately parallel to the direction of the holes. Once a photon traverses the collimator and deposits its energy within the crystal, the resulting light scintillation is detected and augmented by an array of photomultiplier tubes that generate three electrical impulses. The intensities of two of the electrical impulses reflect the location of the scintillation and are determined by the relative scintillation intensity detected by each of the photomultiplier tubes. These two electrical impulses dictate the x and y coordinates for placing a single dot (or count) on the radionuclide image. The intensity of the third electrical impulse generated by the array of photomultiplier tubes is proportional to the total scintillation intensity, which is in turn proportional to the energy deposited in the crystal by the gamma photon. A pulse-height analyzer incorporates into the image only those scintillations which reflect a preset range of gamma energies, thereby excluding radiation from extraneous sources and lower-energy scatter.

The gamma camera has the disadvantage of dead time, which is the time required to detect and process a gamma photon, during which no additional photons may be processed. An alternative is the multicrystal scintillation camera, which has an array of individual scintillation crystals, permitting marked reduction of dead time. The multicrystal camera is better suited than the single-crystal gamma camera for single-pass dynamic studies, which require high count-detection rates to achieve optimal temporal resolution.

An increasingly popular alternative detector is a specially collimated nonimaging probe and associated dedicated microprocessor, which can be positioned over the heart in a manner similar to the gamma camera. Dubbed the "nuclear stethoscope," this device is unable to produce images of the heart, but it can measure the counts within the left ventricle with high precision, thus permitting the assessment of functional parameters on a beat-to-beat basis.

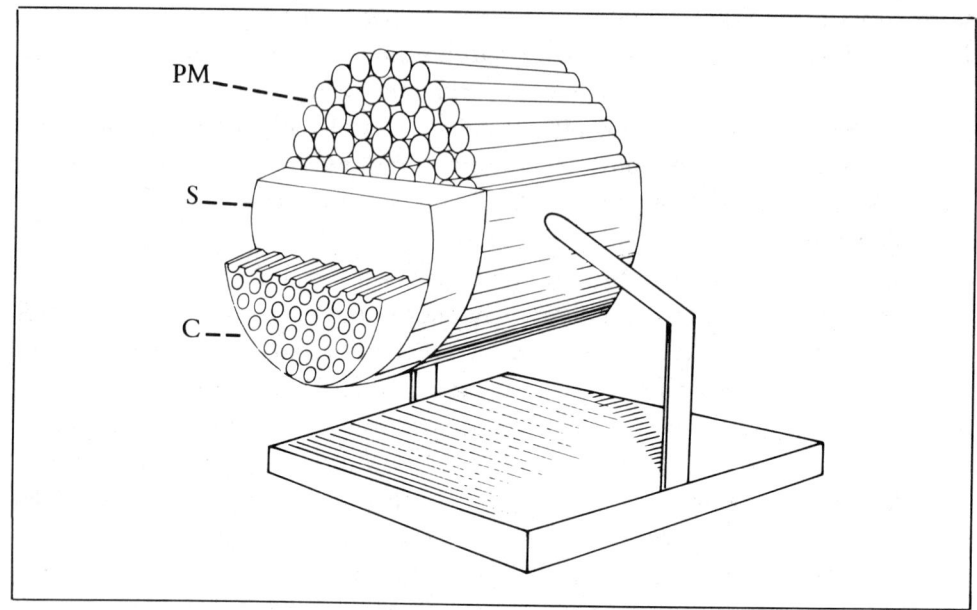

FIGURE 7-1. Schematic representation of a gamma camera. C = collimator, PM = array of photomultiplier tubes, S = sodium iodide scintillation crystal.

TECHNETIUM-99M

Technetium-99m is the isotope used most frequently in cardiac imaging. Its principal gamma energy of 140 keV is sufficiently high to largely escape tissue absorption and sufficiently low to permit a high efficiency of absorption by standard scintillation crystals. Its physical half-life of 6.04 hours is long enough to permit fairly stable concentrations during equilibrium studies and to permit multiple repeated studies over several hours, but is short enough to prevent excessive radiation exposure. It does not emit beta radiation, which would greatly increase radiation exposure. The isotope is a decay product of the more stable molybdenum-99 (half-life 3 days) and is readily available in the form of sodium pertechnetate ($NaTcO_4$) by elution with saline from a molybdenum-technetium column (generator).

METHODS OF RADIONUCLIDE VENTRICULOGRAPHY

There are two basic radionuclide methods by which ventriculography is performed; the first-pass method and the equilibrium-gated method. For the first-pass method [5, 6], a bolus of radiotracer (usually sodium pertechnetate) is injected rapidly into an antecubital fossa vein. Multiple sequential cardiac images (frames) are obtained at a rapid framing rate (e.g., 20 frames/sec) during the initial passage of the radiotracer bolus through the heart and lungs. The imaging device, either a gamma camera or a multicrystal scintillation camera, is interfaced to a computer, where the images are stored on a magnetic disk to permit subsequent analysis.

After completing the study acquisition, the borders of the right and left ventricles may be identified either manually or by computer algorithm, and the computer plots the radioactivity detected within the ventricular "region of interest" against time. The ventricular ejection fraction may be calculated from the sum of activity within several end-systolic frames and the sum of activity within several corresponding end-diastolic frames.

For the second method of radionuclide ventriculography, equilibrium-gated scanning [3], a large stable intravascular concentration of radiotracer must be achieved. For this purpose, technetium-99m may be bound to human serum albumin in vitro or to the patient's red blood cells either in vitro or in vivo [2]. In vivo red blood cell labeling, the usual method, is achieved by intravenously injecting a source of stannous ion (a reducing agent), followed in 20 minutes by technetium-99m–pertechnetate, which binds to red blood cell membranes. The efficiency of labeling is quite high, and the bond is stable over time. After achieving an equilibrium intravascular tracer concentration, a gated cardiac scan is performed by interfacing the gamma camera-computer system to an electrocardiographic monitor, which senses the QRS complex. Each cardiac cycle is divided into a series of segments by the computer, and counts from corresponding segments of multiple heart beats are summated. The result is a study composed of many frames, each frame representing a single segment of the cardiac cycle derived from multiple cycles. In order to separate the two ventricles, a left anterior oblique projection must be used. A 30-degree caudally-tilted slant-hole collimator may be used to maximize separation between the ventricles and the atria and to visualize the left ventricle perpendicular to its long axis. As with the first-pass study, the ventricular ejection fraction is calculated from a time-activity curve, which is generated following identification of the ventricular region of interest (Fig. 7-2).

Both the first-pass method and the equilibrium-gated method of radionuclide ventriculography have advantages:

Advantages of the first-pass method
1. Visualization of the right heart and of the left heart are temporally separated. Ventricular function may be studied in any projection without impairment by overlap of the other ventricle.
2. There is minimal background activity. With the equilibrium-gated method, there is a considerable amount of background activity within the lungs and chest wall. The necessity of estimation and subtraction of background activity is a potential source of error.
3. The study may be completed in under 30 seconds, minimizing artifacts due to patient motion.

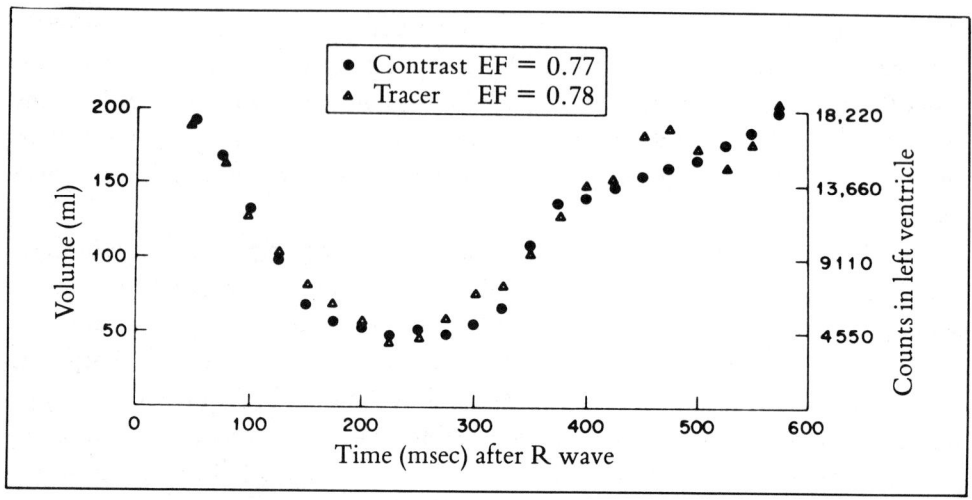

FIGURE 7-2. Left ventricular time-activity curve derived from an equilibrium-gated radionuclide ventriculogram, and time-volume curve derived from a contrast ventriculogram in the same patient. Note the close agreement between the two curves and between the ejection fractions (*EF*) calculated using the two techniques. (From RD Burow et al: Analysis of left ventricular function from multiple gated acquisition cardiac blood pool imaging. *Circulation* 56:1024, 1977, by permission of the American Heart Association, Inc.)

Advantages of the equilibrium-gated method
1. Information from numerous cardiac cycles is integrated. Excessively long or short cycles may be excluded from the study. One or two premature beats may ruin a first-pass study.
2. Time-activity curves comprise a greater number of points, affording greater temporal resolution and facilitating calculation of ejection times and rates as well as ejection fraction.
3. Assessment of regional ventricular function is facilitated by count rates significantly higher than those achieved with the first-pass method.
4. Studies may be repeated frequently over a short time period and without additional radiotracer administration. Multiple views may be obtained.

Evaluation of Left Ventricular Function

GLOBAL FUNCTION

When the frames of the radionuclide ventriculogram, performed either by the first-pass or the equilibrium-gated technique, are viewed in rapid sequence, the resulting radionuclide cineangiogram (Fig. 7-3) is an excellent tool for subjective evaluation of global left ventricular systolic function. In addition, the technique affords an opportunity to objectively evaluate global function from images ob-

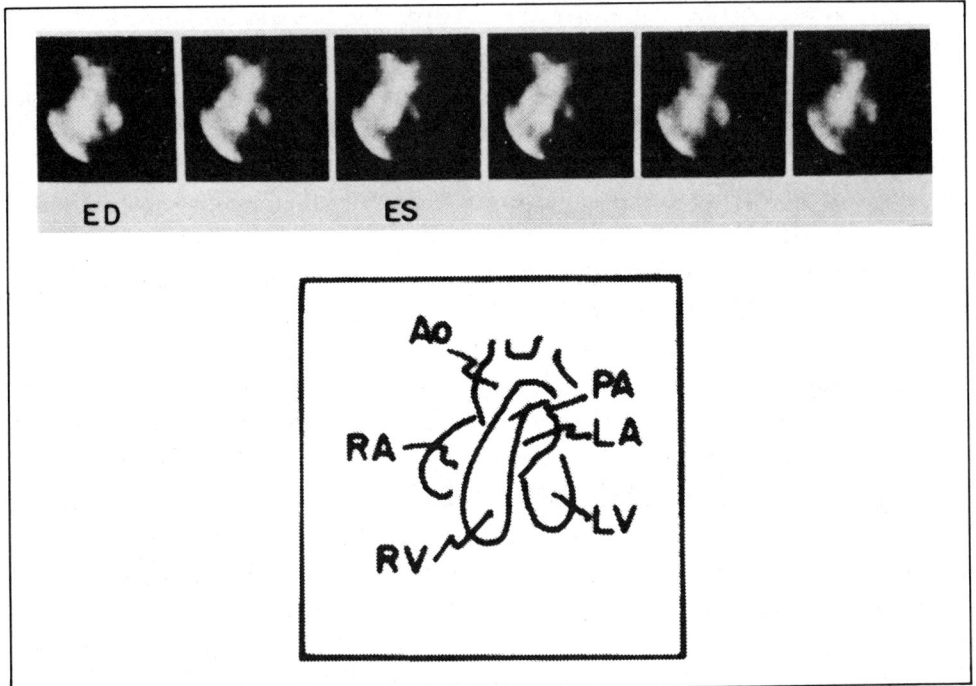

FIGURE 7-3. *Top,* Selected sequential frames from a left anterior oblique equilibrium radionuclide ventriculogram. *Bottom,* Schematic representation of the cardiac chambers and great vessels, as seen in the radionuclide study. *Ao* = aorta, *ED* = end-diastole, *ES* = end-systole, *LA* = left atrium, *LV* = left ventricle, *PA* = pulmonary artery, *RA* = right atrium, *RV* = right ventricle. (Reprinted by permission from JS Borer et al: *N Engl J Med* 296:840, 1977.)

tained in a single projection, since changes in ventricular count rate with time are proportional to changes in intracavitary volume [7, 8]. This relationship between activity and volume permits calculation of objective parameters of systolic function, such as ejection fraction, without resorting to the geometric assumptions needed for interpretation of contrast ventriculograms.

The ejection fraction is the most frequently used indicator of left ventricular systolic function. It is the fraction of the end-diastolic volume ejected during each heart beat. Since it is a *ratio* of volumes, the ejection fraction may be calculated without a knowledge of the absolute end-systolic and end-diastolic volumes. Because count rate is proportional to volume during the cardiac cycle, ejection fraction may be expressed as

$$\text{Ejection fraction} = \frac{\text{end-diastolic activity} - \text{end-systolic activity}}{\text{end-diastolic activity}}$$

Several investigators, using either the first-pass or the equilibrium-gated technique, have found excellent correlation between radionuclide left ventricular ejection fraction and ejection fraction measured at cardiac catheterization by contrast ventriculography [3, 8–11]. In addition, the radionuclide ejection fraction has been shown to be highly reproducible and is, therefore, an ideal parameter for assessing the effect of an intervention such as exercise or drug therapy on left ventricular function [8, 11, 12].

The normal range for resting left ventricular ejection fraction is approximately 0.50 to 0.75 [13–15]. The ejection fraction is an indicator of ventricular systolic function but is influenced not only by intrinsic myocardial contractility, but also by the end-diastolic fiber length (preload) and by systolic wall stress (afterload). As described by the Frank-Starling relation, a modest increase in preload, which is reflected in the intact heart as an increase in left ventricular end-diastolic pressure or volume, results in augmentation of systolic function, reflected by an increased ejection fraction. With an increase in preload beyond a certain end-diastolic pressure, approximately 18 mm Hg in normal humans, ejection fraction increases only minimally and may, in fact, decline. At a constant state of preload and ventricular contractility, an increase in afterload, or systolic wall stress, results in a reduction in ejection fraction. The influence of preload and afterload on the ejection fraction must be considered when interpreting the radionuclide ventriculogram in such disease states as mitral or aortic regurgitation (abnormal preload) and aortic stenosis or systemic hypertension (abnormal afterload).

Absolute left ventricular volumes may be measured by equilibrium-gated radionuclide ventriculography with reasonable accuracy, as indicated by excellent correlation with end-systolic and end-diastolic volumes calculated from contrast ventriculograms [16, 17]. The geometric method for volume measurement, conceptually identical to the method used with contrast ventriculography, entails tracing the border of the left ventricle and calculating the volume based on geometric assumptions and on a knowledge of the relationship between image length and true length. Most often, calculation of ventricular volume by the geometric method is based on the formula for the volume of an ellipsoid

$$\text{Volume} = \frac{4\pi}{3} \times \frac{L}{2} \times \frac{M}{2} \times \frac{N}{2}$$

where L, M, and N are the lengths of the three axes. If a single projection is used, M and N are assumed to be equal. The major disadvantage of the geometric approach is the the assumptions regarding ventricular shape are not always valid, particularly at end-systole and with configurational aberrations, as occur following myocardial infarction and with ventricular aneurysms.

The activity method for volume measurement entails comparing the activity measured within the ventricle at end-systole and end-diastole with the activity measured within a known volume of the patient's blood, drawn at the time of the radionuclide ventriculogram acquisition. After correction for counting efficiency, ventricular volume may be calculated as

$$\text{Volume} = \frac{\text{ventricular activity}}{\text{activity per ml of blood}}$$

Although the activity method has the advantage of not relying on geometric assumptions, error may result from variation in left ventricular counting efficiency due to differences in patient body habitus and in ventricular size and configuration. The need to subtract background from the ventricular region of interest imposes an additional source of error.

The end-diastolic volume is an indicator of the degree of volume loading, or preloading, of the ventricle. End-diastolic volume is enlarged most commonly when there is excessive diastolic filling, as with mitral or aortic regurgitation or ventricular septal defect, or when there is inadequate systolic emptying, as with dilated cardiomyopathy or myocardial infarction.

In recent years, the left ventricular end-systolic volume (indexed for body surface area) has become recognized as an important parameter of ventricular systolic function. Its lack of dependence on preload provides an advantage over ejection fraction in judging ventricular performance, particularly in the presence of valvular regurgitation (see below). The rise in end-systolic volume with increased afterload has led to analysis of the left ventricular end-systolic pressure-volume relation and to calculation of the ratio of peak arterial pressure (measured by cuff) to radionuclide end-systolic volume, as a measure of ventricular contractility independent of preload and incorporating afterload [18, 19]. The equilibrium-gated radionuclide ventriculogram is an excellent means for noninvasively monitoring the end-systolic volume in response to therapeutic agents.

Measurement of left ventricular volumes permits calculation of stroke volume (end-diastolic volume minus end-systolic volume) and left ventricular minute output (stroke volume times heart rate) [20]. Measurement of left ventricular output by the activity method does not require background subtraction, since background cancels out when end-systolic counts are subtracted from end-diastolic counts (assuming background counts remain fairly constant throughout the cardiac cycle). Left ventricular output calculated in this manner has been found to correlate well with cardiac output measured at catheterization by the Fick technique, in the absence of mitral or aortic regurgitation or left-to-right shunt [20]. Noninvasive left ventricular output measurement is of great clinical value, particularly to evaluate the efficacy of pharmacologic therapy in congestive heart failure, where a reduction in cardiac output is a major cause of incapacity and where improvement in cardiac output is a major therapeutic goal.

Since the stroke volume, over time, should be equal from the right and left ventricles, a comparison of biventricular stroke counts may be used to assess valvular regurgitation. Mitral or aortic regurgitation leads to an elevation of the output of the left ventricle, since both forward and regurgitant flow are ejected. By comparing the ratio of stroke counts, additional parameters of left ventricular systolic function that may be measured using radionuclide ventriculography include the first-third ejection fraction (the percent of end-diastolic volume ejection during the first third of systole) [21], systolic time intervals (preejection period, ejection time) [22], mean ejection rate, and peak ejection rate [5, 6, 23]. Left ventricular ejection rate has been found to correlate with ejection fraction. Like the ejection fraction, the mean systolic ejection rate is influenced by change in afterload as well as ventricular contractility, but it is relatively independent of preload and therefore has potential clinical value.

REGIONAL FUNCTION

The radionuclide ventriculogram is an excellent means of evaluating systolic wall motion for individual regions of the left ventricle. Regional wall motion analysis may be performed by examining the motion of left ventricular segments and by comparing the locations of these segments at end-diastole and at end-systole (wall motion method). If this method is used, images in at least two projections must be taken in order to adequately examine segmental motion for the entire ventricle. The ventricular wall may be divided into anterolateral, apical, and inferior segments in the anterior projection and into septal, apical-inferior, and posterior segments in the left anterior oblique projection (Fig. 7-4) [24]. Alternatively, the ventricular cavity may be divided into regions, and the change in counts (indicating the change in blood volume) from end-diastole to end-systole for each region may be determined (counts methods). Analysis by the counts method is facilitated by use of the modified left anterior oblique projection (30-degree caudal tilt) in which the ventricular cavity may be divided into anteroseptal, inferoposterior, and apical regions (Fig. 7-5) [15, 25]. It is more difficult to compare a regional analysis by contrast angiography with an analysis performed by the radionuclide counts method than with one performed by the radionuclide wall motion approach. Regions into which the left ventricular cavity is divided by the counts method do not strictly correspond to segments of the ventricular wall as defined by either contrast angiography or the radionuclide wall motion method. Nevertheless, several studies have shown reasonable correlation between regional wall motion measured by either of the radionuclide methods and by contrast angiography [15, 24].

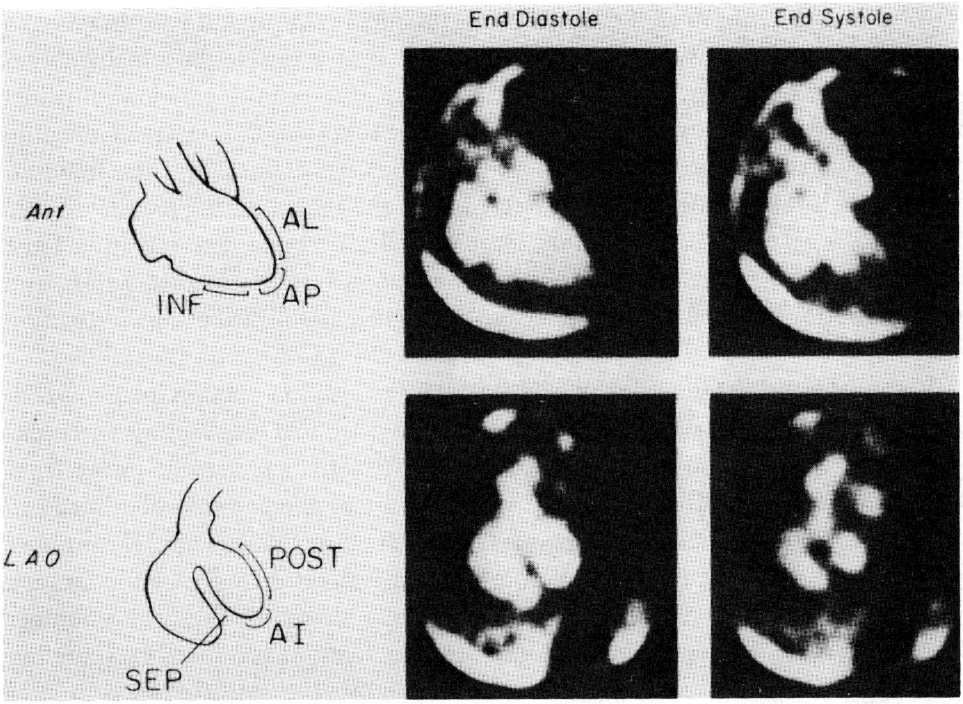

FIGURE 7-4. Anterior (*Ant*) (*top*) and left anterior oblique (*LAO*) (*bottom*) images from an equilibrium-gated radionuclide ventriculogram, with schematic drawings demonstrating regions of the left ventricular wall. *AI* = apical-inferior, *AL* = anterolateral, *AP* = apical, *INF* = inferior, *POST* = posterior, *SEP* = septal. (From [24].)

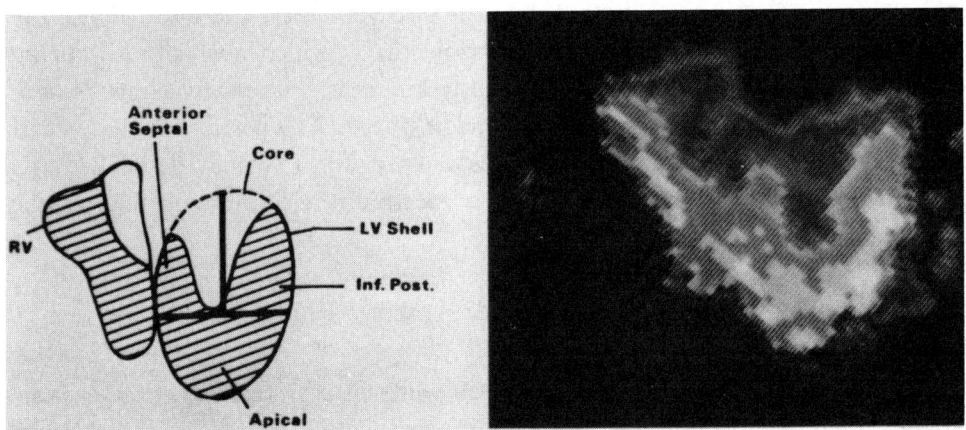

FIGURE 7-5. An ejection fraction image derived from a modified left anterior oblique radionuclide ventriculogram with schematic drawing demonstrating segments of the left ventricular (*LV*) cavity. *Inf Post* = inferoposterior, *RV* = right ventricle. (From [25].)

Motion of a ventricular segment may be classified as normal if it contracts to a normal extent during systole, hypokinetic if its contraction is abnormally abbreviated, akinetic if it fails to contract, or dyskinetic if it expands paradoxically during systole. Using a counts analysis, the systolic function of a ventricular region may be quantified more objectively by measuring the regional ejection fraction, which equals the number of counts ejected from the region during systole divided by the regional end-diastolic counts. A separate background determination must be made for each ventricular region. Normal ranges for anteroseptal, apical, and inferoposterior regional ejection fractions have been established at our institution [15].

Regional ejection fraction may be depicted by an ejection fraction image, which is a computer-generated functional image created by first subtracting the background-corrected counts in each picture element of the end-systolic image from the counts in each corresponding picture element of the end-diastolic image to create a stroke counts image (analogous to stroke volume) [25]. Then, the number of stroke volume counts in each picture element is divided by the counts in each corresponding picture element of the end-diastolic image. The resulting number for each picture element represents the ejection fraction for the corresponding small region of the left ventricular cavity. Each number is translated by computer into a corresponding light intensity or color in order to generate a picture from which regional ejection fraction may be analyzed by inspection (Fig. 7-5).

A dyskinetic segment may be identified by inspection of a paradox image, which is generated by computer subtraction of the end-diastolic image from the end-systolic image (Fig. 7-6) [26]. Normally, the paradox image should be dark (indicating the absence of paradox) over the two ventricles, and light (indicating an increase in counts) over the left and right atria, which normally fill during ventricular systole. A region of ventricular dyskinesis is indicated by a light region, signifying systolic expansion, on the paradox image. The paradox image is particularly well suited to identify a ventricular aneurysm that may be defined as a discrete area of dyskinesis surrounded by myocardium with more normal systolic motion.

Abnormalities of the Left Ventricle: Resting Function
Myocardial Infarction

As discussed above, a reduction in global left ventricular systolic function, as indicated by a reduced ejection fraction, may occur as a result of reduced contractility due to myocardial disease or due to an increase in afterload. The most common cause of a reduced ejection fraction is diminished contractility due to recent or old myocardial infarction. During myocardial infarction, a reduction in myocardial blood supply to a level insufficient to meet myocardial oxygen demands results in

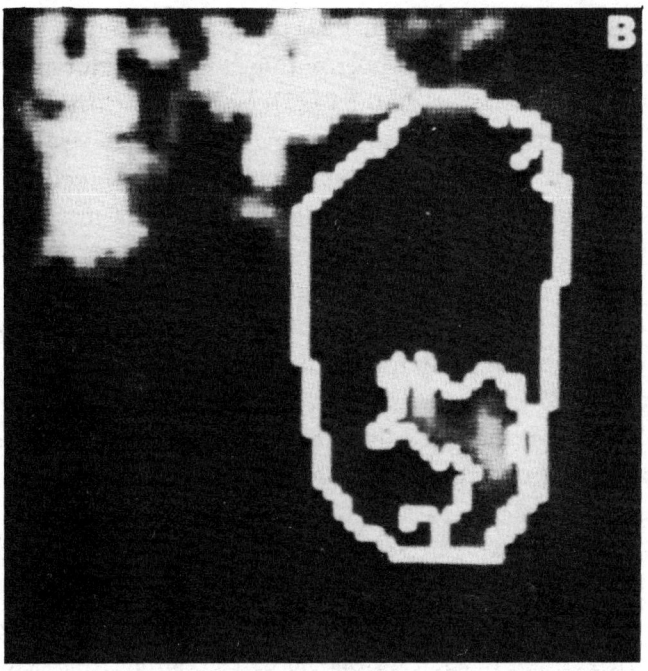

FIGURE 7-6. A paradox image derived from a modified left anterior oblique radionuclide ventriculogram. The light region within the left ventricle represents a localized area of inferoapical dyskinesis. (From [26].)

necrosis of myocardial cells and ischemia of cells in a surrounding zone (border zone). Both the total loss of contractile function of the necrotic cells and the diminution in contractile function of the cells within the border zone contribute to the decline in global systolic function. Depending on the relationship between blood supply and metabolic demand during the hours and days following the initial acute infarction, variable portions of the border zone will become necrotic, will remain ischemic, or will recover completely. The relative sizes of the fractions of the border zone with each of these three fates influences the ultimate effect of the myocardial infarction on global ventricular performance. Aside from the mere reduction in contractile capacity due to infarction, additional reduction in global ejection fraction may eventually result from ventricular wall thinning leading to a localized increase in myocardial compliance (following an initial decrease in compliance). A portion of the contractile effort of the remaining viable myocardium may serve to paradoxically expand the infarcted zone, thus diminishing forward flow and ejection fraction.

When studied within 24 hours of a first myocardial infarction, the majority of patients have a decreased left ventricular ejection fraction. In one study, 96 percent of patients with acute anterior and 61 percent with acute inferior myocardial infarction had ejection fractions less than 0.54 [27]. Some investigators have found the first-third ejection fraction to be more sensitive than the standard ejection fraction for detecting left ventricular dysfunction, observing a reduction in first-third ejection fraction (less than 0.25) in all patients with acute myocardial infarction [21].

The extent and location of infarction may be delineated by radionuclide ventriculography (Fig. 7-7). Using a count analysis method for studying regional ejection fraction, we found that following an initial myocardial infarction, left ventricular wall motion abnormality frequently extended beyond the region of expected involvement as indicated by electrocardiography [28]. This discrepancy between impairment of systolic function and electrocardiographic abnormality was particularly apparent in patients wtih anterior infarction and with severe pump failure and may be explained either by electrocardiographic underestimation of the extent of infarction or by ongoing ischemia in noninfarcted zones.

The radionuclide ventriculogram is frequently useful in guiding therapy for severe left ventricular failure and cardiogenic shock complicating acute myocardial infarction. Cardiogenic shock may be caused by a specific mechanical abnormality such as disruption of the ventricular septum causing left-to-right shunting, and left ventricular volume overload as may be seen with rupture of a papillary muscle causing severe mitral regurgitation. If left ventricular systolic function, as judged by radionuclide ventriculography, is relatively preserved in the presence of cardiogenic shock, the diagnoses of acute ventricular septal defect or papillary muscle rupture should be considered. Furthermore, these lesions may be quantified by comparing left and right ventricular stroke volumes (see p. 183). The detection of severe left ventricular dysfunction decreases the likelihood that ventricular septal defect or mitral regurgitation is contributing substantially to the patient's condition or that the patient will benefit from emergency surgery. As will be discussed later, an additional cause of cardiogenic shock that may be diagnosed by radionuclide ventriculography in severe right ventricular infarction (see p. 187). Radionuclide indexes of ventricular function may be followed as a means of monitoring the efficacy of medical therapy, such as vasodilator administration, in cardiogenic shock.

Radionuclide ventriculography has been used as a prognostic indicator following myocardial infarction. A markedly reduced left ventricular ejection fraction immediately after a first myocardial infarction is associated with a high early mortality. One study showed 55 percent mortality in patients with ejection fractions less than 0.30, as opposed to only one in-hospital death among 45 patients with

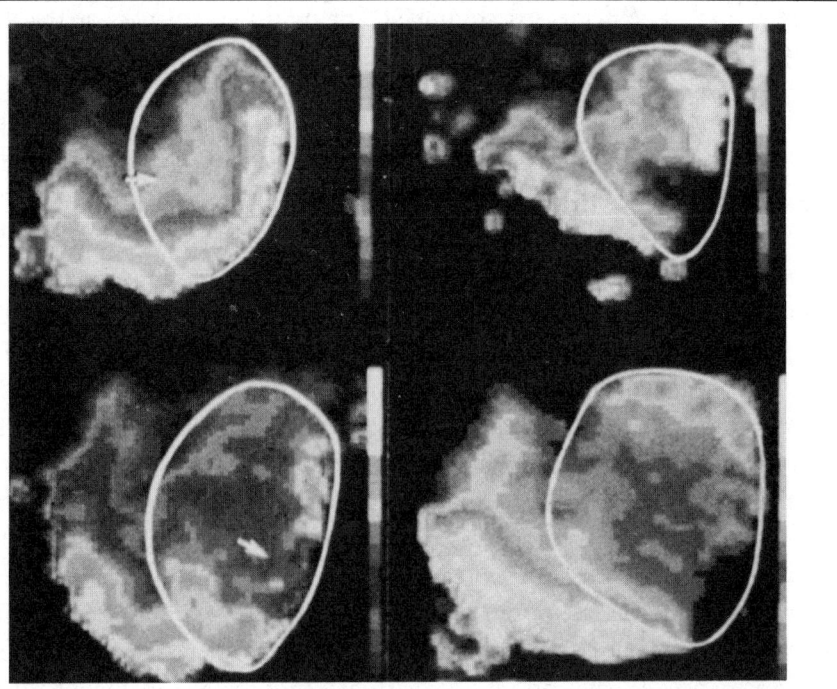

FIGURE 7-7. Ejection fraction images derived from modified left anterior oblique radionuclide ventriculograms in four patients showing various left ventricular wall motion abnormalities due to myocardial infarction. *Top left,* Anteroseptal hypokinesis (*arrow*); *top right,* apical akinesis and anteroseptal hypokinesis (dark region); *bottom left,* inferoapical hypokinesis (*arrow*); *bottom right,* diffuse abnormality (dark region). From [25].)

ejection fractions greater than 0.30 [21]. Patients with an abnormal ejection fraction have a lower one-year survival rate and a higher incidence of congestive heart failure than patients with ejection fractions in the normal range [21]. The higher mortality in patients with reduced ejection fractions probably represents a combination of greater loss of viable myocardium and larger areas of ongoing ischemia compared to patients with higher ejection fractions.

CONGESTIVE HEART FAILURE

Symptoms of congestive heart failure, including paroxysmal nocturnal dyspnea and orthopnea, may be caused by a variety of etiologies but typically result from a single mechanism: elevation of the pulmonary venous and therefore the pulmonary capillary pressures. The two major causes of elevated left heart filling pressures (in the absence of mitral stenosis) are systolic dysfunction with impaired efficiency of the pumping ability of the heart, and diastolic dysfunction with increased stiffness of the left ventricular wall, requiring a higher pressure to achieve adequate filling. The decreased compliance or increased stiffness of the ventricle typically results from increased myocardial wall thickness due to hypertrophy or infiltration. The radionuclide ventriculogram can substantially contribute to the differentiation between the various causes of pulmonary congestion, thereby aiding in designing a course of therapy and in determining prognosis.

The radionuclide ventriculogram in a patient with systolic dysfunction and pump failure reveals enlargement of the left ventricle during diastole and systole, with reduction of systolic wall motion (Fig. 7-8). These abnormalities may be quantified by measuring left ventricular end-diastolic and end-systolic volumes, ejection fraction, and other parameters of systolic function. The most common cause of depression of left ventricular contractile performance is coronary artery disease in which one or more previous myocardial infarctions has resulted in large areas of left ventricular scarring. Left ventricular systolic dysfunction may also be of hypertensive, inflammatory, toxic, or metabolic etiologies, or may be idiopathic. A similar condition may result from left ventricular damage due to chronic volume overload from aortic regurgitation or mitral regurgitation.

The radionuclide ventriculogram can often aid in differentiating left ventricular dysfunction due to prior myocardial infarctions from other forms of impaired systolic performance. In the case of coronary artery disease, ventricular function is not usually uniformly depressed. Abnormal function is limited to regions of infarction, where systolic wall motion may be diminished (hypokinetic), absent (akinetic), or paradoxical (dyskinetic). In some patients, a ventricular aneurysm may be detected, an observation which is facilitated by examination of the paradox image [26]. Noninfarcted areas may be hyperkinetic as a compensatory mechanism. A common pattern in the presence of multiple infarctions is a large confluent zone of abnormal wall motion with normal (or hypercontractile) motion present only in the basilar portion of the left ventricle, i.e., a circumferential zone adjacent to the aortic and mitral valves. The basilar region is least vulnerable to infarction, since it derives its blood supply from proximal branches of the coronary arteries. On the other hand, most other causes of pump dysfunction besides coronary artery disease tend to uniformly depress left ventricular systolic function.

In those cases where the ventricle is abnormally stiff, systolic function is typically preserved. Hypertrophic cardiomyopathy is one such disease whose hallmark is abnormal diastolic behavior. It is an idiopathic, often familial, disease that results in abnormal left ventricular hypertrophy, often preferentially involving the septum. Ventricular wall thickness becomes excessive and, if the abnormality involves the subaortic aspect of the ventricular septum, obstruction to ventricular outflow may occur ("idiopathic hypertrophic subaortic stenosis"). Diminished diastolic compliance due to myocardial hypertrophy results in elevation of left

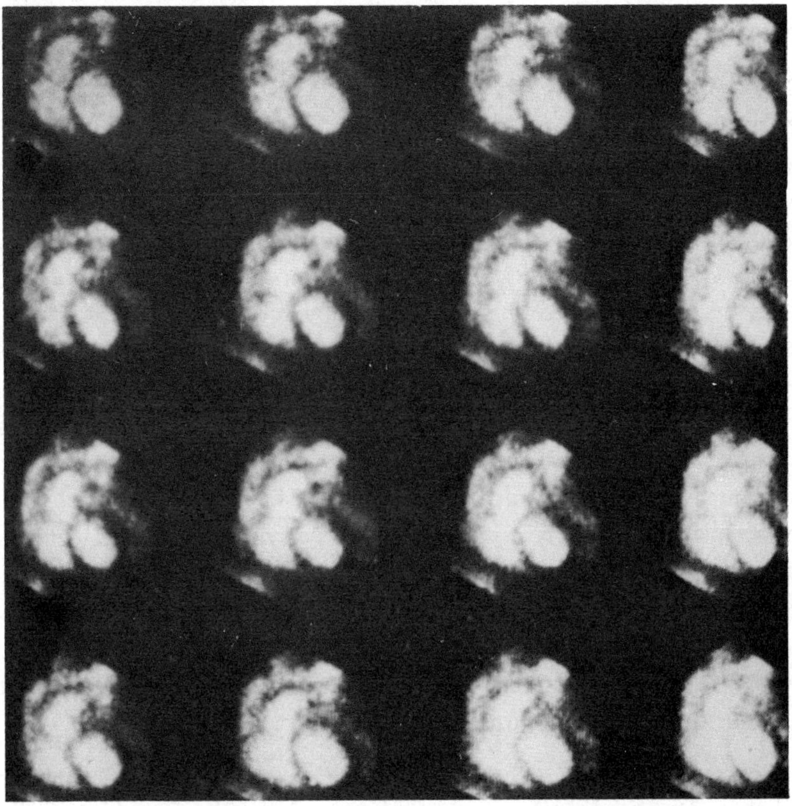

FIGURE 7-8. Sequential frames from a left anterior oblique equilibrium-gated radionuclide ventriculogram in a patient with the dilated form of cardiomyopathy. Note the left ventricular dilatation and global reduction in systolic wall motion. (From RD Burow et al: Analysis of left ventricular function from multiple gated acquisition cardiac blood pool imaging. *Circulation* 56:1024, 1977, by permission of the American Heart Association, Inc.)

ventricular end-diastolic pressure and symptoms of congestive heart failure. Radionuclide ventriculography usually demonstrates a normal or supernormal (hyperkinetic) left ventricular ejection fraction. The area of hypertrophy may be identified as a thickened, count-deficient zone, most often in the region of the ventricular septum. Restrictive cardiomyopathy occurs in disorders such as amyloidosis and hemochromatosis, where infiltration of the myocardium results in impairment of both right and left ventricular filling. The diagnosis should be suspected when there is evidence of congestive heart failure, particularly with predominance of right ventricular failure, in the presence of normal biventricular systolic function as demonstrated by radionuclide ventriculography. Restrictive cardiomyopathy may be difficult to differentiate from constrictive pericarditis, even with cardiac catheterization.

ABNORMAL AFTERLOAD

Left ventricular systolic function, as measured by the radionuclide ejection fraction, may be impaired by abnormally high afterload in the presence of normal intrinsic myocardial contractility. Afterload, or systolic wall stress, is proportional to ventricular systolic pressure and to internal ventricular systolic dimension and is inversely related to wall thickness. Causes of increased left ventricular afterload include systemic hypertension, valvular, subvalvular, or supravalvular aortic stenosis, and coarctation of the aorta. In the presence of compensatory left ventricular hypertrophy, these conditions may not result in impairment of systolic function, since wall stress will remain normal despite abnormally high systolic pressure. The radionuclide ventriculogram demonstrates normal or hyperkinetic left ventricular wall motion, although there may be localized apical hypokinesis. Left ventricular hypertrophy can be detected as a symmetric count-deficient band surrounding the left ventricular cavity. If ventricular hypertrophy is minimal or absent, an elevated systolic pressure results in elevation of systolic wall stress and depression of systolic ejection. In the latter circumstance, the radionuclide ventriculogram will demonstrate global symmetric reduction in left ventricular systolic wall motion and a diminished ejection fraction.

INCREASED SYSTOLIC FUNCTION

There are several causes of increased left ventricular systolic function. Left ventricular contractility is augmented in hypermetabolic states such as hyperthermia and thyrotoxicosis. A similar effect on left ventricular function is seen in the presence of increased catecholamine stimulation as in pheochromocytoma or, more commonly, where catecholamine release is secondary to diminished peripheral oxygen delivery, as in hypoxemia, anemia, or hypovolemia. These conditions are manifested on radionuclide ventriculography by increased left ventricular ejection fraction and ejection rate, decreased end-systolic volume, and normal or decreased end-diastolic volume. Left ventricular minute output is increased except in hypovolemia, where a reduction in cardiac output is the cause of depressed peripheral oxygenation. As noted above, left ventricular contractility, and therefore radionuclide ejection fraction, is also often increased in aortic stenosis when sufficient compensatory ventricular hypertrophy is present, and in many cases of hypertrophic cardiomyopathy. These conditions may be associated with markedly reduced left ventricular end-systolic volumes, often with near obliteration of the ventricular cavity.

Increased left ventricular systolic function may also result from abnormally high preload in the presence of normal ventricular contractility. The most common examples are compensated aortic and mitral regurgitation, in which end-diastolic volume is increased, end-systolic volume is normal, and ejection fraction, stroke volume, and left ventricular output are all increased. Mitral or aortic regurgitation may be diagnosed and quantified by radionuclide ventriculography by calculating the ratio of left ventricular to right ventricular stroke volume counts [29–31]. In the absence of pulmonary or tricuspid regurgitation or intracardiac shunt, right ventricular stroke volume equals forward cardiac output per heart beat. Therefore, the ratio of left to right ventricular stroke volume counts is the same as the ratio of left ventricular stroke volume to forward stroke volume. This ratio is normally unity and increases with increasing severity of valvular regurgitation. The stroke counts ratio has been found to correlate with severity of regurgitation on contrast angiography and with regurgitant fraction, calculated at catheterization from cardiac output and angiographic data. In the presence of right ventricular volume overload, such as with tricuspid regurgitation or atrial septal defect, the stroke counts ratio is misleading in grading left-sided valvular regurgitation, since in these cases right ventricular stroke volume exceeds forward stroke volume. When tricuspid or pulmonic regurgitation is present, left-sided regurgitation may be graded by calculating the ratio of radionuclide left ventricular minute output to forward cardiac output, measured at right heart catheterization by the Fick or indicator-dilution method [20]. Neither of these methods involving radionuclide ventriculography can distinguish mitral from aortic regurgitation, and, in the presence of both lesions, neither method can determine which is predominant. However, the major lesion can usually be determined clinically, and the radionuclide ventriculogram can often help, since in mitral regurgitation, left atrial enlargement is often seen, and in aortic regurgitation, aortic root dilatation may be identified.

Abnormalities of the Left Ventricle: Exercise Studies

The radionuclide ventriculogram is an excellent tool for studying the effect of exercise on global and regional left ventricular function. In coronary artery disease, the resting radionuclide ventriculogram will demonstrate an abnormality of systolic function only in the presence of a recent or old myocardial infarction or with ischemia at rest. However, with exercise, radionuclide ventriculography will identify stress-induced ischemic impairment of systolic function, which may be used as a means of diagnosing coronary artery disease.

The normal left ventricular response to exercise is an augmentation of contractility, resulting in a decrease in end-systolic volume, and increases in stroke volume and ejection fraction [13, 14, 32, 33]. The expected change in ejection fraction with exercise in normals is an increase of 5 percent (ejection fraction units). Older patients (over the age of 60) often demonstrate a blunted ejection fraction response to exercise, even in the absence of demonstrable coronary artery disease; this may relate more to a property of aging rather than any particular disease state. In patients with exertional myocardial ischemia, reduction in the luminal diameter of a coronary artery by an atherosclerotic lesion does not significantly reduce myocardial blood flow at rest. During exercise, the increases in heart rate, blood pressure, and contractility cause a rise in myocardial oxygen requirement, which is normally met by a substantial rise in coronary blood flow. In the presence of a hemodynamically significant coronary lesion, blood flow to the region of myocardium served by that vessel fails to increase sufficiently, causing an imbalance between myocardial oxygen supply and demand, and ischemia results. In the ischemic zone, contractility cannot rise further in response to exercise and generally falls. The resulting depression or absence of systolic wall motion can be discerned on the radionuclide ventriculogram and is reflected by a reduction in regional and global left ventricular ejection fraction [13, 14, 34] (Fig. 7-9).

After performing a baseline rest study, the patient is generally exercised using a bicycle ergometer in the supine or sitting position, with stepwise increases in the level of stress. Exercise may be terminated when the patient becomes fatigued or dyspneic or when significant ischemia occurs as indicated by angina, electrocardiographic changes, or a fall in systolic blood pressure. An additional indication for termination of exercise is the appearance of malignant arrhythmias. A patient is said to have exercised adequately if he or she achieves a heart rate equal to at least 85 percent of the maximal heart rate predicted at his or her age. The radionuclide ventriculogram is repeated during peak exertion.

Several studies have demonstrated exercise radionuclide ventriculography to be superior to conventional exercise testing using electrocardiographic monitoring in diagnosing coronary artery disease [13, 35–37], although sensitivity and specificity for each test varies depending on criteria for positivity and the composition of the study population. Of 42 patients with ≥50 percent stenosis of at least one coronary artery, Borer et al found that with exercise, 62 percent developed diagnostic electrocardiographic changes, but 95 percent developed regional left ventricular dysfunction, as demonstrated by radionuclide ventriculography [35]. Of 21 patients with chest pain but normal coronary arteries documented at catheterization, none had regional dysfunction and all had increased global ejection fraction with exercise. Bodenheimer et al found 58 percent sensitivity for exercise electrocardiography, compared with 82 percent for exercise radionuclide ventriculography in 56 patients with ≥75 percent stenosis of at least one coronary artery [36]. In 19 patients with chest pain and normal coronary arteries, specificity was 84 percent for exercise electrocardiography and 79 percent for exercise radionuclide ventriculography.

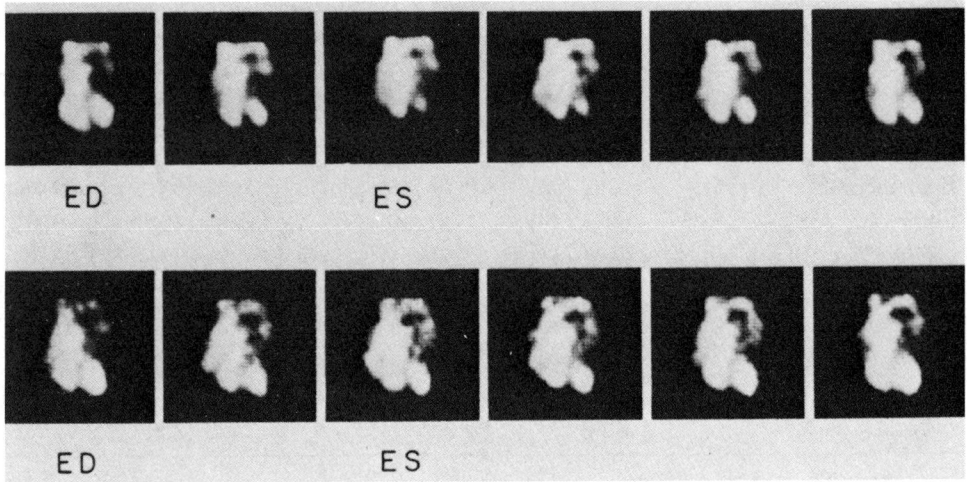

FIGURE 7-9. Selected sequential frames from left anterior oblique equilibrium-gated radionuclide ventriculograms performed at rest (*top*) and during maximal supine bicycle exercise (*bottom*) in a patient with triple-vessel coronary artery disease. At rest, left ventricular function is normal. With the development of myocardial ischemia during exercise there is a marked global reduction in systolic wall motion. ED = end-diastole, ES = end-systole. (Reprinted with permission from JS Borer et al: *N Engl J Med* 296:840, 1977.)

With increasing severity of coronary disease, there is likely to be an increase in the sensitivity of the exercise radionuclide ventriculogram. However, there is evidence that the advantage in sensitivity of the radionuclide study, as compared with exercise electrocardiography, is more marked with single- or double-vessel disease than with more severe involvement [36]. It is uncertain whether exercise radionuclide ventriculography is as sensitive in patients who do not achieve an adequate heart rate and stop because of fatigue as it is in patients who exercise maximally and stop because of angina [13, 35].

Whereas the radionuclide ventriculogram can diagnose coronary artery disease by identifying a functional effect of ischemia (i.e., exercise-induced abnormal systolic wall motion), perfusion scanning using thallium-201 directly analyzes the distribution of myocardial blood flow. Several studies have compared the accuracy of these two imaging techniques [36–43]. Okada et al reviewed data from seven prior studies and concluded that exercise radionuclide ventriculography and thallium-201 imaging have similar sensitivities for detection of coronary disease, but that thallium-201 scanning is more specific [44] (Table 7-1). However, the specificity of radionuclide ventriculography improves if an exercise-induced abnormality in regional wall motion is accepted as a necessary criterion for the diagnosis of coronary disease. Furthermore, Jengo et al found that the exercise radionuclide

TABLE 7-1. Comparison Between Exercise Radionuclide Ventriculography and Thallium-201 Imaging in Coronary Artery Disease

Study	Radionuclide Ventriculography		Thallium-201 Imaging	
	Sens (n)	Spec (n)	Sens (n)	Spec (n)
Bodenheimer et al [36]	0.82 (56)	0.79 (19)	0.82 (56)	0.89 (19)
Borer et al [38]	0.93 (43)	1.00 (10)	0.81 (43)	0.90 (10)
Caldwell et al [39]	0.94 (33)	0.67 (6)	0.91 (33)	1.00 (6)
Johnstone et al [43]	0.77 (26)	1.00 (7)	0.69 (26)	1.00 (7)
Kirshenbaum et al [40]	0.76 (50)	0.55 (11)	0.86 (50)	0.91 (11)
Massie et al [37]	1.00 (10)	1.00 (6)	0.80 (10)	1.00 (6)
Verani et al [41]	0.52 (21)	0.94 (17)	0.81 (21)	1.00 (17)
Total	0.82 (239)	0.84 (76)	0.82 (239)	0.95 (76)

Sens = sensitivity, Spec = specificity.
Adapted from Okada et al: *Am J Cardiol* 46:1188, 1980.

ventriculogram was superior in sensitivity to the thallium-201 scan for detecting significant additional coronary disease in the presence of prior myocardial infarction [42]. Radionuclide ventriculography has the additional advantage that abnormalities are more readily quantified than with thallium-201 scanning, since with the former, the effect of exercise on regional ejection fraction may be measured. When exercise electrocardiography, radionuclide ventriculography, and thallium-201 perfusion imaging are used in some combination, with an abnormality in any one test accepted as indicating coronary disease, the sensitivity increases. Nearly 100 percent of patients with coronary lesions are detected when all three tests are used [36]. However, the use of a combination of these tests markedly decreases specificity.

Considering the expense of an exercise radionuclide study and the small, but present, radiation exposure, it is probably not reasonable to use radionuclide ventriculography as the *initial* diagnostic test in evaluating patients with possible coronary artery disease. This role is more appropriately played by conventional exercise electrocardiography. Becker suggests the following indications for exercise radionuclide imaging [45]: (1) an inadequate exercise electrocardiogram due to fatigue, arrhythmia, or lack of sufficient chronotropic response; (2) an uninterpretable stress electrocardiogram due to baseline abnormalities or conduction disturbances; (3) the result of the exercise electrocardiography being markedly contrary to the clinical suspicion, or lack of suspicion, of significant disease.

In the presence of a normal resting study, exercise radionuclide ventriculography may be useful in eliciting abnormalities of myocardial function not due to coronary disease. There is an abnormal left ventricular response to exercise in hypertrophic cardiomyopathy [46] and in ventricular damage due to aortic regurgitation [47], for example.

Right Ventricular Function

The assessment of right ventricular function by any technique poses several special problems. A geometric approach to right ventricular volume analysis either by radionuclide ventriculography or by contrast angiography is hampered by the complexity of right ventricular geometry and by the coarse trabeculation of the chamber. There is, therefore, a significant advantage in measuring the ejection fraction by radionuclide ventriculography from end-diastolic and end-systolic activity, as described earlier for the left ventricle. Right ventricular function was initially assessed by the first-pass method [48, 49]. Since this method results in temporal separation between visualization of the left and right ventricles, the study may be performed in the right anterior oblique projection, which affords maximal separation between the right atrium and right ventricle. Steele et al found reasonable correlation between right ventricular ejection fraction measured by first-pass radionuclide ventriculography and by contrast angiography [48]. If the equilibrium-gated method is used, the modified left anterior oblique projection, using a caudally-tilted slant-hole collimator, yields maximal separation between the right ventricle and both the right atrium and left ventricle. Several studies have shown good correlation between results using this method and the first-pass approach [50–52]. Since normally the right ventricle is larger than the left ventricle and both have the same stroke volumes, the normal ejection fraction is lower for the right than for the left ventricle and has been found to range from approximately 0.45 to 0.60 [48–52].

The radionuclide ventriculogram is useful in diagnosing right ventricular infarction. The right ventricle derives its blood supply from right ventricular branches of the right coronary artery and from the posterior descending branch of either the right (right-dominant) or circumflex (left-dominant) coronary artery. When hemodynamically significant right ventricular infarction occurs, it generally results from proximal disease of a dominant right coronary artery. The syndrome of severe right ventricular infarction has been described in the setting of acute infarction of the left ventricular inferior wall and may be characterized clinically by shock, distended jugular veins, and clear lung fields. The radionuclide ventriculogram demonstrates marked dilatation of the right ventricle with severely reduced systolic wall motion and ejection fraction. Systolic motion may be preserved in the basilar or outflow portion of the right ventricle, where the blood supply is usually not compromised. Global left ventricular function is often not severely depressed, although dysfunction of the inferior and posterior segments is the rule. Treatment generally consists of fluid administration, which is best guided by monitoring the pulmonary capillary wedge pressure. The use of radionuclide ventriculography has also uncovered lesser degrees of right ventricular dysfunction in the setting of acute myocardial infarction. Reduto et al found that 50 percent of patients with acute inferior wall myocardial infarction had subnormal right ventricular ejection fractions [53]. These findings are likely to represent right ventricular infarction rather than dysfunction due to left ventricular failure, since only one of 13 patients with acute anterior infarction had an abnormally low right ventricular ejection fraction. Acute infarct scintigraphy with technetium-99m-pyrophosphate may also be used to diagnose right ventricular infarction by selective uptake of the radiopharmaceutical by the necrotic myocardium of the right ventricle. Unlike radionuclide ventriculography, however, technetium-99m-pyrophosphate scintigraphy is not easily amenable to quantitating the degree of right ventricular infarction.

In the presence of marked left ventricular dysfunction due to coronary artery disease, resting right ventricular function may be predictive of long-term survival. This observation may indicate that right ventricular abnormality reflects particularly severe left ventricular failure or that in the setting of left ventricular disease, additional primary right ventricular abnormality carries a poor prognosis.

Analysis of right ventricular function with exercise may be useful in diagnosing right coronary artery disease. As with the left ventricle, right ventricular ejection fraction normally increases with exercise. Several studies have shown a correlation between the presence of significant proximal right coronary stenosis and abnormal exercise right ventricular function [54, 55]. In one study, however, right ventricular dysfunction appeared to be more closely related to left ventricular dysfunction than to right coronary artery disease [56]. This issue requires further clarification.

Assessment of both resting and exercise right ventricular function by radionuclide ventriculography appears to be helpful in evaluating patients with right ventricular pressure overload, particularly on the basis of obstructive pulmonary disease. Berger et al showed that of 10 patients with clinically evident cor pulmonale, all had depressed resting right ventricular ejection fractions [49]. More importantly, of nine patients with obstructive lung disease and abnormal right ventricular function but without clinical evidence of cor pulmonale, four developed respiratory decompensation and cor pulmonale within one year following study. None of 12 patients with normal right ventricular function developed clinically evident cor pulmonale within one year. Matthay et al demonstrated a correlation between exercise right ventricular function and both pulmonary function and arterial oxygen saturation in obstructive lung disease [57]. Analysis of both resting and exercise right ventricular systolic function may be helpful in monitoring the efficacy of therapeutic intervention in obstructive lung disease. It may also be useful in other causes of right ventricular pressure overload such as valvular and congenital heart disease, pulmonary emboli, and primary pulmonary hypertension.

Assessment of Drug Therapy

Radionuclide ventriculography is an effective means of noninvasively judging the effect of a pharmacologic intervention on ventricular function. Ejection fraction is the most commonly monitored parameter of systolic function, but mean or peak systolic ejection rate, end-systolic volume, stroke volume, and left ventricular output can also be followed. Radionuclide ventriculography is particularly useful in demonstrating the efficacy of inotropic or vasodilatory agents in patients with congestive heart failure, both acutely and chronically. Both classes of drugs have been shown to decrease left ventricular end-systolic volume, increase ejection fraction and increase left ventricular output. It may be possible to establish whether the major mechanism of action of a particular drug is improvement of contractility or reduction of systolic wall stress by examining the drug's effect on the relationship between left ventricular end-systolic volume (measured by radionuclide ventriculography) and peak systolic pressure (measured by blood pressure cuff).

If the clinician is contemplating administering an agent with a potentially negative inotropic effect such as propranolol or disopyramide to a patient with compromised ventricular reserve, radionuclide ventriculography may be performed before and after initiation of therapy in order to detect a reduction in systolic function prior to the clinical appearance of congestive heart failure. Similarly, radionuclide ventriculography may be used to monitor patients at risk of cardiotoxicity due to the antineoplastic agent doxorubicin (Adriamycin). A fall in the left ventricular ejection fraction by at least 15 percent to a final level of ≤ 45 percent appears to identify patients who, while otherwise asymptomatic, are at risk of developing congestive heart failure if doxorubicin is continued [58]. Late cardiotoxicity may be demonstrated by radionuclide ventriculography in over half of asymptomatic patients treated with customary doses of doxorubicin and may persist for years [59].

Exercise radionuclide ventriculography is useful in evaluating the efficacy of a medical program for the treatment of ischemic heart disease. Improvement in peak exercise ventricular function or a decrease in exercise-induced regional wall motion abnormality indicates improvement in the imbalance between myocardial oxygen supply and demand. For example, such an improvement has been demonstrated following administration of a beta-adrenergic blocking agent, which reduces peak exercise heart rate and left ventricular contractility, thereby decreasing myocardial oxygen requirements.

Determining Indications for Surgery

The radionuclide ventriculogram is a valuable tool in determining the advisability of cardiac surgery. Its use in acute myocardial infarction and cardiogenic shock, where papillary muscle rupture or acute ventricular septal defect are possibilities, has already been discussed. Other settings in which the radionuclide ventriculogram can aid with indication for surgery are (1) consideration of revascularization in coronary artery disease; (2) left ventricular aneurysm; and (3) chronic valvular heart disease.

Coronary Bypass Surgery

When coronary artery bypass surgery is being considered, radionuclide ventriculography can add information in several ways. First, the major determinant of operative risk is left ventricular function. In many institutions, the operative mortality for coronary artery bypass surgery in a patient with normal resting left ventricular function is less than 1 to 2 percent. This risk rises precipitously as ventricular systolic function falls. With the radionuclide ventriculogram, the operative risk based on left ventricular function may be determined without subjecting the patient to contrast ventriculography. The potential benefits of proceeding to coronary angiography and to surgery must be weighed against the high potential risks in a patient with coronary disease who has a substantial reduction in the resting left ventricular ejection fraction, generally due to prior infarction. Although in some patients resting ventricular dysfunction may be partly due to ongoing ischemia that potentially could be reversed by revascularization, bypass surgery has not substantially improved resting ventricular function in the majority of such patients.

It is often difficult to determine the physiologic significance of a coronary arterial lesion from the coronary arteriogram alone. Although coronary angiography is considered the gold standard against which other tests to detect coronary lesions are evaluated, it is merely an anatomical study and is limited in its ability to judge the hemodynamic significance of a lesion or the extent of myocardium in jeopardy. Since the exercise radionuclide ventriculogram measures the functional consequence of ischemia, it may be useful in determining the extent of disease or the significance of a coronary lesion. It is therefore potentially complementary to the coronary angiogram in deciding whether or not to surgically bypass a particular coronary lesion. Further studies are needed to evaluate this potentially important use of exercise radionuclide ventriculography.

Ventricular Aneurysm

The presence of a left ventricular aneurysm following myocardial infarction predisposes the patient to (1) congestive heart failure due to loss of myocardium and

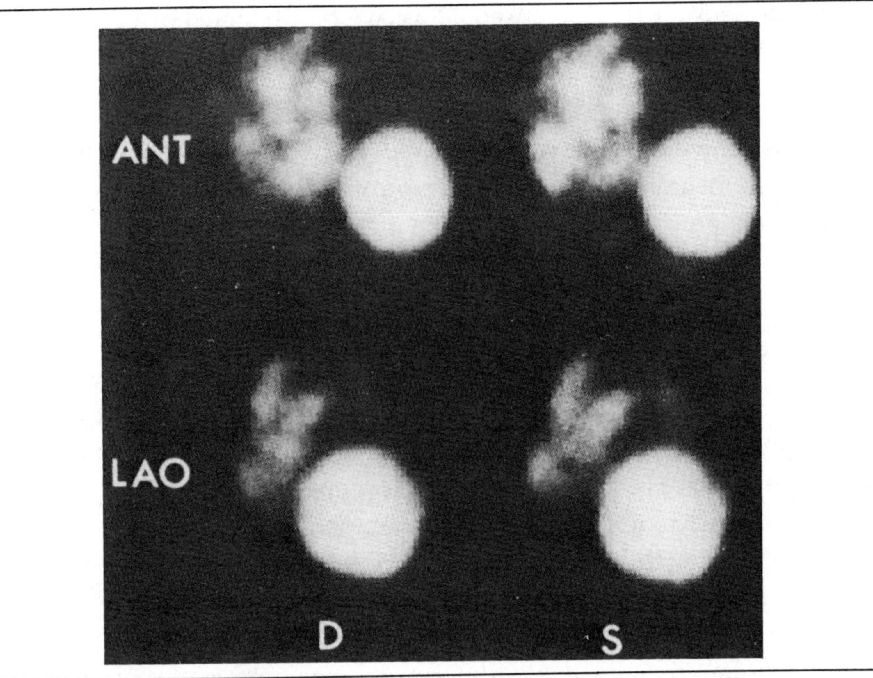

FIGURE 7-10. End-diastolic (*D*) and end-systolic (*S*) frames from anterior (*ANT*) and left anterior oblique (*LAO*) equilibrium-gated radionuclide ventriculograms in a patient with an enormous anterolateral left ventricular aneurysm. (From [61].)

ineffective ejection by the normal myocardium into the dyskinetic aneurysm; (2) systemic embolization due to thrombosis within the aneurysm; and (3) ventricular arrhythmias. A ventricular aneurysm may be diagnosed by radionuclide ventriculography as a discrete area of dyskinesis surrounded by myocardium with more normal systolic motion [60, 61] (Fig. 7-10). As already discussed, the paradox image is particularly useful for identifying ventricular aneurysms [26] (see Fig. 7-6). If an aneurysm is identified in the presence of one of the above complications, consideration may be given to resection. However, several reservations must be stated. There is substantial operative morbidity and mortality for aneurysmectomy. Depending on the extent of the aneurysm and the amount of viable myocardium remaining, there may be difficulty weaning the patient from the cardiopulmonary bypass machine, and postoperatively there may not be substantial improvement in congestive heart failure. With regard to ventricular arrhythmias, resection of the aneurysm may not resolve the problem, and several groups have utilized electrocardiographic mapping techniques to localize the origin of the arrhythmia and to direct the resection. Because of these difficulties, medical management for congestive heart failure, systemic embolization, and ventricular arrhythmias should usually be attempted first, even when an aneurysm is identified by radionuclide ventriculography.

Chronic Valvular Heart Disease

The usefulness of radionuclide ventriculography in determining the optimum time for valve replacement in mitral and aortic regurgitation is being increasingly recognized. As noted previously, because of the increase in preload, well-compensated regurgitant lesions are associated with increased left ventricular systolic function, indicated by increased ejection fraction, stroke volume, and left ventricular output, with an increased end-diastolic volume and normal end-systolic volume. With time, chronic volume overload may lead to gradually increasing ventricular dysfunction. Although the exact timing for surgery remains controversial, it seems reasonable to consider valve replacement when early manifestations of ventricular dysfunction appear, which may be recognized on the radionuclide ventriculogram by normalization of the ejection fraction and an increase in end-systolic volume. It is often useful in this regard to obtain serial studies, since otherwise it may not be recognized that a single ejection fraction within the usual normal limits actually indicates a decline in systolic function of a volume overloaded left ventricle. If surgery is delayed, the abnormality may progress to a grossly cardiomyopathic picture, with markedly elevated end-diastolic and end-systolic volumes and a severely reduced ejection fraction. At this point, operative mortality is extremely high and the potential benefit from surgery is reduced. Exercise radionuclide ventriculography may also be helpful in eliciting abnormalities of ventricular function that may not be evident on a resting study [47].

In aortic stenosis, the radionuclide ventriculogram is less helpful in determining the timing of surgery. Depending on the degree of ventricular hypertrophy, stenosis of a given severity may be associated with varying levels of left ventricular systolic wall stress and therefore may result in varying levels of systolic function ranging from supernormal to severely depressed. With surgical relief of severe aortic stenosis, even a ventricle with a severely reduced ejection fraction is likely to improve [62].

Shunt Scintigraphy

The first-pass method of blood pool imaging may be used to assess the presence, severity, and location of left-to-right cardiac shunts. The radioactive agent is injected in as compact a bolus as is feasible, often by injection into an external jugular vein. The passage of the radioindicator through first the right side of the heart, followed by the lungs and finally the left side is recorded and stored by a gamma camera/computer system. A computer-derived region of interest is placed over the lung, and the computer plots the counts that pass through the region over time. In normal individuals, this pulmonary time-activity curve shows an initial

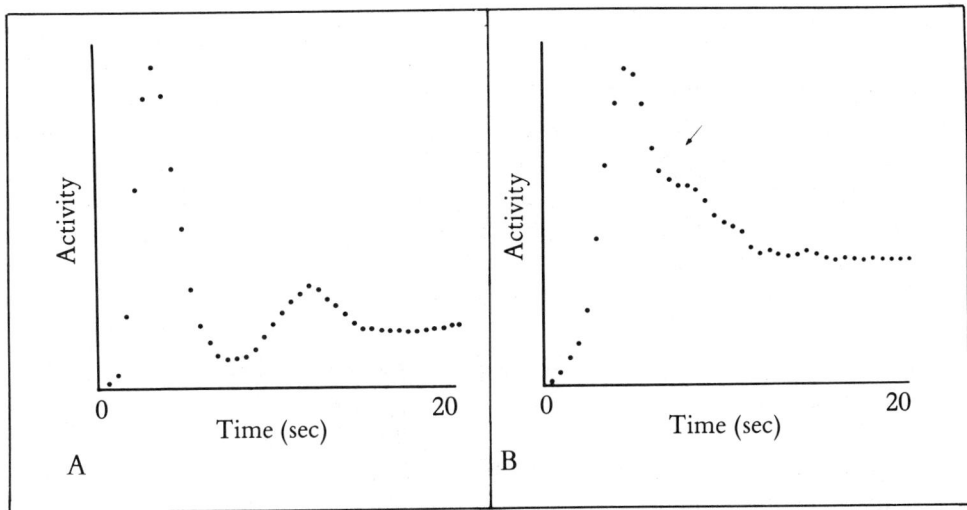

FIGURE 7-11. Pulmonary time-activity curves, which were obtained at 2 frames/sec. (A) Normal curve with taller initial appearance curve and shallower recirculation curve. (B) Curve in left-to-right shunt, with early recirculation (*arrow*). (From SL Treves, JA Parker: Detection and quantification of intracardiac shunts. In HW Strauss, B Pitt (eds): *Cardiovascular Nuclear Medicine*. 2nd ed. St Louis: CV Mosby Co, 1979, pp 148–161.)

peak as the bolus passes through the lungs, to be followed later by a smaller secondary peak due to recirculation as part of the bolus reappears in the lungs after having travelled to the systemic circuit. With a left-to-right shunt, the recirculation curve is abnormally early and unusually prominent, resulting from the early reappearance of radiotracer that took a "short circuit" through the shunt (Fig. 7-11). By computer curve fitting of the pulmonary time-activity curves, it is possible to calculate the ratio of pulmonary-to-systemic blood flow ($\dot{Q}p/\dot{Q}s$), although absolute blood flow cannot be determined directly. Ordinarily, a $\dot{Q}p/\dot{Q}s$ of $\geq 2:1$ is considered an indication for repair of an otherwise uncomplicated intracardiac shunt. Agreement with cardiac catheterization has been excellent, particularly for shunts with $\dot{Q}p/\dot{Q}s$ of 1.2:1.0 to 3.0:1.0 [63]. Determining the level of the shunt is more problematic. By comparing the time-activity curves obtained from over the right atrium, right ventricle, and lungs, it may be possible in some patients to localize the site of the shunt to the chamber just proximal to wherever the abnormal $\dot{Q}p/\dot{Q}s$ ratio first appears.

Technical considerations are critical with shunt scintigraphy, and a poor injection of the radiotracer with fractionation of the bolus may simulate an intracardiac shunt. Severe valvular regurgitation or ventricular dysfunction may also simulate a shunt. On the other hand, a normal shunt study effectively excludes an intracardiac left-to-right shunt of any significance.

References

1. Anger HO: Scintillation camera. *Rev Sci Instrum* 29:23, 1959
2. Pavel DG, Zimmer AM, Patterson VN: In vivo labeling of red blood cells with ^{99m}Tc: A new approach to blood pool visualization. *J Nucl Med* 18:305, 1977
3. Strauss HW, Zaret NL, Hurley PJ, Natarajan TK, Pitt B: A scintiphotographic method for measuring left ventricular ejection fraction in man without cardiac catheterization. *Am J Cardiol* 28:575, 1971
4. Pitt B, Strauss HW: Evaluation of ventricular function by radioisotopic techniques. *N Engl J Med* 296:1097, 1977
5. Marshall RC, Berger HJ, Costin JC, Freedman GS, Wolberg J, Cohen LS, Gottschalk A, Zaret BL: Assessment of cardiac performance with quantitative radionuclide angiocardiography. *Circulation* 56:820, 1977
6. Van Dyke D, Anger HO, Sullivan RW, Velter WR, Yano Y, Parker HG: Cardiac evaluation from radioisotope dynamics. *J Nucl Med* 13:585, 1972
7. Green MV, Ostrow HG, Scott RN, Douglas MA, Bailey JJ, Johnson GS: A comparison of simultaneous measurements of systolic function in the baboon by electromagnetic flowmeter and high frame rate ECG-gated blood pool scintigraphy. *Circulation* 60:312, 1979
8. Burow RD, Strauss HW, Singleton R, Pond M, Rehn T, Bailey IK, Griffith LC, Nickoloff E, Pitt B: Analysis of left ventricular function from multiple gated acquisition cardiac blood pool imaging. Comparison to contrast angiography. *Circulation* 56:1024, 1977
9. Federman J, Brown ML, Tancredi RG, Smith HC, Wilson DB, Becker GP: Multiple-gated acquisition cardiac blood-pool isotope imaging. Evaluation of left ventricular function correlated with contrast angiography. *Mayo Clin Proc* 53:625, 1978
10. Parker JA, Uren RF, Jones AG, Maddox DE, Zimmerman RE, Neill JM, Holman BL: Radionuclide left ventriculography with the slant hole collimator. *J Nucl Med* 18:848, 1977
11. Slutsky R, Karliner J, Battler A, Pfisterer M, Swanson S, Ashburn W: Reproducibility of ejection fraction and ventricular volume by gated radionuclide angiography after myocardial infarction. *Radiology* 132:155, 1979
12. Marshall RC, Berger HJ, Reduto LA, Gottschalk A, Zaret BL: Variability in sequential measures of left ventricular performance assessed with radionuclide angiocardiography. *Am J Cardiol* 41:531, 1978
13. Berger HJ, Reduto LA, Johnstone DE, Borkowski H, Sands JM, Cohen LS, Langou RA, Gottschalk A, Zaret BL, Pytlik L: Global and regional left ventricular response to bicycle exercise in coronary artery disease. Assessment by quantitative radionuclide angiocardiography. *Am J Med* 66:13, 1979
14. Borer JS, Bacharach SL, Green MV, Kent KM, Epstein SE, Johnston GS, Mack B: Real-time radionuclide cineangiography in the noninvasive evaluation of global and regional left ventricular function at rest and during exercise in patients with coronary artery disease. *N Engl J Med* 296:840, 1977

15. Maddox DE, Wynne J, Uren R, Parker JA, Idoine J, Siegel LC, Neill JM, Cohn PF, Holman BL: Regional ejection fraction: A quantitative radionuclide index of regional left ventricular performance. *Circulation* 59:1001, 1979
16. Dehmer GJ, Lewis SE, Hillis LD, Twieg D, Falkoff M, Parkey RW, Willerson JT: Nongeometric determination of left ventricular volumes from equilibrium blood pool scans. *Am J Cardiol* 45:293, 1980
17. Slutsky R, Karliner J, Ricci D, Kaiser R, Pfisterer M, Gordon D, Peterson K, Ashburn W: Left ventricular volumes by gated equilibrium radionuclide angiography: A new method. *Circulation* 60:556, 1979
18. Nivatpumin T, Katz S, Scheuer J: Peak left ventricular systolic pressure/end-systolic volume ratio: A sensitive detector of left ventricular disease. *Am J Cardiol* 43:969, 1979
19. Slutsky R, Karliner J, Gerber K, Battler A, Froelicher V, Gregorates G, Peterson K, Ashburn W: Peak systolic blood pressure/end systolic volume ratio: Assessment at rest and during exercise in normal subjects and patients with coronary heart disease. *Am J Cardiol* 46:813, 1980
20. Konstam MA, Wynne J, Holman BL, Brown EJ, Neill JM, Kozlowski J: Quantitation of left ventricular output in patients with and without left-sided valvular regurgitation using equilibrium (gated) radionuclide ventriculography. *Circulation* 64:578, 1981
21. Battler A, Slutsky R, Karliner J, Froelicher V, Ashburn W, Ross J: Left ventricular ejection fraction early after acute myocardial infarction: Value for predicting mortality and morbidity. *Am J Cardiol* 45:197, 1980
22. Qureshi S, Wagner HN, Alderson PO, Housholder DF, Douglas KH, Lotter MG, Nickoloff EL, Tanabe M, Knowles LG: Evaluation of left-ventricular function in normal persons and patients with heart disease. *J Nucl Med* 19:135, 1978
23. Steele P, Lefree M, Kirch D: Measurement of left ventricular mean circumferential fiber shortening velocity and systolic ejection rate by computerized radionuclide angiocardiography. *Am J Cardiol* 37:388, 1976
24. Okada RD, Pohost GM, Nichols AB, McKusick KA, Strauss HW, Boucher CA, Block PC, Rosenthal SV, Dinsmore RE: Left ventricular regional wall motion assessment by multigated and end-diastolic, end-systolic gated radionuclide left ventriculography. *Am J Cardiol* 45:1211, 1980
25. Maddox DE, Holman BL, Wynne J, Idoine J, Parker JA, Uren R, Neill JM, Cohn PF: Ejection fraction image: A noninvasive index of regional left ventricular wall motion. *Am J Cardiol* 41:1230, 1978
26. Holman BL, Wynne J, Idoine J, Zielonka J, Neill J: The paradox image: A noninvasive index of regional left-ventricular dyskinesis. *J Nucl Med* 20:1237, 1979
27. Shah PK, Pichler M, Berman DS, Singh BN, Swan HJC: Left ventricular ejection fraction determined by radionuclide ventriculography in early stages of first transmural myocardial infarction. Relation to short-term prognosis. *Am J Cardiol* 45:542, 1980
28. Wynne J, Sayres M, Maddox DE, Idoine J, Alpert JS, Neill J, Holman BL: Regional

left ventricular function in acute myocardial infarction: Evaluation with quantitative radionuclide ventriculography. *Am J Cardiol* 45:203, 1980
29. Bough HW, Gandsman AJ, North DL, Shulman RS: Gated radionuclide angiographic evaluation of valve regurgitation. *Am J Cardiol* 46:423, 1980
30. Rigo P, Alderson PO, Robertson RM, Becker LC, Wagner HN: Measurement of aortic and mitral regurgitation by gated cardiac blood pool scans. *Circulation* 60:306, 1979
31. Sorensen SG, O'Rourke RA, Chaudhuri T: Noninvasive quantitation of valvular regurgitation by gated equilibrium radionuclide angiography. *Circulation* 62:1089, 1980
32. Slutsky R, Karliner J, Ricci D, Scheuler M, Pfisterer M, Peterson K, Ashburn W: Response of left ventricular volume to exercise in man assessed by radionuclide equilibrium angiography. *Circulation* 60:565, 1979
33. Rerych SK, Scholz PM, Sabiston DC, Jones RH: Effects of exercise training on left ventricular function in normal subjects: A longitudinal study by radionuclide angiography. *Am J Cardiol* 45:244, 1980
34. Pulido JI, Doss J, Twieg D, Blomqvist GC, Faulkner D, Horn V, Debates D, Tobey M, Parkey RW, Willerson JT: Submaximal exercise testing after acute myocardial infarction: Myocardial scintigraphic and electrocardiographic observations. *Am J Cardiol* 42:19, 1978
35. Borer JS, Kent KM, Bacharach SL: Sensitivity, specificity, and predictive accuracy of radionuclide cineangiography during exercise in patients with coronary artery disease. Comparison with exercise electrocardiography. *Circulation* 60:572, 1979
36. Bodenheimer MM, Banka VS, Fooshee CM, Helfant RH: Comparative sensitivity of the exercise electrocardiogram, thallium imaging and stress radionuclide angiography to detect the presence and severity of coronary heart disease. *Circulation* 60:1270, 1979
37. Massie B, Botvinick E, Shames D, Brundage B: Correlation of myocardial perfusion with global and segmental ventricular function during exercise: Increased sensitivity of exercise blood pool scintigraphy for coronary disease. *Am J Cardiol* 43:343, 1979
38. Borer JS, Bacharach SL, Green MV: Sensitivity of stress radionuclide cineangiography and stress thallium perfusion scanning in detecting coronary artery disease. *Am J Cardiol* 43:431, 1979
39. Caldwell J, Sorensen S, Ritchie J, Hamilton G, Kennedy JW: Exercise radionuclide ventriculography and thallium imaging: Comparison of sensitivity and specificity. *Am J Cardiol* 43:432, 1979
40. Kirshenbaum HE, Okada RD, Kushner FG: The relation of global left ventricular function with exercise to thallium-201 exercise scintigrams. *Clin Res* 27:180, 1979
41. Verani MS, Del Ventura L, Meller RR: Radionuclide ventriculograms during dynamic and isometric exercise in coronary artery disease: Comparison with exercise thallium-201 scintigrams. *Clin Res* 27:211, 1979
42. Jengo JA, Freeman R, Brizendine M, Mena I: Detection of coronary artery disease: Comparison of exercise stress radionuclide angiocardiography and thallium stress perfusion scanning. *Am J Cardiol* 45:535, 1980

43. Johnstone DE, Sands JM, Berger HJ, Reduto LA, Lachman AS, Wackers FJT, Cohen LS, Gottschalk A, Zaret BL, Pytlik L: Comparison of exercise radionuclide angiocardiography and thallium-201 myocardial perfusion imaging in coronary artery disease. *Am J Cardiol* 45:1113, 1980
44. Okada RD, Boucher CA, Strauss HW, Pohost GM: Exercise radionuclide imaging approaches to coronary artery disease. *Am J Cardiol* 46:1188, 1980
45. Becker LC: Diagnosis of coronary artery disease with exercise radionuclide imaging: State of the art. *Am J Cardiol* 45:1301, 1980
46. Borer JS, Bacharach SL, Green MV, Kent KM, Maron BJ, Rosing DR, Seides SF, Epstein SE: Obstructive vs. nonobstructive asymmetric septal hypertrophy: Differences in left ventricular function with exercise. *Am J Cardiol* 41:379, 1978
47. Bonow RO, Borer JS, Rosing DR, Henry WL, Pearlman AS, McIntosh CL, Morrow AG, Epstein SE: Preoperative exercise capacity in symptomatic patients with aortic regurgitation as a predictor of postoperative left ventricular function and long-term prognosis. *Circulation* 62:1280, 1980
48. Steele P, Kirch D, Lefree M, Battock D: Measurement of right and left ventricular ejection fraction by radionuclide angiocardiography in coronary artery disease. *Chest* 70:51, 1976
49. Berger HJ, Matthay RA, Loke J, Marshall RC, Gottschalk A, Zaret BL: Assessment of cardiac performance with quantitative radionuclide angiocardiography: Right ventricular ejection fraction with reference to findings in chronic obstructive pulmonary disease. *Am J Cardiol* 41:897, 1978
50. Maddahi J, Berman DS, Matsuoka DT, Waxman AD, Stankus KE, Forrester JS, Swan HJC: A new technique for assessing right ventricular ejection fraction using rapid multiple gated equilibrium cardiac blood pool scintigraphy. *Circulation* 60:581, 1979
51. Slutsky R, Hooper W, Gerber K, Battles A, Froelicher V, Ashburn W, Karliner J: Assessment of right ventricular function at rest and during exercise in patients with coronary artery disease: A new approach using equilibrium radionuclide angiography. *Am J Cardiol* 45:63, 1980
52. Holman BL, Wynne J, Zielonka JS, Idoine JD: A simplified technique for measuring right ventricular ejection fraction using the equilibrium radionuclide angiogram and the slant-hole collimator. *Radiology* 138:429, 1981
53. Reduto LA, Berger HJ, Cohen LS, Gottschalk A, Zaret B: Sequential radionuclide assessment of left and right ventricular performance after acute transmural myocardial infarction. *Ann Intern Med* 89:441, 1978
54. Johnson LL, McCarthy DM, Sciacca R, Cannon PJ: Right ventricular ejection fraction during exercise in patients with coronary artery disease. *Circulation* 60:1284, 1979
55. Maddahi J, Berman DS, Matsuoka DT, Waxman AD, Forrester JS, Swan HJC: Right ventricular ejection fraction during exercise in normal subjects and in coronary artery disease patients: Assessment by multiple-gated equilibrium scintigraphy. *Circulation* 62:133, 1980

56. Berger HJ, Johnstone DE, Sands JM, Gottschalk A, Zaret BL: Response of right ventricular ejection fraction to upright bicycle exercise in coronary artery disease. *Circulation* 60:1292, 1979
57. Matthay RA, Berger HJ, Davies RA, Loke J, Mahler DA, Gottschalk A, Zaret BL: Right and left ventricular exercise performance in chronic obstructive pulmonary disease: Radionuclide assessment. *Ann Intern Med* 93:234, 1980
58. Alexander J, Dainiak N, Berger HJ, Goldman L, Johnstone D, Reduto L, Duffy T, Schwartz P, Gottschalk A, Zaret BL: Serial assessment of doxorubicin cardiotoxicity with quantitative radionuclide angiocardiography. *N Engl J Med* 300:278, 1979
59. Gottdiener JS, Mathisen DJ, Borer JS, Bonow RO, Myers CE, Barr LH, Schwartz DE, Bacharach SL, Green MV, Rosenberg SA: Doxorubicin cardiotoxicity: Assessment of late left ventricular dysfunction by radionuclide cineangiography. *Ann Intern Med* 94:430, 1981
60. Rigo P, Murray M, Strauss HW, Pitt B: Scintiphotographic evaluation of patients with suspected left ventricular aneurysm. *Circulation* 50:985, 1974
61. Winzelberg G, Strauss HW, Bingham JB, McKusick KA: Scintigraphic evaluation of left ventricular aneurysm. *Am J Cardiol* 46:1138, 1980
62. Carabello BA, Wynne J, Holman BL: Assessment of left ventricular function early after aortic valve replacement. *Circulation* 90(Suppl II):193, 1979
63. Askenasi J, Ahnberg D, Korngold E, LaFarge CG, Maltz DL, Treves SL: Quantitative radionuclide angiocardiography: Detection and quantitation of left-to-right shunts. *Am J Cardiol* 37:382, 1976

Chapter 8

Myocardial Perfusion and Infarct Imaging

Edward J. Brown, Jr., and Joshua Wynne

Myocardial Perfusion Imaging with Thallium-201

With the proliferation of new and sophisticated treatment regimens for patients with ischemic heart disease, the ability to accurately detect, localize, and quantitate the extent of coronary artery disease is becoming increasingly important. Thallium-201 myocardial perfusion imaging is a valuable technique that can supplement information obtained from the history, physical examination, and other cardiac diagnostic techniques and allow the physician to detect and characterize coronary artery disease with greater accuracy than has been possible in the past.

This section will review the historical development of thallium-201 imaging, the biologic and physical properties of thallium-201, the clinical experience with this technique in various disease states, and finally, the technique of performing and interpreting a thallium-201 study.

DEVELOPMENT OF THALLIUM-201 PERFUSION IMAGING

In 1952, the use of radiotracers to detect regions of decreased myocardial perfusion was first demonstrated using phosphorus-32, since the tracer was found in normal but not infarcted regions [1]. The ability of radioactive potassium to accumulate in normal myocardial cells was demonstrated in 1954 [2]. The possibility of utilizing the accumulation of radioactive potassium (or analogs of potassium) in myocardial cells to measure coronary blood flow was proposed in 1956 [3]. In 1962, using radioactive potassium and rubidium, an analog of potassium, external scintigraphic imaging was utilized to detect the accumulation of radionuclides in the myocardium and to map areas of regional myocardial perfusion, since the amount of tracer uptake was largely proportional to regional blood flow [4, 5]. In 1973, areas of decreased myocardial accumulation of radioactive potassium, which were not present during resting studies, were detected using external imaging after exercise [6]. Thus, the ability to detect transient exercise-induced myocardial perfusion abnormalities was demonstrated. In 1975, thallium-201, an analog of potassium, was introduced [7, 8], and it provided a readily available tracer with physiologic properties suitable for rest and exercise myocardial imaging.

For imaging to be successful, thallium-201 must be injected intravenously, be delivered to the heart, accumulate in the myocardial cells in proportion to the amount of local blood flow, and emit photons that can be detected externally to form an image that accurately reflects the distribution of tracer in the myocardium. Thus, the quality of the image depends on first, the physiologic properties of the tracer; second, the physical properties of the tracer; and third, the characteristics of the imaging devices. Understanding the capabilities and limitations of each of the components involved in obtaining a successful image is important if one is to fully utilize the potential of thallium-201 perfusion imaging.

Physiologic Properties of Thallium-201

Ideal and Actual Properties

Table 8-1 compares the physiologic properties of the ideal radionuclide with those of thallium-201. An ideal radionuclide should have no pharmacologic effects and injection of the radionuclide should not produce any hemodynamic derangements. Thallium-201 fulfills this property well and does not perturb the cardiovascular system when injected. The ideal tracer would deliver as much radionuclide as possible to the heart, with little or no delivery to other organs. When all organs receive a portion of the injected radionuclide, greater amounts must be injected in order to achieve myocardial levels adequate for imaging, and thus a larger radiation dose must be delivered to the patient. A second problem with delivery to organs other than the heart is the difficulty of differentiating myocardial radiation from radiation emitted from nearby organs. This potentially contaminating radiation is referred to as "background" and is an important consideration when interpreting perfusion images of the heart. Thallium-201 is delivered to all organs in proportion to the amount of blood flow they receive. The heart receives 4 percent of the cardiac output and thus 4 percent of an injected dose of thallium-201. The amount of thallium-201 accumulated by the myocardium, however, depends not only on the amount delivered in the blood but also on the amount the myocardial cells extract from the blood. Normally, the heart is very efficient and extracts 80 to 90 percent of the thallium-201 delivered to it. Although other organs extract slightly less, the end result is that the myocardium receives only 3 to 4 percent of the total injected dose of thallium-201, with the major portion accumulating in other organs.

Ideally, the radionuclide should clear from the blood rapidly, with all of the radionuclide being extracted in a single passage through the heart. Such a property would allow the measurement of perfusion at a single point in time (for example, perfusion at peak exercise). Thallium-201 fulfills this requirement well, with 80 to 90 percent of the agent extracted on the first pass of blood through the coronary arteries. A short physiologic half-life is also desirable. Rapid breakdown

TABLE 8-1. Physiologic Properties of an Ideal Radionuclide vs. Thallium-201

Ideal	Thallium-201
No pharmacologic effects	No pharmocologic effects
Delivery only to the heart	Delivered to all organs in proportion to blood flow
Rapid blood clearance	Rapid blood clearance
Short physiologic $t_{1/2}$	Very long $t_{1/2}$
Accumulation in proportion to regional blood flow	Accumulation in proportion to regional blood flow at physiologic flows
Low cost and easy availability	Expensive and not always easily obtained

and excretion would permit serial injections and measurements of myocardial perfusion over the time course of minutes to hours. The physiologic half-life of thallium-201, unfortunately, exceeds the already long 72-hour physical half-life. Thus, serial measurements of myocardial perfusion over a short time span are not possible with thallium-201.

Fifth, regional accumulation of the radionuclide should be proportionate to regional perfusion. Regional accumulation of thallium-201 is directly proportionate to regional blood flow in the normal physiologic range of coronary blood flow; however, at very high or very low flows thallium-201 accumulation is not proportionate to myocardial perfusion. Finally, the ideal radionuclide should be inexpensive and easily available. Thallium-201 is expensive and procurement can be difficult.

Physiology of Initial Distribution: The Initial Image

Initial images of thallium-201 uptake are obtained as soon as possible after tracer injection. Whether thallium-201 is injected at peak exercise during exercise testing and an image is obtained immediately following exercise, or an image is obtained following a rest injection, the physiology of initial distribution is the same. Approximately 4 percent of intravenously injected thallium-201 is delivered to the heart, carried in the 4 percent of cardiac output normally received by the heart. The myocardial cells extract 80 to 90 percent of the thallium-201 delivered by the coronary arteries (called the extraction fraction) [9], and thus 3 to 4 percent of the injected dose accumulates in the myocardium. The myocardial extraction fraction remains constant at varying heart rates, in the presence of acidosis, hypoxemia, and drugs such as propranolol and acetylstrophanthidin [9]. A linear relationship between myocardial uptake and regional myocardial blood flow is found in dogs when perfusion measured by thallium-201 is compared to perfusion measured by microspheres [10, 11]. Thus, the regional accumulation of thallium-201 as recorded on the initial image following injection is an indicator of regional myocardial perfusion.

Physiology of Redistribution: The Delayed Image

Initial observations suggested that once thallium-201 accumulated in the myocardium it would remain there several hours [7]. Although these observations may be valid for the total uptake of thallium-201 by the heart, regional distribution in the heart is not constant but changes within a period of minutes to a few hours following the initial objection. This phenomenon was observed in patients who received injections of thallium-201 at peak exercise and were found to have perfusion defects on images obtained immediately following exercise that corresponded to exercise-induced areas of inadequate perfusion. Delayed images obtained several hours following the initial images, however, showed a filling-in of the initial perfusion defects [10, 12]. Similar observations were made in animals when thallium-201 was injected during coronary occlusion. Delayed images obtained following release of the coronary occlusion demonstrated a filling-in of the initial perfusion defects found during occlusion [13].

While the pathophysiologic explanation for this redistribution effect is not completely understood, it is clear that the effect may occur in the absence of apparent changes in regional myocardial perfusion [14–16]. Redistribution appears to be the result of loss of thallium-201 from normal areas and accumulation in previously ischemic regions.

A compartmental model is helpful for describing the changes that occur during redistribution [17]. Three compartments are considered: the blood, the heart, and other tissues of the body. Immediately following an intravenous injection of thallium-201, distribution is confined to the blood (Fig. 8-1A). Thallium-201 is next carried by the blood to the organs of the body in an amount proportional to the amount of blood each organ receives. Each organ then extracts thallium-201 from the blood. Accumulation of thallium-201 in the heart is determined by multiplying the 4 percent of cardiac output which the heart receives by the 85 percent extraction efficiency of the heart; thus, 3 to 4 percent of injected thallium-201 accumulates in the heart (Fig. 8-1B). The pattern of uptake within the heart reflects the health or disease of the coronary vessels. If, for example, a critical left circumflex artery stenosis limits blood flow at rest, the myocardium it perfuses will accumulate less thallium-201 than the myocardium supplied by the normal left anterior descending coronary artery. An image obtained at this point would reveal a perfusion defect in the myocardium supplied by the left circumflex coronary artery. Thallium-201 that is not taken up by the heart accumulates in other organs of the body, with only small amounts remaining in the blood. Thus,

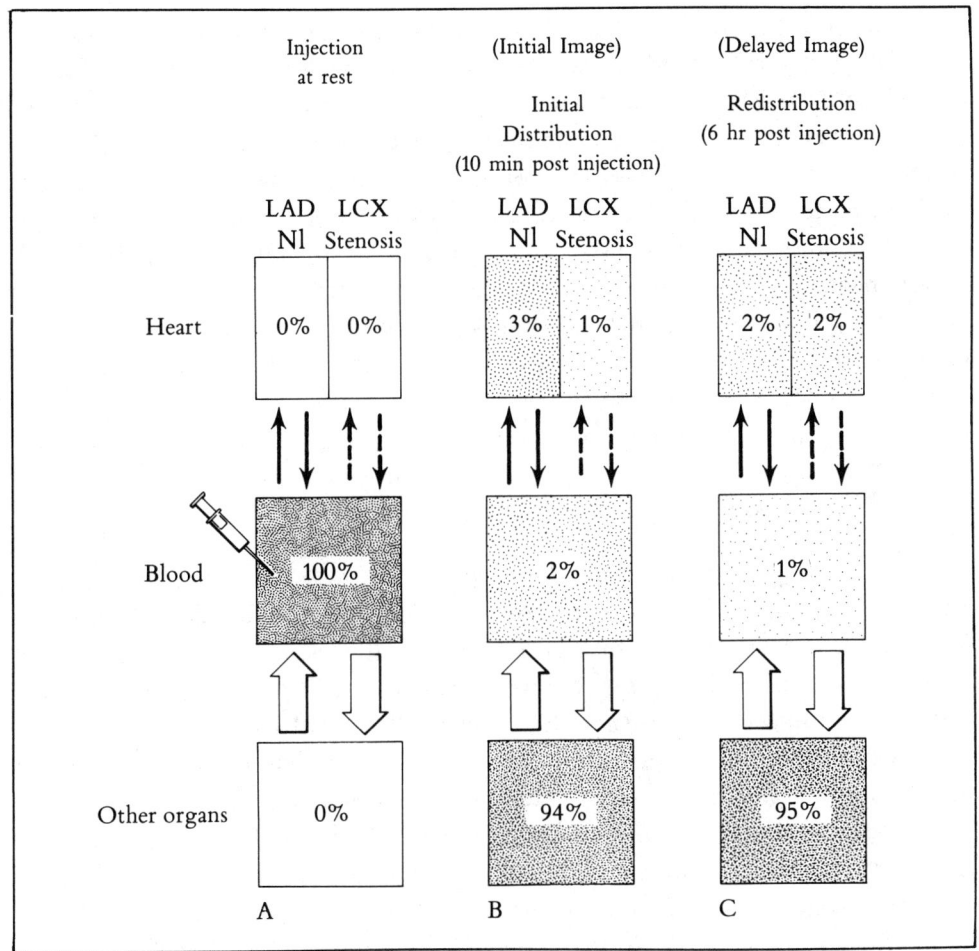

FIGURE 8-1. Schematic depiction of thallium-201 compartmental distribution during injection (A), immediately following injection (B), and 6 hours after injection (C). The left circumflex coronary artery (*LCX*) is assumed to be severely stenotic and limiting flow at rest. The flow in the left anterior descending coronary artery (*LAD*) is assumed to be normal (Nl).

initial images of thallium-201 distribution reflect regional perfusion at the time of injection.

Immediately following initial distribution, redistribution begins. There is a continuous turnover of the thallium-201 pool, with movement of ions between the various compartments. For any given compartment or region within a compartment, the amount of thallium-201 present is a function of the balance between the inflow of thallium-201 and its washout. If the movement into a region is equal to the movement out, no net change in thallium-201 distribution occurs between initial and delayed images. If there is a net gain or loss of thallium-201 from any organ or region of an organ, the accumulation of thallium-201 will differ from initial to delayed images. Figure 8-1C shows how redistribution can fill in a perfusion defect noted on an initial image. Between the time of the initial image and the delayed image, thallium-201 ions are concentrated by the myocardium perfused by the stenotic coronary artery, at least partly because of the positive concentration gradient between it and the thallium-201 in the blood. Simultaneously, the region supplied by the normal coronary artery registers a net loss in the amount of thallium-201 ions [13]. The resulting delayed image shows disappearance of the perfusion defect observed on the initial image. Thus, unlike the initial image, which reflects perfusion and extraction, the delayed image reflects not only perfusion but a more complex relationship with final thallium-201 accumulation depending on a balance between influx and washout of thallium-201 from individual myocardial regions.

Clinical Utility of the Redistribution Phenomenon
Viable myocardial cells capable of concentrating thallium-201 are required for redistribution. Scar tissue is unable to extract thallium-201 and thus will not fill in. Redistribution allows one to differentiate ischemic but viable tissue from scar with a single injection. Perfusion defects that fill in on delayed images represent viable but underperfused myocardium, while perfusion defects that do not fill in on delayed images represent scar tissue or acutely infarcted myocardium.

The optimal time to obtain a delayed image depends on the rate of redistribution. Redistribution begins to occur soon after injection with rapid filling in typically occurring between 5 and 90 minutes. Most filling in occurs from 2 to 4 hours post injection; by 6 hours the phenomenon is complete, and thallium-201 concentration in different regions of the myocardium is in equilibrium [14]. Thus, initial images should be obtained as soon after injection as possible and delayed images 4 to 6 hours following injection, although in practice delayed images may be obtained at 2 to 4 hours after injection.

Physical Properties of Thallium-201
Ideal and Actual Properties
Table 8-2 compares the physical properties an ideal radionuclide would possess with the actual physical properties of thallium-201. An ideal radionuclide would emit energy between 100 kev and 200 kev in the form of photons with little or no beta or other particulate radiation. This permits easy collimation and efficient detection by the scintillation camera crystal, and it minimizes radiation exposure to the patient. The low energy of thallium-201 photons results in interactions of the photons with other tissues as they are emitted from the heart. This process,

TABLE 8-2. Physical Properties of an Ideal Radionuclide vs. Thallium-201

Ideal	Thallium-201
Energy emitted as photons between 100 kev and 200 kev	Most abundant energy emitted as photons at 80 kev
Short $t_{1/2}$ (ca 30 min)	Long $t_{1/2}$ (72 hr)

called attenuation, produces considerable degradation of image quality and renders quantitative analysis of thallium-201 concentration quite problematic. A short half-life is useful because it allows several measurements to be taken over a short time span, although the longer half-life of thallium-201 has the advantage of longer storage. The optimum half-life should be as short as possible to allow serial masurements and yet long enough to permit easy availability. Availability depends on where and how the radionuclide is manufactured and the ease of delivery.

Thallium-201 is typically produced by a cyclotron, and then shipped to the user. It is thus unlike technetium-99m, which can be eluted from a generator, and once procured from the supplier thallium-201 must be used or it is lost by decay. Its relatively long half-life of 72 hours ensures reasonable shelf-life.

Instrumentation

The various components of a gamma scintillation camera have been reviewed in the previous chapter (p. 166). Effective collimation is of particular importance in thallium-201 scintigraphy because of its low energy and significant degradation of the image by attenuation.

CLINICAL EXPERIENCE WITH THALLIUM-201 MYOCARDIAL PERFUSION IMAGING

Although it has been suggested that thallium-201 scintigraphy may be useful in a wide variety of clinical situations, the ultimate utility of this technique remains to be established; many of the potential applications listed in Table 8-3 are of more theoretical interest than clinical usefulness.

Evaluation of Patients with Known or Suspected Coronary Artery Disease

Thallium-201 myocardial perfusion imaging, most frequently used in conjunction with exercise stress testing to evaluate patients with suspected coronary artery disease, should supplement rather than replace other diagnostic cardiac techniques. This imaging technique is uniquely able to detect relative differences in myocardial perfusion in different regions of the myocardium. It does not delineate the *results* of ischemia, as does the electrocardiogram, for example, but rather is a more direct measure of decreased perfusion itself. Similarly, the exercise radionuclide ventriculogram detects wall motion abnormalities that are the result

TABLE 8-3. Clinical Indications for Thallium-201 Perfusion Imaging

Evaluation of patients with known or suspected coronary artery disease
    Evaluation of asymptomatic patients for the presence of coronary artery disease
    Evaluation of resting perfusion abnormalities in patients with severe coronary artery disease
    Evaluation of patients with abnormal resting electrocardiograms or uninterpretable exercise tests*
    Selection of patients with severe left ventricular dysfunction likely to benefit from coronary artery bypass graft surgery
    Localization of coronary artery disease
    Evaluation of coronary artery stenoses noted on coronary angiography of uncertain hemodynamic significance*
Evaluation of patients with myocardial infarction
    Diagnosis of myocardial infarction
    Localization of myocardial infarction
    Sizing myocardial infarctions
    Evaluation of shock associated with myocardial infarction
    Evaluation of patients during postmyocardial infarction rehabilitation*
Evaluation of the results of coronary artery bypass graft surgery
Evaluation of patients with right ventricular pressure or volume overload
Evaluation of patients with coronary artery spasm
Evaluation of patients with cardiomyopathies
    Dilated cardiomyopathies
    Hypertrophic cardiomyopathies
Evaluation of patients with myocardial infiltrative diseases

*Major accepted uses of thallium-201 scintigraphy.

of ischemia. Coronary angiography visualizes stenoses but is not a precise guide to the hemodynamic significance of the lesions. By combining these techniques, one can visualize the coronary anatomy (coronary angiography), detect any perfusion abnormalities beyond an area of stenosis (thallium-201 imaging), and determine whether or not a stenosis and perfusion abnormality is severe enough to cause ischemia (electrocardiography, radionuclide ventriculography).

SENSITIVITY AND SPECIFICITY OF EXERCISE THALLIUM-201 STUDIES. The abilities of the exercise electrocardiogram and thallium-201 study to detect significant coronary artery disease are frequently compared. Considered separately, thallium-201 exercise imaging is reported to have a sensitivity as high as 85 to 90 percent and a specificity of 90 percent or greater [18]. The sensitivity and specificity of exercise electrocardiography are generally found to be lower, typically in the 65 to 70 percent range. The value of combining these two diagnostic techniques has been demonstrated in a multicenter study that evaluated thallium-201 imaging and electrocardiography in 190 patients, 148 of whom had significant coronary artery disease [19]. Electrocardiography detected 73 percent of the patients with significant coronary artery disease, while thallium-201 imaging detected 76 percent. Thus, the sensitivities were similar. Specificity was also found to be similar — 86 percent for electrocardiography and 88 percent for thallium-201 imaging. However, when the two studies were combined, sensitivity significantly improved to 91 percent, better than either test alone. Specificity was not improved by combining the two techniques.

The diagnostic value of exercise electrocardiography decreases when the resting electrocardiographic complex is abnormal. In these instances, thallium-201 imaging can greatly improve the clinician's diagnostic abilities. In 65 patients with significant (>75 percent) coronary stenosis undergoing exercise thallium-201 imaging and exercise electrocardiography, thallium-201 imaging was found to be more sensitive (85 percent vs. 67 percent), more specific (89 percent vs. 63 percent), and more accurate (87 percent vs. 65 percent) than exercise electrocardiography in patients with normal isoelectric ST segments at rest. However, in patients with abnormal resting ST segments (due to left bundle branch block, left ventricular hypertrophy, digoxin), the differences in accuracy were even greater (89 percent vs. 53 percent) [20].

USE OF THALLIUM-201 IMAGING IN THE EVALUATION OF ASYMPTOMATIC PATIENTS. As discussed on page 59, the utility of any diagnostic test depends not only on its sensitivity and specificity but also on the disease prevalence in the population under study. With these considerations in mind, we do not advocate the routine testing of asymptomatic individuals for the presence of coronary artery disease. On the other hand, with the present popularity of fitness programs, increasing numbers of asymptomatic individuals are undergoing screening exercise electrocardiography (ECG). A proportion of such individuals have positive exercise ST-segment changes [21] and present the physician with a difficult dilemma. Thallium-201 imaging in this subgroup of patients can be helpful in separating patients with falsely positive exercise ECGs from those with significant but asymptomatic coronary artery disease. In one study, 35 patients with either no chest pain or atypical chest pain and positive exercise electrocardiograms (≥ 1.0 mm horizontal or downsloping ST segments) underwent thallium-201 myocardial perfusion imaging and cardiac catheterization. Twenty-four of the 35 patients with a positive exercise ECG had negative thallium-201 scans, and 23 of the 24 patients did not have significant coronary artery disease. Among the group of 11 patients with abnormal thallium-201 images, 10 were found to have significant coronary artery stenosis [22]. In a second study, nine asymptomatic patients with greater than 1 mm of ST-segment depression during exercise testing underwent resting and exercise thallium-201 myocardial perfusion imaging and coronary angiography. Seven patients had positive thallium-201 scans, and all of these patients had >50 percent stenosis demonstrated by coronary angiography. In the remaining two patients, both thallium-201 images and coronary angiograms were normal [23].

These two reports demonstrate the utility of thallium-201 imaging to differentiate true-positive from false-positive exercise ECGs in asymptomatic patients. Although thallium-201 imaging is not as definitive as coronary angiography in identifying individuals with and without coronary artery disease, a negative thallium-201 image in an asymptomatic patient with a positive exercise ECG is reassuring and together with other information from the history, physical examination, and other noninvasive diagnostic studies may obviate coronary angiography. Conversely, a positive thallium-201 scan under the same circumstances makes significant but asymptomatic coronary artery disease more likely, prompting further appropriate diagnostic and therapeutic measures.

EVALUATION OF RESTING PERFUSION ABNORMALITIES IN PATIENTS WITH SEVERE CORONARY ARTERY DISEASE. In patients with severe coronary artery disease, it is generally believed that resting coronary blood flow is normal in the absence of angina pectoris or an acute myocardial infarction. However, some defects appearing on initial images following resting injections in such patients fill in on delayed images, suggesting decreased perfusion at rest [14, 15, 24]. Segments filling in with time are usually supplied by severely stenotic vessels.

In most patients with severe coronary artery disease, the decreased resting coronary blood flow has little or no effect on myocardial function. Most of the segments with decreased perfusion demonstrate normal or only slightly hypokinetic wall motion [14, 15, 24]. Thallium-201 imaging can detect perfusion abnormalities when flow is decreased by approximately 40 percent of normal [25]. To decrease perfusion to this extent, a long segment of 40 to 60 percent stenosis is necessary [26]. Shorter lesions must be more severely stenosed to produce a decrease in perfusion. Wall motion abnormalities cannot be detected until resting flow is decreased by more than 50 percent [27]. Thus, thallium-201 perfusion imaging may be able to detect decreases in flow before they are severe enough to cause evidence of ischemia as manifested by abnormalities in wall motion. On the other hand, only a small number of patients with severe coronary artery disease demonstrate this abnormality, and its significance in the general population of patients with ischemic heart disease remains to be established.

The prognosis for patients with resting perfusion abnormalities is not clear, but such patients would likely benefit from intensive medical therapy or revascularization surgery. Experience with this group of patients does suggest caution when interpreting thallium-201 scans. Initial defects that fail to completely fill in over several hours may not invariably indicate scar tissue. In this case, a separate thallium-201 injection at rest at a subsequent visit (a week or more later) should be considered. Defects that persist on follow-up may be presumed to represent scar tissue rather than ischemic myocardium.

EVALUATION OF PATIENTS WITH ABNORMAL RESTING ELECTROCARDIOGRAMS. In patients with left bundle branch block, intraventricular conduction defects, left ventricular hypertrophy, mitral valve prolapse, and Wolff-Parkinson-White syndrome, evaluation of ST-segment changes with exercise is often not feasible. In this group of patients, exercise thallium-201 imaging can be particularly useful in the evaluation of patients for the presence of significant coronary artery disease.

SELECTION OF PATIENTS WITH SEVERE LEFT VENTRICULAR DYSFUNCTION FOR CORONARY ARTERY BYPASS GRAFT SURGERY. Patients with severe left ventricular dysfunction due to diffuse coronary artery disease are not generally recommended for coronary artery bypass graft (CABG) surgery, particularly if they have no angina pectoris, because of the high mortality and minimal therapeutic benefit. Coronary angiography and left ventriculography usually reveal severe triple-vessel coronary artery disease with diffuse left ventricular wall motion abnormalities. How much of the left ventricular dysfunction is due to scar and how much may be due to reversible ischemia is not easily determined. A thallium-201 perfusion scan that reveals perfusion defects that fill in over time suggests reversible ischemia. If significant areas of ischemic tissue can be demonstrated, CABG surgery may be of benefit in these patients [28]. In most patients, however, differentiation of ischemic from irreversible left ventricular dysfunction may be gleaned from the clinical history. Patients without angina pectoris who manifest typical symptoms of left ventricular power failure (e.g., paroxysmal nocturnal dyspnea, orthopnea) are not usually benefited by CABG surgery, and their operative risk is high. On the other hand, patients who have symptoms of transient ischemia, typically in the form of angina pectoris, usually respond favorably to surgery, even if they have significant left venticular dysfunction. The risk in these patients is somewhat higher than in patients with normal left ventricular function but not inordinately so, and we recommend surgery in this subgroup of patients if their symptoms of angina pectoris are unacceptable to the patient. Thallium-201 scans may be of use in the minority of these patients in whom the history does not provide decisive criteria for differentiating ischemic symptoms from failure symptoms.

LOCALIZATION OF CORONARY ARTERY DISEASE. The ability to noninvasively localize the site of coronary stenoses can be helpful in certain clinical situations. Thallium-201 myocardial perfusion imaging can in part fulfill this role [29, 30]. Anterior, 40-degree left anterior oblique (LAO), and 60-degree LAO thallium-201 images obtained in 133 patients with coronary artery disease demonstrated an association between perfusion defects in certain segments and coronary artery stenoses, as shown in Figure 8-2 [31]. Correlation is not complete. Overlap of regions per-

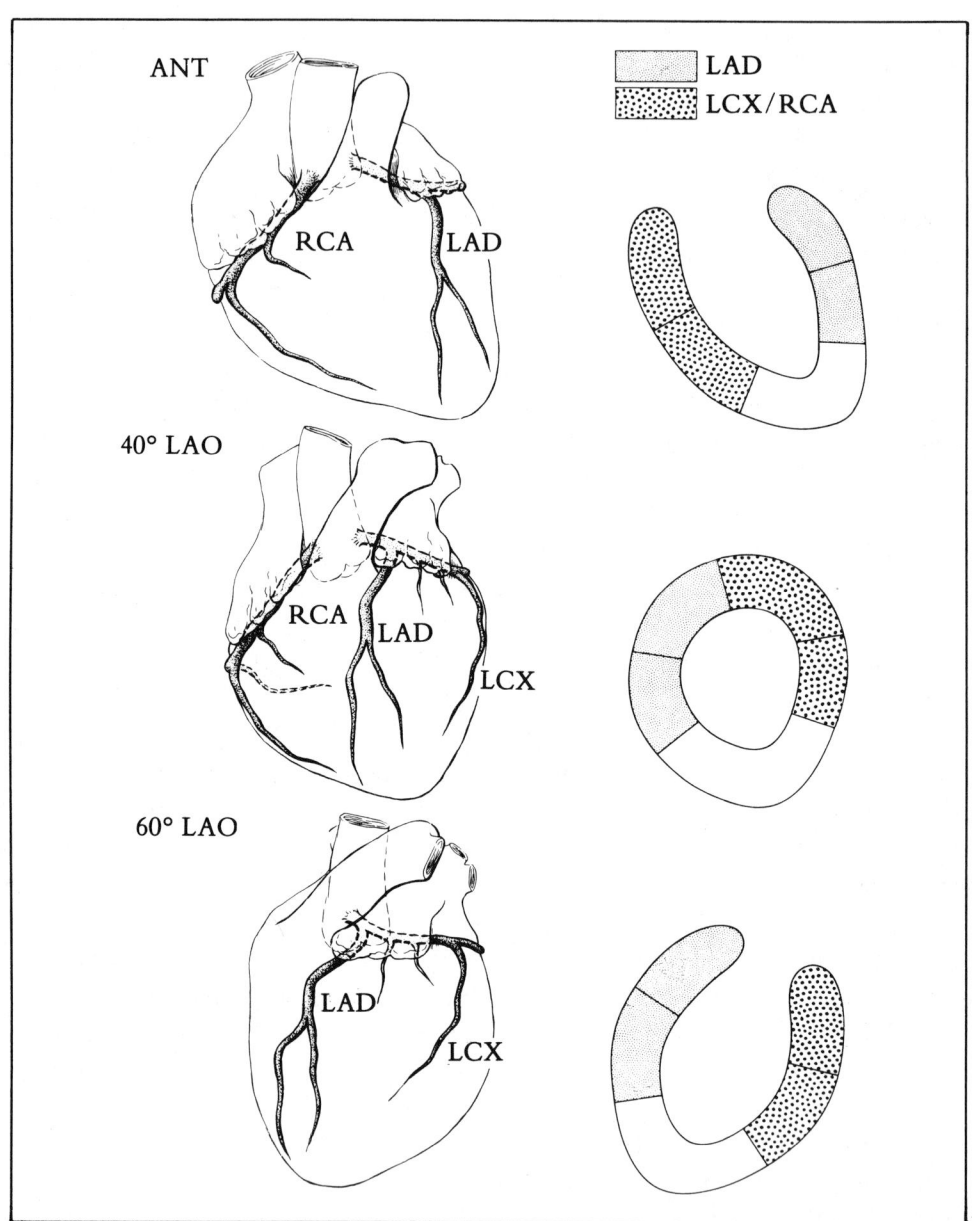

FIGURE 8-2. Diagrammatic depiction of the association of perfusion defects with specific coronary artery lesions. Due to vessel overlap, apical perfusion defects are not helpful in localizing involved coronary arteries. ANT = anterior, LAD = left anterior descending coronary artery, LAO = left anterior oblique, LCX = left circumflex coronary artery, RCA = right coronary artery.

fused by different coronary arteries and variable coronary anatomy limit the accuracy of this technique. Because perfusion imaging detects relative differences in myocardial perfusion, the ability to differentiate single from multiple vessel disease is not good [32]. Perfusion defects appear in the most severely underperfused regions, while regions supplied by less severely compromised vessels appear normal. Since the common consensus is that symptomatic patients with left main coronary artery stenoses should undergo surgery, it had been hoped that thallium-201 imaging might be able to distinguish patients with left main coronary artery disease. Thus far, this has not been possible.

Thallium-201 scanning may be quite useful, however, in the evaluation of a stenosis of uncertain hemodynamic significance noted on coronary angiography. A lesion of 40 to 60 percent may or may not limit flow with exercise. A corresponding thallium-201 perfusion defect with exercise would support the hemodynamic significance of the lesion, while a negative scan would be good evidence that the lesion was not responsible for flow limitations, or, by inference, ischemia.

Evaluation of Patients with Myocardial Infarction

Myocardial perfusion imaging with thallium-201 can be helpful in the care of certain patients with suspected or proven myocardial infarction.

DIAGNOSIS OF MYOCARDIAL INFARCTION. The decision to admit a patient with chest discomfort to a coronary care unit is usually based on an assessment of the nature of the chest pain, past history of cardiac disease, risk factors, and the appearance of the electrocardiogram. Patients with crushing substernal chest pain and an injury current (that is, ST-segment elevation) on the electrocardiogram do not present a decision-making problem. However, some patients present with atypical chest pain and nondiagnostic electrocardiograms. In this group of patients, thallium-201 imaging can supplement information obtained from the history and physical examination and may allow the physician to make a more reliable diagnosis.

Ischemic and necrotic myocardial cells associated with acute myocardial infarction do not accumulate thallium-201 and thus appear as perfusion defects on the thallium image. Wackers and coworkers administered thallium-201 to 200 patients with acute myocardial infarctions as soon as possible after the onset of symptoms [33]. All 44 patients in the group imaged at rest within 6 hours of the onset of symptoms demonstrated perfusion defects. Defects were found in only 72 percent of patients imaged later than 24 hours after the onset of symptoms. The reason for the decreased sensitivity with time is not known but may be caused by a decrease in the size of the ischemic area, perhaps due to increased collateral flow. Similar results were obtained in a multicenter study involving 111 patients with acute myocardial infarction [19]. Images were obtained an average of 5 days following the onset of infarction, and thallium-201 perfusion defects were detected in 81 percent of these patients.

Old myocardial scar, new necrotic tissue, and ischemic tissue cause similar perfusion defects on the resting image; however, delayed images may be helpful in differentiating acute from old lesions [34]. In one study, patients with suspected acute myocardial infarction but nondiagnostic initial electrocardiograms and cardiac enzyme levels were imaged with thallium-201 within 6 hours of the onset of symptoms. Postinjection resting and delayed images were obtained. On the basis of subsequent clinical courses, four groups of patients were defined. The first group had unstable angina pectoris with no subsequent electrocardiographic or enzyme evidence of myocardial infarction. In this group, initial resting thallium-201 defects were not present on delayed images 3 hours later. The second group had unstable angina pectoris that evolved to myocardial infarction. This group's thallium-201 images showed initial perfusion defects that varied but persisted on delayed images. A third group had remote myocardial infarctions with new acute infarction. Thallium-201 images revealed resting perfusion defects that did not change on delayed images. In the fourth group of patients with chest pain of noncardiac origin, normal thallium-201 images at rest remained normal on delayed images. Thus, by combining resting and 3-hour delayed images, valuable information can be obtained that may allow the physician to assess the severity of disease more accurately and thus better utilize coronary care units. In actual clinical practice, however, thallium-201 scanning is rarely available to assist in triage decisions. The majority of patients are scanned only *after* being admitted to the coronary care unit, since most physicians would not deprive a patient with possible myocardial infarction of the monitoring and life support facilities available in the unit by sending the patient directly to the nuclear medicine unit prior to admission. Serum creatine kinase (CK) levels are positive within 12 hours in most patients with myocardial infarction, so the actual impact of thallium-201 scanning in admission or triage decisions is minimal.

It must be remembered that thallium-201 imaging can be negative in the presence of an acute myocardial infarction. Small infarcts, subendocardial infarcts, and scans performed late (>24 hours) after the onset of symptoms are all reasons for negative scans. Like any other diagnostic information, thallium-201 images must be interpreted along with other data before making clinical decisions. However, in certain instances, thallium-201 imaging can supply the clinician with information helpful in the diagnosis of acute myocardial infarction.

LOCALIZATION OF MYOCARDIAL INFARCTION. Once a diagnosis of myocardial infarction is made and the patient is in the coronary care unit, thallium-201 imaging can continue to have a role in diagnostic and therapeutic decisions. Because of differences in prognosis, pacemaker indications, and treatment strategies between anterior and inferior myocardial infarctions, it may be important to localize the site of infarction. The electrocardiogram is not always helpful in localizing infarction, particularly in the presence of left bundle branch block or other intraventricular conduction delays. In such instances, the use of a resting thallium-201 injection can be helpful. Localization of perfusion defects in the septum in anterior myocardial infarctions or inferoposterior wall in inferior myocardial infarctions is reliable and correlates well with localization by electrocardiography [35–41], ventriculography [41, 42], and postmortem studies [40].

SIZING MYOCARDIAL INFARCTIONS. Estimates of infarct size can be made from the physical examination, electrocardiogram, and hemodynamic parameters. Gallops, diffuse injury currents, and low cardiac output in the presence of normal or elevated left ventricular filling pressure all indicate a large area of infarction. More accurate sizing of infarction is useful to the clinician for several reasons. Knowledge of infarct size allows more accurate prognostication; thus, patients more likely to develop congestive heart failure, arrhythmias, and sudden death can be identified. Therapeutically, knowledge of infarct size can assist in decisions about length of time in the coronary care unit, assist in the formulation of rehabilitation programs, and guide the decision about frequency of follow-up visits. With increasing interest in hemodynamic, mechanical, and pharmacologic interventions designed to reduce infarct size [43], accurate sizing of infarction is necessary to evaluate the results of these interventions.

Thallium-201 imaging has been used successfully to size infarctions. The size of thallium-201 perfusion defects correlates well with the size of infarction in postmortem studies in patients [44] and in animals undergoing experimental coronary occlusion [45, 46]. Thallium-201 perfusion defect size also correlates well with infarct size as estimated by CK release [47] and the amount of abnormal wall motion following an acute myocardial infarction [42].

The size of a thallium-201 perfusion defect reflects not only new necrotic myocardial tissue but also old scar and potentially salvageable ischemic tissue. Because scar, ischemic tissue, and necrotic tissue all have an adverse effect on myocardial function, it is not surprising that large defect size is related to a high mortality [48]. Because initial perfusion defects represent both necrotic and ischemic tissue, initial postinfarction perfusion defect size can be compared to defect size on scans several days after infarction to determine the fate of the ischemic areas. Nitroglycerin given to patients post myocardial infarction results in smaller thallium-201 perfusion defects one week after infarction than does placebo [49], suggesting that border zone ischemic areas in patients given nitroglycerin are less likely to go on to infarction.

EVALUATION OF SHOCK ASSOCIATED WITH MYOCARDIAL INFARCTION. Patients with acute myocardial infarction and shock present the clinician with a challenging problem. Although the most common cause is destruction of large amounts of myocardium, other causes such as a ruptured papillary muscle, a ruptured ventricular septum, and right ventricular infarction can also lead to shock in the presence of only small amounts of myocardial damage. The more refined medical and surgical methods become (e.g., valve replacement for a ruptured papillary muscle), the more important it is to know the specific etiology of shock in order to provide appropriate therapy. Although the history, physical examination, and hemodynamic monitoring often make the diagnosis clear, there are instances when further information can be of value. Although radionuclide ventriculography is usually the scintigraphic procedure of first choice for evaluating shock in the setting of an acute myocardial infarction (p. 178), thallium-201 scanning may be indicated when radionuclide ventriculography is unavailable, since thallium-201 scanning does not require the gating equipment and computer necessary for the blood pool study.

Right ventricular infarction as a cause of shock should be suspected when there is hemodynamic evidence of right ventricular dysfunction in the presence of an acute inferior myocardial infarction. Diagnosis of this condition is important because intravascular volume expansion and treatment with agents that reduce pulmonary vascular resistance can often be helpful. Thallium-201 imaging, although not specific for this condition, can be suggestive when small perfusion defects of the left ventricle are seen in the presence of shock, suggesting the amount of ischemic or necrotic myocardium is too small to cause shock. A more specific diagnosis can be made by combining technetium-99m-pyrophosphate imaging (p. 222) with thallium-201 imaging [44]. In the 45-degree LAO view, thallium-201 is injected and used to define the location of the interventricular septum. Following an injection of technetium-99m-pyrophosphate (a radionuclide taken up by infarcted myocardial cells), the heart is scanned, and any uptake of technetium-99m-pyrophosphate in the area of the right ventricle is due to right ventricular infarction.

The sudden onset of a systolic murmur and shock during the course of a myocardial infarction suggests either a ruptured papillary muscle and mitral regurgitation, or a ruptured ventricular septum and left-to-right shunting of blood. Both are amenable to surgical correction, although the timing of surgery remains controversial. The value of thallium-201 imaging in these two disorders is to assess the amount of remaining viable myocardium. A small, well-localized defect indicates a small amount of damaged myocardium and thus a low operative mortality and a good prognosis, whereas large diffuse defects indicate the opposite. Such information can assist the clinician in decision making when dealing with these acute mechanical problems.

EVALUATION OF PATIENTS DURING POSTMYOCARDIAL INFARCTION REHABILITATION. Decisions in postinfarction patients about exercise programs, how soon to return to work, and advisability of coronary angiography and possible coronary artery bypass surgery can be aided with information from thallium-201 imaging. Thallium-201 imaging may detect patients with residual jeopardized myocardium following infarction. The presence and size of thallium-201 defects appear to have important prognostic significance. When resting scans obtained early after onset of symptoms in one study were subjected to computer analysis, a quantitative score appeared to be more predictive of ultimate patient prognosis than routine variables [48]. Exercise thallium-201 scans obtained several weeks after infarction may provide additional prognostic information and may identify patients at high risk of complications [50].

Evaluation of the Results of Coronary Artery Bypass Graft Surgery

Thallium-201 imaging can provide the clinician with valuable information when evaluating patients for coronary artery bypass surgery. Although coronary angiography precisely localizes coronary artery lesions, no information is provided about the functional significance of a given lesion. Minimal stenoses of less than 50 percent or severe stenoses of greater than 90 percent do not present management problems. However, many lesions of moderate severity are of unknown functional significance, and in these patients thallium-201 imaging can be more useful than additional angiographic views. A patient with angina pectoris, a severe proximal right coronary artery lesion, and a moderate proximal left anterior descending coronary artery lesion might be treated differently depending on whether or not a thallium-201 perfusion defect appears in the myocardium supplied by the left anterior descending coronary artery. For the patient with no perfusion defect beyond the moderate left anterior descending coronary lesion, more intensive medical therapy might be appropriate, whereas surgery might be indicated in the patient with a perfusion defect, since this would suggest that the left anterior descending coronary artery lesion was producing hemodynamic compromise.

Symptomatic results following coronary artery bypass surgery do not always predict graft patency. Patients can improve as the result of a placebo effect [51] or perioperative infarction [52]. The patency of bypass grafts can be evaluated with thallium-201 imaging. Perfusion defects that fill in with time, indicating viable but ischemic myocardium preoperatively, can be reassessed postoperatively. Absence of the perfusion defects indicates successful bypass grafting, while a persistence of the defects indicates graft closure or perhaps a perioperative infarction [15, 53].

Evaluation of Patients with Right Ventricular Pressure or Volume Overload
Right ventricular hypertrophy as a result of right ventricular pressure overload (due to pulmonary outflow obstruction or pulmonary hypertension) or right ventricular volume overload (due to a left-to-right intracardiac shunt or tricuspid regurgitation) cannot be uniformly detected by the electrocardiogram, chest x-ray, or echocardiogram. Detection of right ventricular hypertrophy by thallium-201 is possible and appears to be more sensitive than the other noninvasive techniques [54, 55]. In resting thallium-201 images, the normal right ventricle is not visualized, owing to its thin wall and low blood flow. In the presence of a right ventricular pressure or volume overload, the right ventricle performs increased work, which leads to right ventricular hypertrophy. The hypertrophied right ventricular myocardium has increased blood flow, which results in increased thallium-201 accumulation and therefore is visualized in the resting image [56]. In right ventricular hypertrophy secondary to left ventricular pressure or volume overload, both ventricles typically have thickened walls.

Evaluation of Patients with Coronary Artery Spasm
Resting thallium-201 studies in patients with known or suspected variant angina pectoris can provide useful diagnostic information. Injections of thallium-201 during chest pain in patients with variant angina pectoris result in perfusion defects that correspond in location to areas identified by ST-segment elevation [57]. Thallium-201 studies can be particularly useful in the diagnosis of variant angina pectoris and localization of involved vessels in patients with abnormal resting electrocardiograms.

Evaluation of Patients with Cardiomyopathies
DILATED CARDIOMYOPATHIES. Ischemic cardiomyopathy and idiopathic dilated cardiomyopathy both present with congestive heart failure and large, poorly functioning left ventricles. The two are differentiated by the presence of severe coronary artery disease in the former and normal coronary arteries in the latter. In patients with silent coronary artery disease, the two cardiomyopathies cannot be differentiated clinically, and often coronary angiography is necessary. Thallium-201 imaging provides a noninvasive method of differentiating these two cardiomyopathies [58]. Resting images in ischemic cardiomyopathies reveal multiple large perfusion defects, while scans of patients with idiopathic cardiomyopathies show homogeneous thallium-201 myocardial distribution or only rare small perfusion defects.

Once a patient with ischemic cardiomyopathy is identified, thallium-201 may provide useful information for therapeutic decisions. Patients with severe left ventricular dysfunction and no angina pectoris do not ordinarily benefit from coronary artery bypass surgery. Coronary angiography in these patients will demonstrate coronary stenosis but will not provide information about the viability of myocardium beyond the coronary stenoses. Thallium-201 images allow the clinician to locate and quantitate areas of reversible ischemia. Patients with large areas of reversible ischemia (large perfusion defects that fill in with time) can improve functionally following coronary artery bypass surgery. Patients with little or no reversibly ischemic myocardium would not likely benefit from bypass surgery.

HYPERTROPHIC CARDIOMYOPATHY. Thallium-201 scans may help to identify the asymmetric septal hypertrophy seen in hypertrophic cardiomyopathy, particularly if echocardiography is technically unsatisfactory. Scintigraphy with thallium-201 appears to be less useful in assessing patients with chest pain and hypertrophic cardiomyopathy, since abnormal stress thallium-201 defects that fill in have been noted in these patients despite normal coronary arteriograms.

Evaluation of Patients with Myocardial Infiltrative Diseases

Perfusion defects on thallium-201 images are not always due to coronary artery disease. Infiltration due to parasites (Chagas' disease), tumors, or granulomas will also result in an absence of flow, and therefore perfusion defects may appear in the myocardium. In sarcoidosis, granulomatous infiltration into the myocardium is frequently detected at autopsy but is difficult to diagnose during life. Thallium-201 imaging in patients with sarcoidosis and myocardial involvement demonstrates multiple left ventricular perfusion defects [59]. The ability to make a premortem diagnosis of myocardial granulomas in patients with sarcoidosis allows closer follow-up for possible cardiac complications and provides a means to evaluate the results of therapy.

ACQUIRING AND INTERPRETING A THALLIUM-201 STUDY

Preparation

If a thallium-201 exercise study is to be performed, the same precautions observed for an exercise electrocardiogram apply. Patients with unstable angina pectoris, congestive heart failure, or physical limitations that make exercise difficult or unsafe must be excluded. During exercise, electrocardiographic monitoring for arrhythmias and ST-segment depression as well as monitoring of the blood pressure and pulse rate is necessary, as is a defibrillator and other resuscitative equipment. An intravenous line must be inserted to allow injection of the thallium-201 at peak exercise. The patient should fast for 12 hours prior to the study. This decreases splanchnic blood flow and the resulting lower liver and spleen blood flow results in less thallium-201 accumulation in these organs and less background activity, which interferes with imaging of the myocardium.

Exercise

For an exercise study, any form of exercise can be used, most commonly treadmill testing and bicycle ergometry. Cardiac pacing and isometric exercise have also been employed. Treadmill exercise is the most desirable form, since it places the patient under maximal physiologic stress. It is usual to exercise a patient to the same end points used in exercise electrocardiography, stopping when the patient experiences chest pain or fatigue. At peak exercise, 1.5 to 2.0 mCi of thallium-201 is injected as an intravenous bolus. Exercise must then be continued for an additional 30 to 60 seconds to allow time for several complete circulations of thallium-201 and thus to insure initial thallium-201 distribution in proportion to the amount of blood flow.

Imaging

Redistribution begins quickly; therefore, initial images must be obtained immediately post exercise. Because redistribution is insignificant in the first 10 to 15 minutes following initial distribution, all initial images should (ideally) be obtained within this time period. In general, three views are obtained: anterior, 45-degree left anterior oblique, and left lateral view. The left lateral view is obtained with the patient supine, lying on the right side, to avoid artifactual inferoposterior defects due to attenuation by the diaphragm. Collections are usually made to a predetermined number of counts, usually 200,000 to 400,000 counts, a number designed to give adequate resolution over a short time span. Image display can be accomplished in the simplest system as an unprocessed analog image collected on Polaroid film. More advanced systems include computer processing of images, which can subtract background and enhance the myocardial images. Color combinations representing numbers of counts can be included to make visual interpretation easier. Each system differs, and each institution must become familiar with and validate its own equipment. Imaging is repeated 3 to 4 hours later to assess the presence of redistribution.

Interpretation of Images

In a normal image (Fig. 8-3), there is nearly homogeneous thallium-201 distribution. At the apex, there may be slightly less thallium-201 accumulation owing to a thinning of the wall in this area [60]. Normal resting images will show mild heterogeneity, although no obvious perfusion defects will be seen. This heterogeneity is not present on exercise images. In the center of the ventricle, an area of decreased concentration corresponds to the cavity of the ventricle. If perfusion

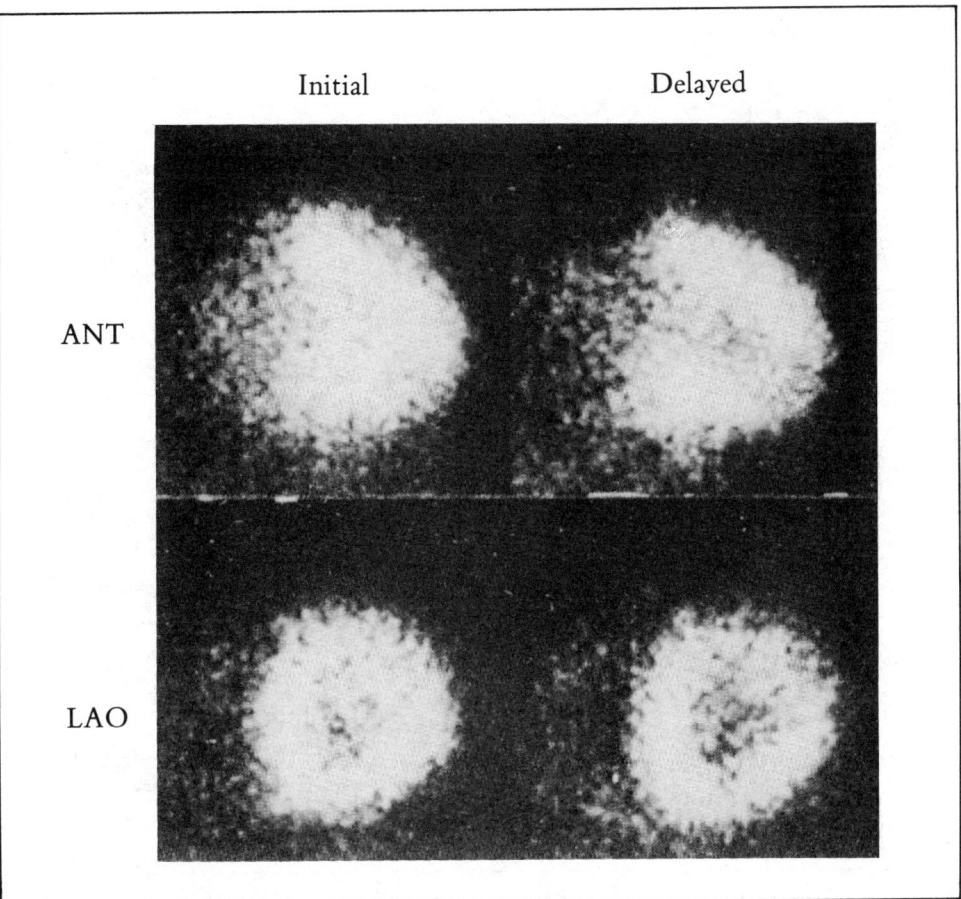

FIGURE 8-3. Anterior (*ANT*) and 45° left anterior oblique (*LAO*) images of a normal thallium-201 study. There is normal homogeneous distribution of the tracer in a U-shaped configuration in the anterior and a circular configuration in the left anterior oblique projections. The cavity of the left ventricle is responsible for the region of reduced activity in the center of the images. There is no significant change in the tracer distribution between initial and delayed images. (From GM Pohost et al: Radionuclide imaging. In RA Johnson, E Haber, WG Austen [eds]: The Practice of Cardiology. Boston: Little, Brown, 1980.)

defects are present, they are localized to the apex, anteroseptal, inferior or posterolateral regions (Fig. 8-4).

The wall thickness and myocardial cavity size are noted. Cavity size is difficult to quantitate, but with experience, a semiquantitative estimate of size can be made. The absence or presence of the right ventricular myocardium should be noted. In a normal resting study, the right ventricle should not be visualized. Vis-

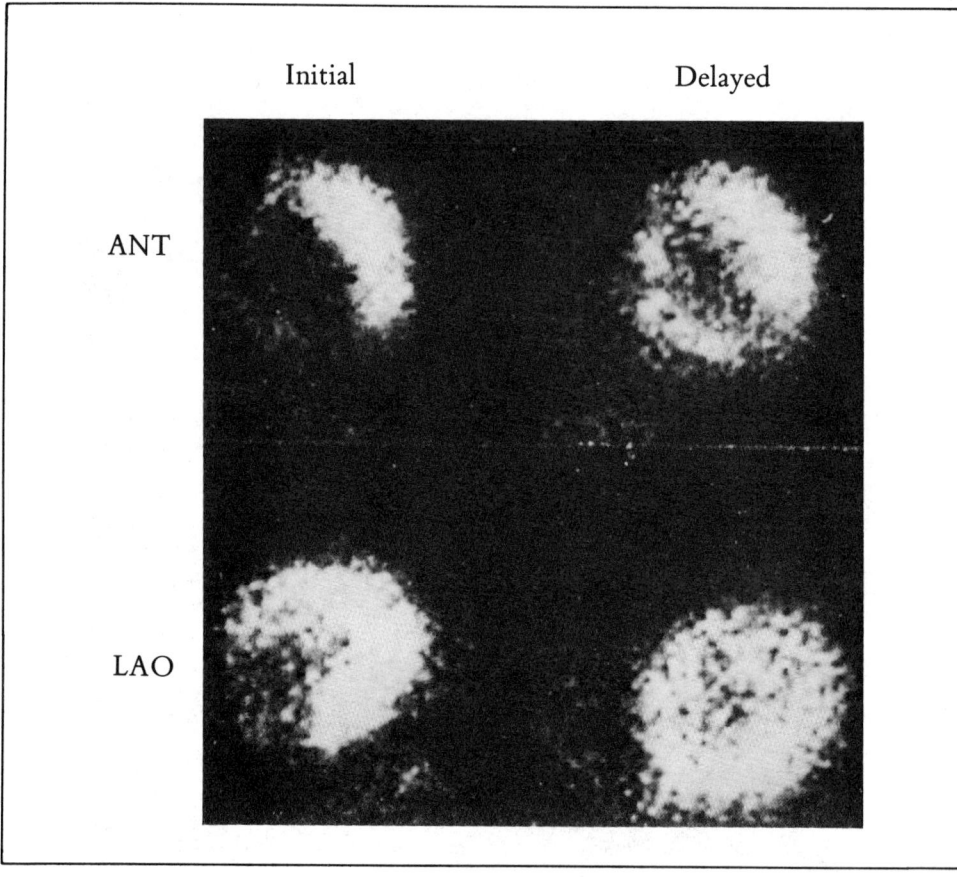

FIGURE 8-4. Anterior (*ANT*) and 45° left anterior oblique (*LAO*) images of an abnormal thallium-201 study. The initial anterior view demonstrates a large defect involving the inferior and apical segments whereas the anterolateral segment appears to have relatively normal thallium-201 content. On the delayed image (obtained 2 1/2 hours later), partial filling in of thallium-201 activity into the inferior segment has occurred, but the apical defect persists. The initial LAO view demonstrates a large defect involving the septal and apical inferior segments, whereas the posterior segment appears to have relatively normal thallium-201 activity. On the delayed image, the septal and apical-inferior segments fill in nearly completely. These images are consistent with exercise-induced ischemia of the inferior, septal, and apical-inferior segments, and probably myocardial scar involving the apical segment. (From GM Pohost et al: Radionuclide imaging. In RA Johnson, E Haber, WG Austen [eds]: The Practice of Cardiology. Boston: Little, Brown, 1980.)

ualization at rest suggests right ventricular hypertrophy. If the image is obtained during exercise or during tachycardia, the right ventricular myocardium normally is visualized.

Any pulmonary uptake of thallium-201 should be noted during exercise studies. Compared to the delayed image, thallium-201 pulmonary activity on initial

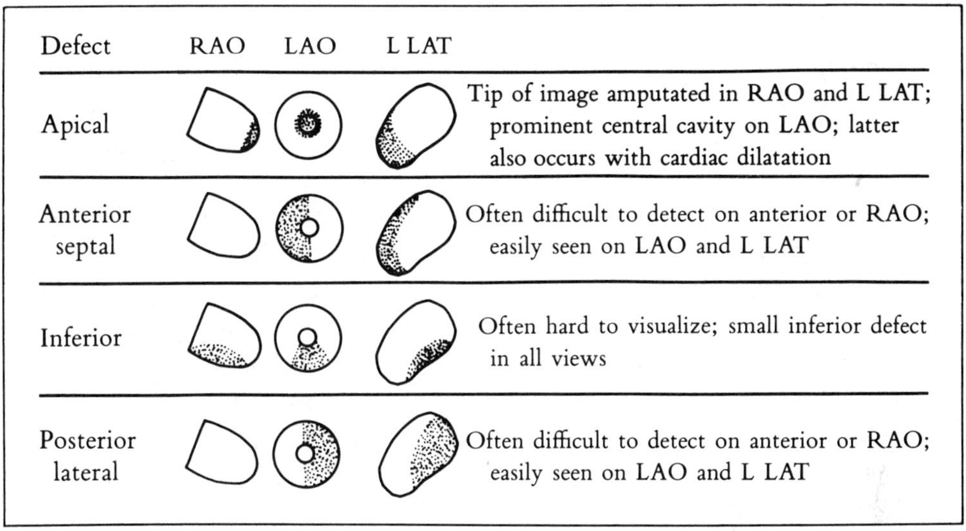

Defect	RAO	LAO	L LAT	
Apical				Tip of image amputated in RAO and L LAT; prominent central cavity on LAO; latter also occurs with cardiac dilatation
Anterior septal				Often difficult to detect on anterior or RAO; easily seen on LAO and L LAT
Inferior				Often hard to visualize; small inferior defect in all views
Posterior lateral				Often difficult to detect on anterior or RAO; easily seen on LAO and L LAT

FIGURE 8-5. Schematic drawing illustrates typical image defects in the major coronary artery distribution beds. Note that all but apical defects are identified best in the left anterior oblique (*LAO*) view. The anterior view (not pictured) is similar to the right anterior oblique (*RAO*) view. *LLAT* = left lateral view. (From JL Ritchie et al: *Radiology* 121:131, 1976.)

images following exercise is increased in patients with significant coronary artery disease [61]. Similar increases in activity are seen in any condition that delays pulmonary transit time or increases left atrial pressure. Differences in pulmonary uptake are best appreciated with computer processing, but increases noted visually on initial images suggest impaired left ventricular function.

Perfusion defects should be found in a pattern consistent with coronary artery anatomy and are usually seen in multiple views (Figs. 8-4 and 8-5). However, a definite defect localized to the distribution pattern of a single coronary artery should not be disregarded merely because it is seen only in one view. It must be remembered, however, that the low energy of thallium-201 makes it highly susceptible to artifactual "defects" due to attenuation by diaphragm, soft tissue, or breasts.

As with radionuclide ventriculography and electrocardiographic stress testing, a thallium-201 scan should not be considered negative unless the patient has exercised maximally. We generally require that the patient achieve at least 85 percent of maximal predicted heart rate or a double product (peak heart rate times systolic blood pressure) of 25,000 or greater. One major advantage of thallium-201 scanning over electrocardiographic stress testing is that the scan may be positive at a level of exercise that is insufficient to result in an abnormal electrocardiogram.

Myocardial Infarct Imaging

In acute infarct scintigraphy, radiopharmaceuticals are sequestered by acutely necrotic myocardium, resulting in regions of *increased* radiotracer uptake. This technique has emerged in recent years as an independent, noninvasive technique to aid in the detection, localization, and quantification of myocardial necrosis. Over the last 20 years, a variety of radiopharmaceuticals have been evaluated for their ability to be sequestered by acutely infarcted myocardium, including radioiodine, mercury 203-chlormerodrin, tetracycline analogs, and radiomercurifluorescein [62]. While the ideal agent has not yet been found, a vast experience has been gained with the myocardial infarct imaging agent technetium-99m–stannous pyrophosphate, an agent used previously in bone scanning [63–73]. At least in principle, technetium-99m-pyrophosphate is taken up by infarcted myocardium but not by normal or ischemic myocardium, thus yielding a scintigraphic image of a "hot spot" of radioactivity.

Mechanism of Pyrophosphate Uptake

In 1974, based on the observation that irreversibly damaged myocardial cells accumulate calcium ions, Bonte et al proposed the use of technetium-99m–stannous pyrophosphate for imaging myocardial infarction [74]. The two most important determinants of uptake of pyrophosphate are the extent of myocardial necrosis and the amount of residual coronary blood flow into the damaged area. One mechanism for pyrophosphate deposition in infarcted cells appears to be through formation of complexes with deposits of calcium. Damage to the myocardial cell results in the influx of calcium and phosphates (including pyrophosphate from the blood, at least in areas with adequate degrees of perfusion). The incoming ions complex with a variety of organic constituents of the cell, and pyrophosphate is adsorbed in several tissue calcium stores. While the uptake of pyrophosphate is limited primarily to sites with elevated calcium levels, a consistent linear relationship between total tissue calcium concentration and the pyrophosphate level has not been demonstrated. Pyrophosphate also appears to bind to organic macromolecules in the damaged tissues [75]. Since deposition of calcium in damaged tissues plays a major role in eventual pyrophosphate uptake, it is clear why the residual blood flow to an infarcted region is so important. Maximal uptake of pyrophosphate occurs in regions with 30 to 40 percent of normal myocardial blood flow [76]. The central area of maximal necrosis typically demonstrates very reduced flow (less than 30 percent) and shows little in the way of calcific deposits; presumably as a result, pyrophosphate deposition is less. In more peripheral zones (with flows over 40 percent), less tissue necrosis results and thus less pyrophosphate uptake. These observations explain the so-called doughnut pattern, which may be observed in patients with large infarcts; there is a central defect with little pyrophosphate uptake as a result of low flow and a zone of high activity at the more peripheral margins of the infarct (corresponding to infarcted regions with 30–40 percent of normal regional myocardial blood flow) [73]. In some patients, the doughnut pattern results from such extensive infarction that the left ventricular cavity itself is imaged as the central cold region.

Imaging Technique and Interpretation

As shown in Figure 8-6A, a normal pyrophosphate image demonstrates no activity in the region of the heart. Since pyrophosphate is a bone imaging agent, the ribs, sternum, and vertebral column are evident. Figure 8-6B–D shows patients with several different types of myocardial infarctions. Note the prominent uptake of the radiopharmaceutical by the heart. Two general types of uptake are found. The first, demonstrated in this figure, is focal uptake in one or more anatomic regions of the heart. The second type, diffuse uptake, is not limited to any specific anatomic region, and in some cases is due to persistent radioactivity within the blood pool within the left ventricular chamber.

Patients with suspected myocardial infarction may be imaged at the bedside in the coronary care unit using a portable scintillation camera. Scans usually first become positive 12 to 24 hours after infarction, although occasional patients may have uptake visible within 4 hours. Maximal uptake is observed between 48 to 72 hours, and many scans revert to normal within 7 to 14 days. Thus, a normal scan a week after chest pain does not exclude a recent myocardial infarction. Imaging may be performed 90 minutes after injection of the radiopharmaceutical, although we have found that a 180-minute delay results in even better images owing to further clearance of the radionuclide from the bloodstream. Myocardial localization is aided by obtaining scans in multiple views, generally the anterior, left anterior oblique, and left lateral projections. Many patients demonstrate persistently positive scans for weeks or months after an infarct, unlike the usual course, which is a fading of the uptake by 7 to 14 days, with disappearance of uptake by 14 days. The cause of persistently positive scans may be related to ongoing cellular necrosis or aneurysm formation.

Clinical Applications

Positive scans are detected in most patients with acute infarcts who are imaged at 2 to 3 days after infarction. A single scan is positive in about 90 percent of patients with transmural infarcts, although nontransmural infarcts are not detected as reliably [62]. Small infarcts (apparently less than 3 gm in weight) are often not imaged, but a negative scan is quite unusual with a large transmural infarct. Serial scanning over several days may improve the detection of acute infarction to some degree.

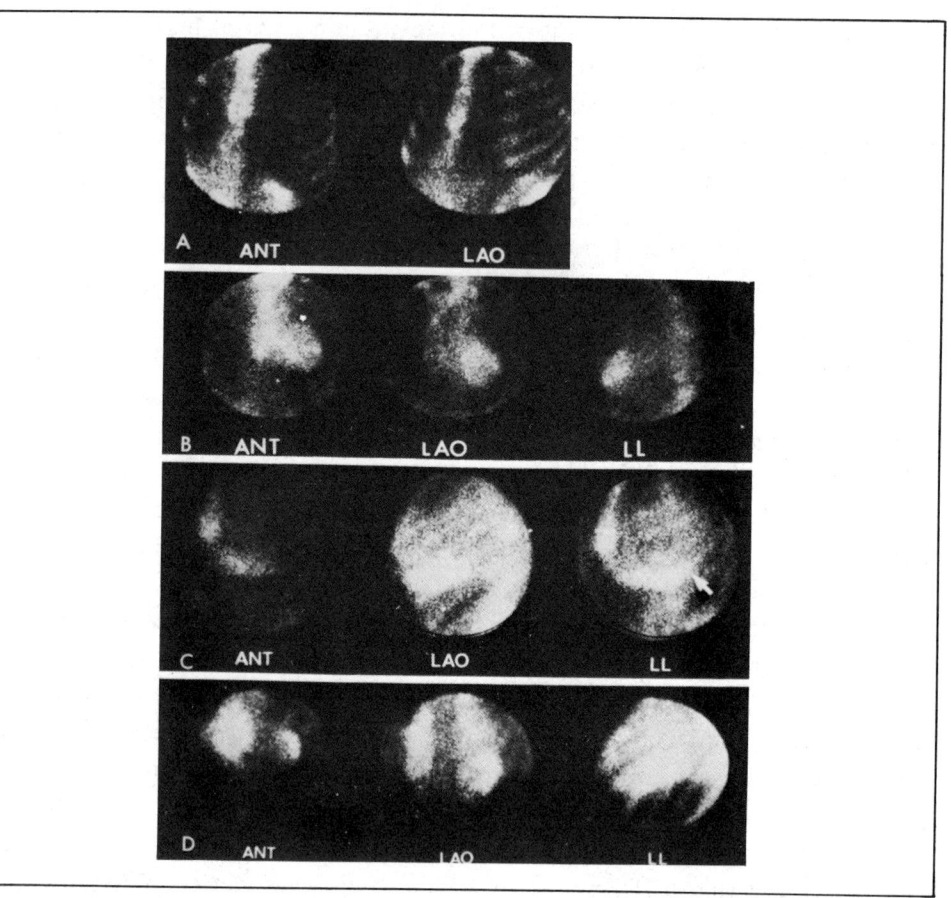

FIGURE 8-6. (A) Normal myocardial scintigram with technetium-99m-pyrophosphate, showing uptake by sternum, ribs, and vertebrae. (B) Myocardial scintigraphy in a patient with an acute anterior myocardial infarct. (C) Myocardial scintigraphy in a patient with an acute inferior myocardial infarct. There is involvement of the posterior left ventricular wall (*arrow*). (D) Myocardial scintigraphy in a patient with an acute lateral myocardial infarct. *ANT* = anterior, *LAO* = left anterior oblique, *LL* = left lateral view. (From BL Holman, J Wynne: Infarct avid (hot spot) myocardial scintigraphy. *Radiol Clin N Am* 18:487, 1980.)

A variety of conditions other than myocardial infarction may result in positive scans, as noted in Table 8-4. Extracardiac causes such as rib fractures and skeletal muscle damage can usually be distinguished from cardiac uptake by the use of multiple views. More troublesome are cardiac causes of positive scans other than infarction, particularly unstable angina pectoris. In some patients, there is diffuse activity within the heart due to persistence of the radiopharmaceutical within the bloodstream, the so-called blood pool effect. In other cases, there may be areas of

TABLE 8-4. Causes of Technetium-99m-Pyrophosphate Uptake

Focal	Diffuse
Acute myocardial infarction	Acute myocardial infarction (subendocardial)
Recent myocardial infarction	Unstable angina pectoris
Breast tumors	Cardiomyopathy
Left ventricular aneurysms	Left ventricular aneurysms (if secondary to blood pool activity)
Rib fractures	Persistent blood pool activity
Skeletal muscle damage	
Cardioversion (secondary to skeletal muscle as well as myocardial damage) (unusual)	
Valvular calcification (unusual)	
Myocardial contusion	
Skin lesions	
Calcified costal cartilage	

subclinical infarction, but it is likely that at least in some cases, pyrophosphate uptake is occurring in ischemic but not necrotic cells.

Pyrophosphate scintigraphy is normal in over 85 percent of patients without myocardial infarction, although 40 percent or more of patients with unstable angina pectoris may demonstrate abnormal scans, usually of the diffusely positive type [62].

Although successful sizing of infarcts by pyrophosphate scintigraphy has been reported, not all studies are in agreement as to its accuracy [62]. With routine two-dimensional imaging, it is necessary to view the largest area of scintigraphic activity. Thus, only anterior transmural infarcts can be sized. While tomographic imaging may be of benefit with inferior and nontransmural infarcts, these methods are still preliminary and experimental [77]. Even with adequate imaging, the relationship between pyrophosphate uptake and extent of necrosis is complex. Although infarct sizing is difficult and hazardous, the size of the pyrophosphate uptake during an acute infarction does predict inhospital and after-discharge prognosis [72]. As shown in Figure 8-7, both inhospital and long-term complications, including cardiogenic shock, ventricular arrhythmias, extension of or development of a new infarction, development of unstable angina pectoris, and death increase in frequency as a function of the size of pyrophosphate uptake.

The majority of patients admitted to a coronary care unit with suspected acute myocardial infarction do not require pyrophosphate imaging. Electrocardiographic and especially enzymatic data are usually definitive when obtained within the first 24 to 48 hours after suspected infarction. Scintigraphy may be useful in patients

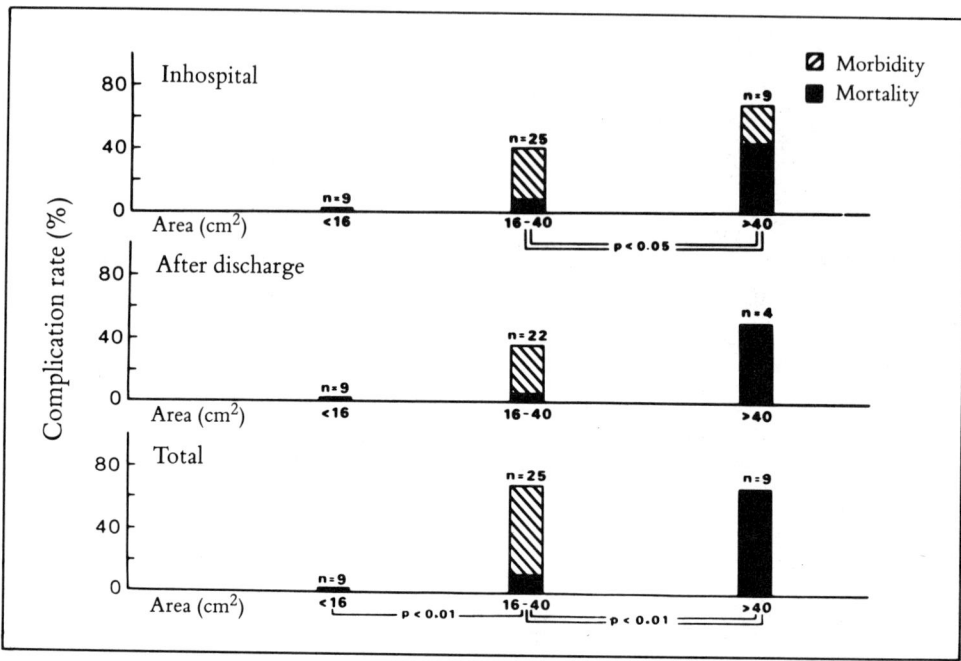

FIGURE 8-7. Complication rate compared to the area of technetium-99m-pyrosphate uptake in patients with acute myocardial infarction and focal uptake. *Single bracket* = complication rate, *double bracket* = mortality. (From BL Holman et al: The prognostic implications of acute myocardial infarct scintigraphy with ^{99m}Tc-pyrophosphate. *Circulation* 57:320, 1978, by permission of the American Heart Association, Inc.)

presenting several days after an acute event, by which time the electrocardiogram and enzyme levels are nondiagnostic. Pyrophosphate imaging may also be useful if the initial evaluation yields equivocal or contradictory results. Imaging may permit recognition of uptake in the right ventricle in the setting of right ventricular infarction. While radionuclide ventriculography is the preferred scintigraphic method of assessing right ventricular infarction, pyrophosphate imaging may be indicated in those hospitals where blood pool scanning cannot be performed in the coronary care unit.

Pyrophosphate scintigraphy may also be particularly useful in the diagnosis of myocardial infarction after cardiac surgery [70]. Since chest pain, enzyme elevation, and electrocardiographic changes are common after cardiac surgery, pyrophosphate imaging may help clarify whether or not infarction has occurred. Some patients with abnormal preoperative myocardial scintigrams demonstrate improvement in the scans after successful coronary artery bypass surgery. Other indications for scintigraphy include evaluation of atypical chest pain in patients with equivocal enzyme or electrocardiographic changes; suspected infarction in patients with left bundle branch block and similar abnormalities that limit the diagnostic utility of the electrocardiogram; new infarcts or infarct extension in patients with old or recent myocardial infarcts; and myocardial contusion [77].

A variety of new radiopharmaceuticals have been investigated to evaluate their utility as infarct-avid agents. One interesting approach utilizes purified labeled antibody against cardiac myosin. Following the intravenous injection of radioiodine-labeled fragments of cardiac myosin-specific antibody, increased activity could be detected within infarcts of experimental animals [78]. The clinical utility of these newer agents remains to be established.

References

1. Yates WK: Experimental location of myocardial infarction using radioisotopes. *US Armed Forces Med J* 3:1597, 1952
2. Love WD, Romney RB, Burch GE: A comparison of the distribution of potassium and exchangeable rubidium in the organs of the dog, using rubidium-86. *Circ Res* 2:112, 1954
3. Sapirstein LA: Fractionation of the cardiac output of rats with isotopic potassium. *Circ Res* 4:689, 1956
4. Carr EA Jr, Beierwaltes WH, Patno ME, Bartlett JD Jr, Wegst AV: The detection of experimental myocardial infarcts by photoscanning. *Am Heart J* 64:650, 1962
5. Carr EA Jr, Gleason F, Shaw J, Krontz B: The direct diagnosis of myocardial infarction by photoscanning after administration of cesium-131. *Am Heart J* 68:627, 1964
6. Zaret BL, Strauss HW, Martin ND, Wells HP Jr, Flamm JD Jr: Noninvasive regional myocardial perfusion with radioactive potassium. Study of patients at rest, with exercise, and during angina pectoris. *N Engl J Med* 288:809, 1973
7. Bradley-Moore PR, Lebowitz E, Green MW, Atkins HL, Ansari AN: Thallium-201 for medical use. II. Biologic behavior. *J Nucl Med* 16:156, 1975
8. Lebowitz E, Green MW, Fairchild R, Bradley-Moore PR, Atkins HL, Anasi AN, Richards P, Belgrave E: Thallium-201 for medical use. *J Nucl Med* 16:151, 1975
9. Weich H, Strauss HW, Pitt B: The extraction of thallium-201 by the myocardium. *Circulation* 56:188, 1977
10. Pohost GM, Zir LM, Moore RH, McKusick KA, Guiney TE, Beller GA: Differentiation of transiently ischemic from infarcted myocardium by serial imaging after a single dose of thallium-201. *Circulation* 55:294, 1977
11. Strauss HW, Harrison K, Langan JK, Lebowitz E, Pitt B: Thallium-201 for myocardial imaging. Relation of thallium-201 to regional myocardial perfusion. *Circulation* 51:641, 1975
12. Blood DK, McCarthy DM, Sciacca RR, Cannon PJ: Comparison of single-dose and double-dose thallium-201 myocardial perfusion scintigraphy for the detection of coronary artery disease and prior myocardial infarction. *Circulation* 58:777, 1978
13. Beller GA, Watson DD, Ackell P, Pohost GM: Time course of thallium-201 redistribution after transient myocardial ischemia. *Circulation* 61:791, 1980

14. Gewitz H, Beller GA, Strauss HW, Dinsmore RE, Zir LM, McKusick KA, Pohost GM: Transient defects of resting thallium scans in patients with coronary artery disease. *Circulation* 59:707, 1979
15. Berger BC, Watson DD, Sipes JN, Pohost GM, Teates CD, Beller GA: Redistribution of thallium at rest in patients with coronary disease (Abstract). *J Nucl Med* 19:680, 1978
16. Pohost GM, O'Keefe DD, Gerwitz H, Strauss HW, Beller GA, Newell JB, Chaffin JS, Daggett WM: Thallium redistribution in the presence of severe fixed coronary stenosis (Abstract). *Clin Res* 26:260A, 1978
17. Beller GA, Watson DD, Pohost GM: Kinetics of thallium distribution and redistribution: clinical applications in sequential myocardial imaging. In Strauss HW, Pitt B (eds): *Cardiovascular Nuclear Medicine.* 2nd ed. St Louis: CV Mosby, 1979, p 225
18. Pitt B, Strauss HW: Clinical application of myocardial imaging with thallium. In Strauss HW, Pitt B (eds): *Cardiovascular Nuclear Medicine.* 2nd ed. St Louis: CV Mosby, 1979, p 243
19. Ritchie JL, Zaret BL, Strauss HW, Pitt B, Berman DS, Schelbert HR, Ashburn WL, Berger HJ, Hamilton GW: Myocardial imaging with thallium-201: A multicenter study in patients with angina pectoris or acute myocardial infarction. *Am J Cardiol* 42:345, 1978
20. Botvinick EH, Taradash MR, Shames DM, Parmley WW: Thallium-201 myocardial perfusion scintigraphy for the clinical clarification of normal, abnormal and equivocal electrocardiographic stress tests. *Am J Cardiol* 41:43, 1978
21. Froelicher VF, Yanowitz FG, Thompson AJ, Lancaster MC: The correlation of coronary angiography and the electrocardiographic response to maximal treadmill testing in 76 asymptomatic men. *Circulation* 48:597, 1973
22. Guiney TE, Pohost GM, Beller GA, McKusick KA: Differentiating false positive from true positive stress tests by single dose thallium-201 stress-scanning (Abstract). *Am J Cardiol* 39:321, 1977
23. Caralis, DG, Kennedy HL, Bailey IK, Pitt B: Thallium-201 myocardial perfusion scanning in the evaluation of asymptomatic patients with ischemic ST segment depression (Abstract). *Am J Cardiol* 39:320, 1977
24. Wackers FJ, Lie KI, Liem KL, Sokole EB, Samson G, van der Schoot JB, Durrer D: Thallium-201 scintigraphy in unstable angina pectoris. *Circulation* 57:738, 1978
25. Muller TM, Marcus ML, Ehrhardt JC, Chaudhuri T, Abbout FM: Limitations of thallium-201 myocardial perfusion scintigrams. *Circulation* 54:640, 1976
26. Felman RL, Nichols WW, Pepine CJ, Conti CR: Hemodynamic significance of the length of a coronary arterial narrowing. *Am J Cardiol* 41:865, 1978
27. Waters DD, Da Luz P, Wyatt HL, Swan HJC, Forrester JS: Early changes in regional and global left ventricular function induced by graded reductions in regional coronary perfusion. *Am J Cardiol* 39:537, 1977
28. Akins CW, Pohost GM, DeSanctis RW, Block PC: Selection of angina-free patients with severe left ventricular dysfunction for myocardial revascularization. *Am J Cardiol* 46:695, 1980

29. Dunn RF, Freedman B, Bailey IK, Uren RF, Kelly DT: Exercise thallium imaging: Location of perfusion abnormalities in a single-vessel coronary disease. *J Nucl Med* 21:717, 1980
30. Massie BM, Botvinick EH, Brundage BH: Correlation of thallium-201 scintigrams with coronary anatomy: Factors affecting region by region sensitivity. *Am J Cardiol* 44:616, 1979
31. Rigo P, Bailey IK, Griffith LSC, Pitt B, Burow RD, Wagner HN, Becker LC: Value and limitations of segmental analysis of stress thallium myocardial imaging for localization of coronary artery disease. *Circulation* 61:973, 1980
32. Lenaers A, Block P, van Thiel E, Lebedelle M, Becquevort P, Erbsmann F, Ermans AM: Segmental analysis of Tl-201 stress myocardial scintigraphy. *J Nucl Med* 18:509, 1977
33. Wackers FJ, Sokole EB, Samson G, van der Schoot JB, Lie KI, Liem KL, Wellens HJJ: Value and limitations of thallium-201 scintigraphy in the acute phase of myocardial infarction. *N Engl J Med* 295:1, 1976
34. Pond M, Rehn T, Burow R, Pitt B: Early detection of myocardial infarction by serial thallium-201 imaging (Abstract). *Circulation* 56:893, 1977
35. Nishimura A, Gorten R, Kim Y, Williams JF Jr: Dual radionuclide myocardial scanning for diagnosis and location of acute myocardial infarcts. *Circulation* 52(Suppl II):II-223, 1975
36. Wackers FJT, van der Schoot JB, Sokole EB, Samson G, Niftrik GJC, Lie KI, Durrer D, Wellens HJJ: Noninvasive visualization of acute myocardial infarction in man with thallium-201. *Br Heart J* 37:741, 1975
37. Ritchie JH, Trobaugh GB, Hamilton GW, Gould KL, Narahara KA, Murray JA, Williams DL: Myocardial imaging with thallium-201 at rest and during exercise: Comparison with coronary arteriography and resting and stress electrocardiography. *Circulation* 56:66, 1977
38. McLaughlin PR, Martin RP, Dohert P, Daspit S, Goris M, Haskell W, Lewis S, Kriss JP, Harrison DC: Reproducibility of thallium-201 myocardial imaging. *Circulation* 55:497, 1977
39. Hamilton GW, Trobaugh GB, Ritchie JL, Williams DL, Weaver WD, Gould KL: Myocardial imaging with intravenously injected thallium-201 in patients with suspected coronary artery disease. *Am J Cardiol* 39:347, 1977
40. Wackers FJT, Becker AE, Samson G, Sokole EB, van der Schoot JB, Vet A, Lie KI, Durrer D, Wellens H: Location and size of acute transmural myocardial infarction estimated from thallium-201 scintiscans: A clinicopathological study. *Circulation* 56:72, 1977
41. Henning H, Schelbert HR, Rigbetti A, Ashburn WL, O'Rourke RA: Dual myocardial imaging with technetium-99m pyrophosphate and thallium-201 for detecting, localizing and sizing acute myocardial infarction. *Am J Cardiol* 40:147, 1977
42. Niess GS, Logic JR, Russel RO, Rackley CE, Rogers WJ: Usefulness and limitations of thallium-201 myocardial scintigraphy in delineating location and size of prior myocardial infarction. *Circulation* 59:1010, 1979

43. Maroko PR, Braunwald E: Effects of metabolic and pharmacologic interventions on myocardial infarct size following coronary occlusion. *Circulation* 53:1, 1976
44. Wackers FJT, Lie KI, Sokole EB, Res J, van der Schoot J, Durrer D: Prevalence of right ventricular involvement in inferior wall infarction assessed with myocardial imaging with thallium-201 and technetium-99m pyrophosphate. *Am J Cardiol* 42:358, 1978
45. DiCola, VC, Downing SE, Donabedian RK, Zaret BL: Pathophysiologic correlation of thallium-201 myocardial uptake in experimental infarction. *Cardiovasc Res* 11:141, 1977
46. Zaret Bl, Lange RC, Lee JC: Comparative assessment of infarct size with quantitative thallium-201 and technetium-99m pyrophosphate dual myocardial imaging in the dog. *Am J Cardiol* 39:309, 1977
47. Fletcher JW, Rao PS, Witztum KF, Hamilton WP, Donati RM, Mueller HS: Clinical estimation of infarct size by ^{201}thallium perfusion scintigraphy and by creatine kinase-MB in early myocardial infarction. *Clin Cardiol* 3:111, 1980
48. Silverman KJ, Becker LC, Bulkley BH, Burow RD, Mellits DE, Kallman CH, Weisfeldt ML: Value of early thallium-201 scintigraphy for predicting mortality in patients with acute myocardial infarction. *Circulation* 61:996, 1980
49. Becker LC, Bulkley BH, Pitt B, Flaherty JT, Weiss JL, Gerstenblith G, Rehn T, Pond M, Mason S, Silverman K, Wang DG, Weisfeldt ML: Enhanced reduction of thallium-201 defects in acute myocardial infarction by nitroglycerine treatment: Initial results of a prospective randomized trial (Abstract). *Clin Res* 26:219A, 1978
50. Turner JD, Schwartz KM, Logic JF, Sheffield LT, Kansal S, Roitman DI, Mantle JA, Russell RO Jr, Rackley CE, Rogers WJ: The detection of residual jeopardized myocardium three weeks after myocardial infarction by exercise testing with thallium-201 myocardial scintigraphy. *Circulation* 61:729, 1980
51. Cobb LA, Thomas GI, Dillard DH: An evaluation of internal mammary artery ligation by a double blind technique. *N Engl J Med* 260:1115, 1959
52. DiLuzio VD, Roy PR, Sowton E: Angina in patients with occluded aortocoronary vein grafts. *Br Heart J* 36:139, 1974
53. Ritchie JL, Narahara KA, Trobaugh GB, Williams DL, Hamilton GW: Thallium-201 myocardial imaging before and after coronary revascularization. *Circulation* 56:830, 1977
54. Khaja F, Alam M, Goldstein S, Anbe D, Marks D: Diagnostic value of visualization of the right ventricle using thallium-201 myocardial imaging. *Circulation* 59:182, 1979
55. Cohen HA, Baird MG, Rouleau JR, Fuhrmann CF, Bailey IK, Summer WR, Strauss HW, Pitt B: Thallium-201 myocardial imaging in patients with pulmonary hypertension. *Circulation* 54:790, 1976
56. Ohsazu F, Handa S, Kondo M, Yamazaki H, Tsaga T, Kubo A, Takagi Y, Nakamura Y: Thallium-201 myocardial imaging to evaluate right ventricular overloading. *Circulation* 61:620, 1980
57. Maseri A, Parodi O, Severi S, Pesola A: Transient transmural reduction of

myocardial blood flow, demonstrated by thallium-201 scintigraphy, as a cause of variant angina. *Circulation* 54:280, 1976

58. Bulkley BH, Hutchins GM, Bailey I, Strauss HW, Pitt B: Thallium-201 imaging and gated cardiac blood pool scans in patients with ischemic and idiopathic congestive cardiomyopathy. A clinical and pathologic study. *Circulation* 55:753, 1977
59. Bulkley BH, Rouleau JR, Whitaker JQ, Strauss HW, Pitt B: The use of ^{201}thallium for myocardial perfusion imaging in sarcoid heart disease. *Chest* 72:27, 1977
60. Cook DJ, Bailey I, Strauss HE, Rouleau J, Wagner HN, Pitt B: Thallium-201 for myocardial imaging: Appearance of the normal heart. *J Nucl Med* 17:184, 1976
61. Bingham JB, McKusick KA, Strauss HW, Boucher CA, Pohost GM: Influence of coronary artery disease on pulmonary uptake of thallium-201. *Am J Cardiol* 46:821, 1980
62. Wynne J, Holman BL: Acute myocardial infarct scintigraphy with infarct-avid radiotracers. *Med Clin N Am* 64:119, 1980
63. Willerson JT, Parkey RW, Bonte FJ, Meyer SL, Atkins J, Stokely EM: Technetium-99m stannous pyrophosphate myocardial scintigrams in patients with chest pain of varying etiologies. *Circulation* 51:1046, 1975
64. Olson HG, Lyons KP, Aronow WS, Brown WT, Greenfield RS: Follow-up technetium-99m stannous pyrophosphate myocardial scintigrams after myocardial infarction. *Circulation* 56:181, 1977
65. Massie MB, Botvinick EH, Werner JA, Shames D, Chatterjee K, Parmley WW: Myocardial infarction scintigraphy with technetium-99m stannous pyrophosphate: An insensitive test for nontransmural myocardial infarction. *Am J Cardiol* 43:186, 1979
66. Henning H, Shelbert HR, Righetti A, Ashburn WL, O'Rourke R: Dual myocardial imaging with technetium-99m pyrophosphate and thallium-201 for detecting, localizing and sizing acute myocardial infarction. *Am J Cardiol* 40:147, 1977
67. Prasquier R, Taradash MR, Botvinick EH, Shames D, Parmley WW: The specificity of the diffuse pattern of cardiac uptake in myocardial infarction imaging with technetium-99m stannous pyrophosphate. *Circulation* 55:61, 1977
68. Poliner LR, Buja LM, Parkey RW, Bonte F, Willerson JT: Clinicopathologic correlations in 52 patients studied by technetium-99m stannous pyrophosphate myocardial scintigraphy. *Circulation* 59:257, 1979
69. Sharpe DN, Botvinick EH, Shames DM, Schiller NB, Massie BM, Chatterjee K, Parmley WW: The noninvasive diagnosis of right ventricular infarction. *Circulation* 57:483, 1978
70. Platt MR, Parkey RW, Willerson JT, Bonte FJ, Shapiro W, Sugg WL: Technetium stannous pyrophosphate myocardial scintigrams in the recognition of myocardial infarction in patients undergoing coronary artery revascularization. *Ann Thorac Surg* 21:311, 1976
71. Sharpe DN, Botvinick EH, Shames DM: The clinical estimation of acute myocardial infarct size with ^{99m}technetium pyrophosphate scintigraphy. *Circulation* 57:307, 1978
72. Holman BL, Chisholm RJ, Braunwald E: The prognostic implication of acute myo-

cardial infarct scintigraphy with Tc-99m pyrophosphate. *Circulation* 57:320, 1978
73. Ahmad M, Logan KW, Martin RH: Doughnut pattern of technetium-99m pyrophosphate myocardial uptake in patients with acute myocardial infarction: A sign of poor long-term prognosis. *Am J Cardiol* 44:13, 1979
74. Bonte FJ, Parkey RW, Graham KD, Moore J, Stokley EM: A new method for radionuclide imaging of myocardial infarcts. *Radiology* 110:473, 1974
75. Dewanjee MK, Kahn PC: Mechanisms of localization of ^{99m}Tc-labeled pyrophosphate and tetracycline in infarcted myocardium. *J Nucl Med* 17:639, 1976
76. Zaret BL, DiCola VC, Donabedian RK, Puri S, Wolfson S, Freedman GS, Cohen LS: Dual radionuclide study of myocardial infarction. Relationship between myocardial uptake of potassium-43, technetium-99m stannous pyrophosphate, regional myocardial blood flow and creatine phosphokinase depletion. *Circulation* 53:422, 1976
77. Holman BL, Wynne J: Infarct avid (hot spot) myocardial scintigraphy. *Radiol Clin N Am* 18:487, 1980
78. Khaw BA, Beller GA, Haber E: Experimental myocardial infarct imaging following intravenous administration of iodine-131 labeled antibody (Fab^1)$_2$ fragment specific for cardiac myosin. *Circulation* 57:743, 1978

Part IV

Invasive Procedures

Chapter 9

Bedside Hemodynamic Monitoring, Cardiac Catheterization, and Pulmonary Angiography

Blase A. Carabello and William Grossman

This chapter will discuss the roles of bedside hemodynamic monitoring, cardiac catheterization, and pulmonary angiography in general medical practice. While cardiac catheterization and pulmonary angiography are typically performed by specially trained cardiologists or radiologists, bedside hemodynamic monitoring may be performed by other physicians as well. Therefore, our chapter will discuss the indications for all of these procedures but will go into technical detail only for bedside hemodynamic monitoring.

Bedside Hemodynamic Monitoring

In 1970, Swan, Ganz, and Forrester described catheterization of the pulmonary artery with a balloon-tipped catheter at the bedside [1]. This procedure has equipped the physician with a powerful readily available clinical tool — the ability to measure accurately left ventricular filling pressure, as reflected by the pulmonary capillary wedge pressure (PCWP). Advances in catheter technology have also permitted concomitant measurement of cardiac output by thermodilution technique, further enhancing the usefulness of the method. It is therefore not surprising that Swan-Ganz catheterization has gained wide acceptance in the treatment of critically ill patients. In the following pages, we will discuss the indications, methods of insertion, data interpretation, and complications of this useful clinical tool.

INDICATIONS
Complications of Myocardial Infarction
CARDIOGENIC SHOCK. Shock develops in approximately 15 percent of myocardial infarctions (MI) and is a common indication for hemodynamic monitoring. There are many definitions for cardiogenic shock. We shall define it as a systolic blood pressure of ≤ 85 mm Hg and a urinary output of < 20 ml/hr due to low cardiac output secondary to pump failure. A key goal in management of this complication of

MI is the optimization of left ventricular filling pressure. Russell and coworkers studied the relationship of left ventricular filling pressure and cardiac output in acute MI [2]. They found a curvilinear relationship with peak cardiac output occurring at a left ventricular end-diastolic pressure of 20 to 24 mm Hg. Crexells et al, in a similar study, found that maximal stroke work index was reached at a PCWP of 18 mm Hg [3] (Fig. 9-1). Thus, the injured left ventricle needs to make full use of the Frank-Starling compensatory mechanism to maximize its cardiac output. Lower filling pressures result in lower outputs, while excessive filling pressures do not increase cardiac output but do progressively increase the risk of pulmonary edema. The importance of the left ventricular filling pressure in this group of patients was emphasized by Carabello and coworkers [4]. They noted that 43 percent of hypotensive patients following MI treated at the Peter Bent Brigham Hospital had suboptimal PCWP upon initial measurement. This group benefited from volume expansion. The mortality rate in this group was 17 percent compared with 75 percent in a group that was hypotensive despite optimum PCWP. Forrester and coworkers used measured cardiac output and PCWP to classify patients with MI into hemodynamic subsets of severity of pump impairment (Table 9-1) [5]. They found a hospital mortality of 2.2 percent in subset I, and 10.1 percent mortality in subset II, a 22.4 percent mortality in subset III, and 55.5 percent mortality in subset IV. Thus, measurement and proper management of the left ventricular filling pressure is important in maximizing cardiac output, minimizing the risk of pulmonary edema, and in determining prognosis. Unfortunately, estimating the PCWP on clinical grounds alone may be difficult. A third heart sound on physical examination and the chest roentgenogram may offer a guide to the PCWP, but these are not always reliable. Rotman et al found that the PCWP was ≥ 15 mm Hg in two-thirds of patients with a third heart sound [6]. Obviously then, one-third of patients with a third heart sound will have PCWP <15 mm Hg. Therefore, an S_3 is only a rough guide to left ventricular filling pressure. McHugh and coworkers found a good correlation between severity of heart failure on the chest roentgenogram and simultaneous PCWP [7]. However, in most patients, failure was detected on x-ray only when PCWP was greater than 18 mm Hg. As can be seen in Figure 9-2, a wide range of PCWP is present for each radiologic grade of failure. As discussed in Chapter 11 the chest x-ray serves as a valuable but imprecise estimate of PCWP in this group of patients. Furthermore, if diuretics have been employed in a patient's care, PCWP may fall, but the chest x-ray improvement may lag behind this fall considerably [3, 8]. In addition, the central venous pressure as estimated from the jugular venous pulsation by direct measurement does not correlate well with PCWP [9]. Currently, the only reliable way of ascertaining PCWP is to measure it directly with a catheter in the pulmonary artery. This measurement is a valuable key to the management of cardiogenic shock.

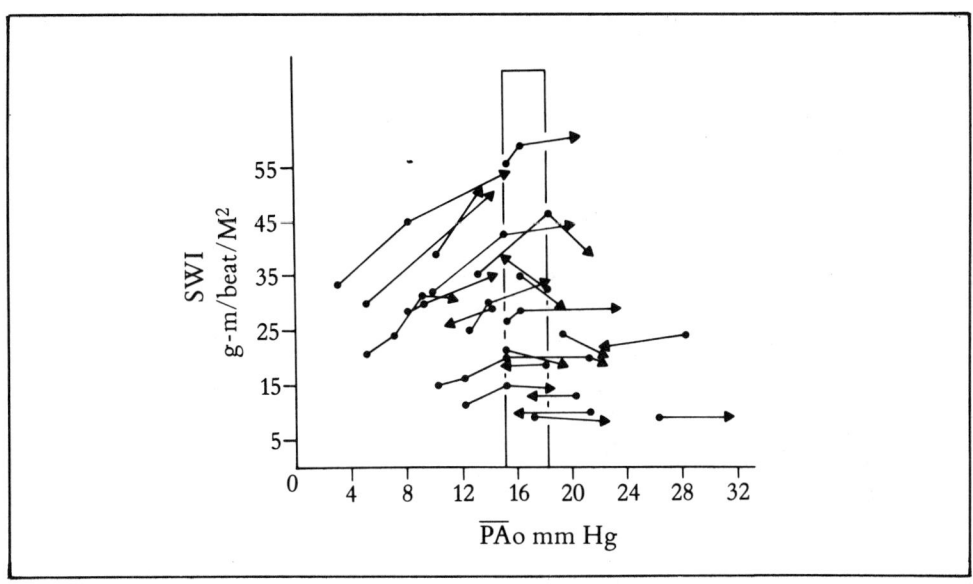

FIGURE 9-1. Relation between stroke work index (*SWI* in gram-meters per beat per square meter of body surface area) and mean pulmonary artery occluded (i.e., wedge) pressure ($\overline{PAo}$) in 21 patients with acute myocardial infarction. The highest level of stroke work index appears to lie in the range of 15–18 mm Hg of $\overline{PAo}$ as indicated by the bars. The direction of change in $\overline{PAo}$ induced by therapy is indicated by the arrows. In all cases, increases in $\overline{PAo}$ were induced by volume loading and decreases in $\overline{PAo}$ by diuresis. (From C Crexells et al: *N Engl J Med* 289:1263, 1973. Reprinted by permission.)

TABLE 9-1. Hemodynamic Subsets in Acute Myocardial Infarction

Clinical Subset	Cardiac Index ($L/min/m^2$)	Pulmonary Capillary Wedge Pressure (mm Hg)	Mortality (%)
I. No pulmonary congestion or peripheral hypoperfusion	2.7 ± 0.5	12 ± 7	2.2
II. Isolated pulmonary congestion	2.3 ± 0.4	23 ± 5	10.1
III. Isolated peripheral hypoperfusion	1.9 ± 0.4	12 ± 5	22.4
IV. Both pulmonary congestion and hypoperfusion	1.6 ± 0.6	27 ± 8	55.5

From JS Forrester et al: Medical therapy of acute myocardial infarction by application of hemodynamic subsets. *N Engl J Med* 295:1404, 1976. Reprinted by permission.

SEPTAL RUPTURE. Septal rupture (acute ventricular septal defect) occurs in approximately 2 percent of acute myocardial infarction [10]. This complication carries with it a high mortality [11] and can be seen in both anterior and inferior MI. The goals of management of acute septal rupture are to minimize left-to-right

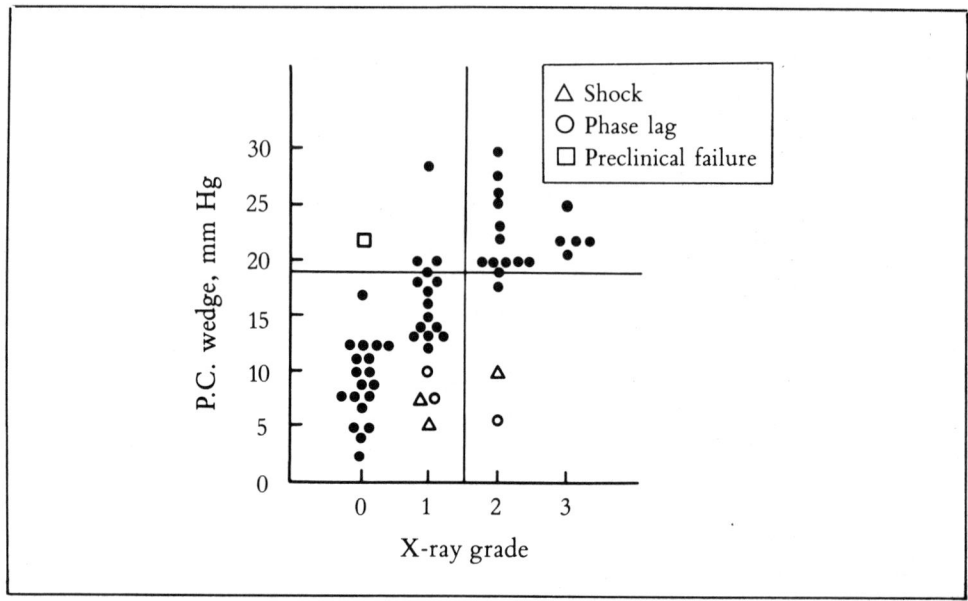

FIGURE 9-2. Relationship between pulmonary capillary (P.C.) wedge pressure and the severity of left ventricular failure on portable chest x-ray. A pulmonary capillary wedge pressure of 18 mm Hg separated patients with absent and mild failure by x-ray (grades zero and one) from those with moderate and severe failure by x-ray (grades two and three) in 86 percent of cases. Discrepancies between the level of pulmonary capillary wedge pressure and degree of failure by x-ray are indicated by open symbols. (From [7].)

shunting, to maximize forward systemic output, and to stabilize the patient for eventual surgical correction. The diagnosis of acute septal rupture is suspected with the appearance of a new murmur following myocardial infarction. The murmur is typically holosystolic and heard on both sides of the sternum. The diagnosis of acute septal rupture can be made by sampling blood in the right atrium, right ventricle, and pulmonary artery, and documenting a step-up in oxygen saturation at the right ventricular level. Although the amount of step-up needed to detect and confirm acute septal rupture will vary depending on systemic blood flow, in general, a step-up of 5 percent saturation is highly suggestive of the diagnosis [12].

The approach to this group of patients is to optimize left ventricular filling pressure to make use of the Frank-Starling mechanism, while minimizing impedance to left ventricular emptying, which tends to reduce left-to-right shunting. This last goal is usually accomplished with systemic vasodilators or intraaortic balloon counterpulsation. The pulmonary artery catheter is quite helpful in monitoring the effects of such therapies. A pulmonary artery catheter with proximal and distal ports from which blood can be sampled is ideal. The proximal port usually resides in the right atrium, while the distal port is located in the pulmonary artery. By simultaneously sampling blood from the right atrium, pulmonary artery, and systemic artery (by systemic arterial puncture or indwelling catheter), one can obtain blood oxygen determinations at these sites. With these data, the pulmonary blood flow to systemic blood flow ratio ($\dot{Q}p/\dot{Q}s$) can easily be calculated by the following formula:

$$\dot{Q}p/\dot{Q}s = \frac{\text{systemic arterial saturation} - \text{right atrial saturation}}{\text{systemic arterial saturation} - \text{pulmonary artery saturation}}$$

Therapeutic maneuvers that increase systemic flow or decrease left-to-right shunting will lower the $\dot{Q}p/\dot{Q}s$ and are generally beneficial. Thus, the results of various therapeutic interventions can be continuously evaluated with this simple technique.

ACUTE MITRAL REGURGITATION. Acute mitral regurgitation due to papillary muscle dysfunction or partial papillary muscle rupture occurs in both anterior and inferior myocardial infarction. Acute severe mitral regurgitation results in a fall in forward cardiac output as up to 60 percent of the left ventricular stroke volume passes backward into the left atrium. In addition, this increased volume in the left atrium increases left atrial and pulmonary venous hydrostatic pressure tending to cause pulmonary edema. This condition is suspected clinically by the appearance of a new holosystolic murmur. Although the murmur is usually heard more toward the cardiac apex than the sternum, it may be impossible to distinguish it clinically from acute septal rupture. Once again, the Swan-Ganz catheter may be quite useful in helping to make the diagnosis in this situation. The diagnosis of acute mitral regurgitation is suggested by the presence of a large v wave in the PCWP tracing (Fig. 9-3). The large v wave is the result of systolic filling of the left atrium from both the pulmonary veins and from the left ventricle by way of the regurgitant mitral valve. Since large v waves can also occur in acute septal rupture due to the increased pulmonary venous return created by the left-to-right shunt, it is important to exclude an oxygen step-up during passage of the pulmonary artery catheter. Although the presence of a large v wave in the PCWP tracing suggests mitral regurgitation, severe mitral regurgitation can also be present in the absence of large v waves.

Intractable Pulmonary Edema

The treatment of classic cardiogenic pulmonary edema usually includes diuretics, oxygen, mechanical occlusion of cardiac venous return, morphine sulfate, and, more recently, vasodilators such as nitroglycerin. Usually, intracardiac hemodynamic monitoring in this setting is neither necessary nor practical, since most

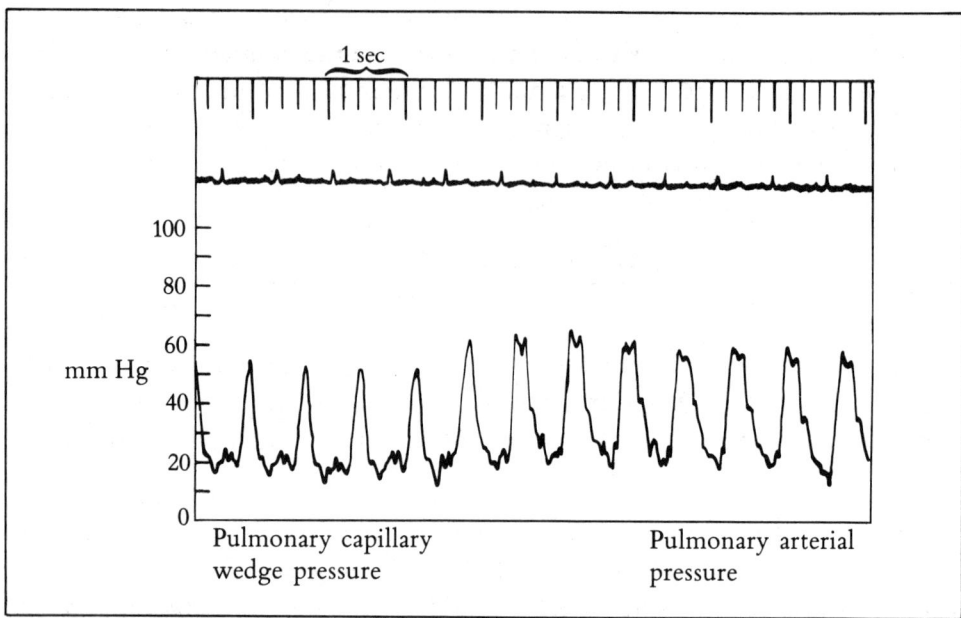

FIGURE 9-3. Acute mitral regurgitation secondary to infarcted papillary muscle in a 45-year-old man. Tracing shows tall v waves in pulmonary capillary wedge tracing. (From JS Alpert, E Braunwald: Pathological and clinical manifestations of acute myocardial infarction. In E Braunwald [ed]: *Heart Disease*. Philadelphia: WB Saunders, 1980, p 1342)

patients respond to conventional therapy adequately and too quickly to allow insertion of a pulmonary artery catheter. However, occasionally patients may not respond to conventional therapy. In some such cases, the lack of response is due to severe cardiac dysfunction, which precludes an adequate diuresis. In other cases, the origin of pulmonary edema may be noncardiac [13]. In these cases, an increase in pulmonary capillary permeability may be responsible for pulmonary edema as opposed to an increase in cardiac filling pressures. Here, lowering of cardiac filling pressure with diuretics or other maneuvers may not be beneficial, since elevation of filling pressure was not implicated in the disease pathogenesis in the first place. In both of these examples, placement of a pulmonary artery catheter may facilitate diagnosis and management. When severe left ventricular dysfunction limits renal blood flow and hence diuresis, lowering of the PCWP to eliminate pulmonary edema must be done cautiously. Excessive lowering of the PCWP will result in greater diminution of already abnormally low cardiac output. In this situation, a pulmonary artery catheter is ideal to gauge the effects of various therapeutic maneuvers and to guide their use. In the case of noncardiac pulmonary edema, a pulmonary artery catheter can be of great diagnostic value. The absence of a relatively high PCWP (>20–25 mm Hg, which is required to produce cardiac pulmonary edema) establishes the diagnosis of noncardiac pulmonary edema and shifts the focus of therapy.

Vasodilator Therapy

Recently, use of venous and arteriolar vasodilators has been demonstrated to be effective in the treatment of congestive heart failure [14]. Drugs that primarily dilate the venous or capacitance vessels help to reduce PCWP and thus symptoms of congestion by blood pooling in the periphery. Drugs that dilate arterioles diminish the impedance to left ventricular emptying and enhance forward cardiac output. Although these drugs can be used empirically, we have found the determination of the patient's hemodynamic profile by Swan-Ganz catheterization prior to institution of vasodilator therapy may be useful in optimizing the results of such therapy. This is particularly true if despite significant left ventricular dysfunction, the PCWP is not grossly elevated prior to therapy. In this case, the addition of a venodilator such as nitroglycerin or prazosin may diminish PCWP even further, thus impeding the Frank-Starling compensatory mechanism. This will result in a fall in cardiac output and often a serious fall in blood pressure. Determination of the patient's hemodynamic status prior to therapy with bedside passage of a Swan-Ganz catheter will allow for a rational choice of vasodilator agents based upon this knowledge and a chance to determine the effects of such therapy. Although we do not feel that every patient who is begun on vasodilator therapy for heart failure must undergo prior hemodynamic evaluation, we do recommend it in patients in whom initial therapy either does not lead to improvement in symptoms or causes symptomatic hypotension.

INSERTION OF THE FLOW-DIRECTED BALLOON-TIPPED PULMONARY ARTERY CATHETER

The standard flow-directed catheter is shown in Figure 9-4. It is constructed from polyvinylchloride and is soft and pliable. The standard catheter has two lumens; the thermodilution catheter has three lumens. One lumen terminates in the tip of the catheter and is used to record PCWP and pulmonary artery pressure. A second lumen ends in the balloon and is the mechanism for balloon inflation and deflation. In thermodilution catheters, a third lumen ends 30 cm proximal from the tip. This is used for iced solution injection in measuring cardiac output. It can also be used to measure pressure and oxygen saturation in the right atrium. The catheters are available in No. 5, 6, and 7 French sizes, but for improved catheter control, we recommend the No. 7 French size in adults.

Inflation of the balloon with air or carbon dioxide causes the tip to become buoyant and hence to float upon the intracardiac blood. In this way, it is carried

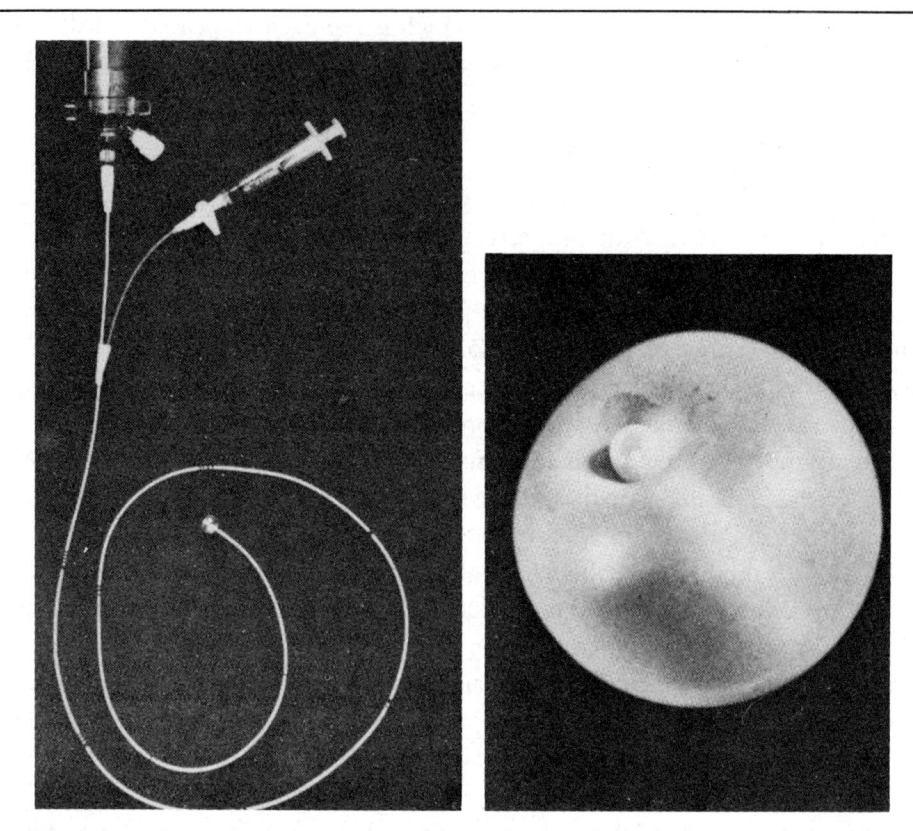

FIGURE 9-4. *Left,* Standard balloon-tipped flow-directed catheter with inflated balloon, closed inflation lumen, and a pressure transducer attached to the large lumen. *Right,* Close-up view of the inflated balloon. (From W Ganz, HJC Swan: Balloon-tipped flow-directed catheters. In W Grossman [ed]: *Cardiac Catheterization and Angiography.* 2nd ed. Philadelphia: Lea & Febiger, 1980, p 79)

in the direction of blood flow by the flow itself. In addition, inflation of the balloon allows the catheter to wedge in a large pulmonary artery. This prevents the tip of the catheter from sensing the pulmonary artery pressure proximal to the balloon, and hence the catheter measures the pressure in the system distal to the balloon, which is essentially left atrial pressure.

The flow-directed pulmonary artery catheter can be inserted from at least three approaches, the brachial vein, internal jugular vein, and femoral vein. Each has its advantages and disadvantages, which will be discussed subsequently. Catheter passage is generally facilitated by fluoroscopic guidance but can be accomplished via pressure monitoring guidance alone. Regardless of the point of insertion, there are a few general guidelines that should be followed. The need for sterile technique in catheter passage is obvious. A wide area around the insertion site should be covered with sterile drapes to prevent inadvertent contamination of both the operator and the catheter. Before proceeding with catheter insertion, the balloon should be inflated with 0.8 ml of air. The inflated balloon is then placed in sterile saline to check for air leaks, which will be detected by the presence of bubbles escaping from the balloon into the water. In the rare event that the patient is suspected of having a right-to-left intracardiac shunt, carbon dioxide should be used for balloon inflation instead of air, for patient safety in case of balloon rupture. This is also true if an atrial septal defect is present and the femoral approach is contemplated for catheter insertion. In such cases, the catheter may pass into the left atrium, where an air embolism from balloon rupture would have serious consequences. This is generally not a concern if ventricular septal rupture is suspected, since inadvertent catheter passage across such a defect is extremely rare.

After the balloon has been checked for air leaks, stopcocks are connected to the pressure lumens of the catheter, and the lumens are flushed with 5 ml of heparinized saline (heparin 3000 U/L). If catheter passage is to be performed without fluoroscopic guidance, we estimate the length of catheter that will be needed to reach the right atrium by placing the catheter on the sterile drapes and tracing its projected course from site of insertion to the right atrium. The catheter is then inserted and advanced to the right atrium by the chosen route using the length previously estimated as a guide. The distal pressure lumen is then connected to a pressure transducer, and right atrial pressure is recorded. If resistance to catheter passage is met prior to reaching the right atrium, force should never be applied. Rather, the catheter is withdrawn 2 or 3 cm from the point where resistance was met, rotated one half-turn clockwise or counterclockwise, and then advanced again. This maneuver may be repeated several times until the obstruction to catheter passage has been successfully negotiated. After right atrial pressure has been recorded, the balloon is inflated and the catheter is advanced first into the right ventricle and then the pulmonary artery. Characteristic pressure tracings are seen in each position and can be used to guide the operator if fluoroscopy is not available. An example of the typical pressure tracing seen is shown in Figure 9-5. When the catheter is advanced across the tricuspid valve into the right ventricle, some ventricular ectopy is likely to occur. This generally subsides with further passage into the pulmonary artery. Ventricular tachycardia or fibrillation is a known, but fortunately rare, occurrence during catheter passage. For this reason, the presence of a cardiac defibrillator is essential during catheter passage. If serious arrhythmia occurs, the balloon is immediately deflated, and the catheter should be withdrawn into the right atrium. Care should be taken that in one's haste to withdraw the catheter, the balloon does not remain inflated, since this may damage the tricuspid valve.

After the pulmonary artery has been successfully entered and the pressure is

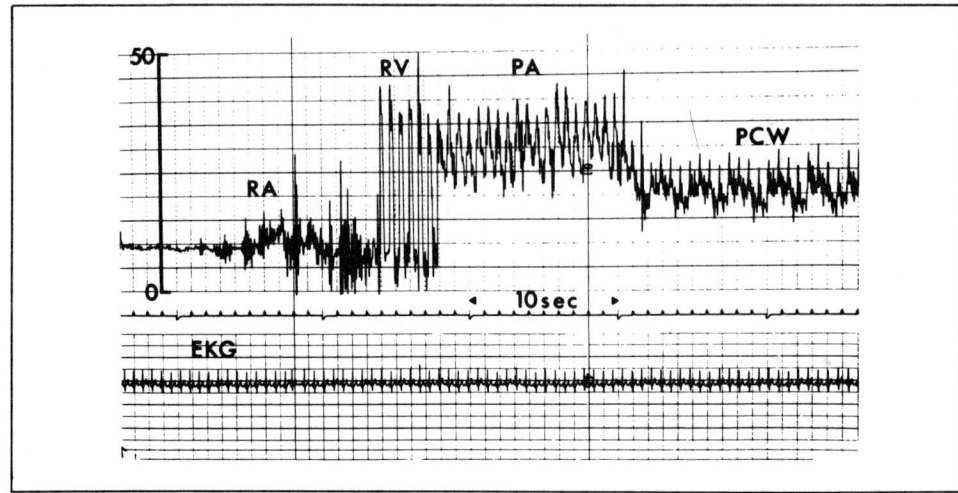

FIGURE 9-5. Pressures recorded during insertion of a balloon-tipped flow-directed catheter. PA = pulmonary arterial pressure, PCW = pulmonary capillary wedge pressure, RA = right atrial pressure, RV = right ventricular pressure. The scale at the left calibrates pressure from 0 to 50 mm Hg. (From W Ganz, HJC Swan: Balloon-tipped flow-directed catheters. In W Grossman [ed]: *Cardiac Catheterization and Angiography.* 2nd ed. Philadelphia: Lea & Febiger, 1980, p 80)

recorded, the catheter is advanced to the pulmonary capillary wedge position. This is always done with the balloon fully inflated, in order to prevent the catheter from advancing into smaller, more distal, pulmonary artery branches where balloon inflation can cause overwedging and even pulmonary artery rupture. This issue will be discussed more thoroughly under Complications.

After the PCWP is recorded, the balloon is deflated, and the catheter is secured at its insertion site and á sterile dressing applied. Pressurized systems are available that permit continuous flushing of the catheter with heparinized dextrose or saline solutions at a rate of 3 to 6 ml/hr. These systems, when combined with occasional manual flushing, serve to prevent catheter clotting.

The Brachial Approach

Insertion of the pulmonary artery catheter via a left or right brachial vein has the advantage that the insertion site is far removed from vital structures, and therefore serious complications of insertion are rare. However, without fluoroscopic guidance, catheter passage around the shoulder into the great veins may be difficult. When fluoroscopy is available, this is our approach site of choice because of its relative safety. Before selecting which arm to use, we prefer to place a tourniquet around each arm to better visualize veins under the skin. If one arm has an easily visualized, medially located vein, it should be used preferentially as the insertion site. After palpating the brachial artery to ascertain its location, local anesthesia is provided by infiltration with 3 to 5 ml of 1% lidocaine. A 3-cm transverse incision is made over the previously identified medial vein 1 cm above the flexor skin crease. If no vein has been identified, a wider, but still medial, skin incision can be made to help facilitate exploration. Medial veins should be chosen for insertion as these usually drain into the basilic system, which is more easily navigated back to the right atrium than the cephalic system, which drains more laterally positioned veins. The vein is exposed by blunt dissection with a curved hemostat at right angles to the incision. The isolated vessel is then tagged proximally and distally by 3-0 silk ties. The chosen vessel should be carefully and lightly palpated to ensure that the structure is not pulsatile, since branches of the brachial artery can be confused with veins. A forceps is then placed under the vein and allowed to spring open gently. This isolates a segment of vein, which facilitates venotomy. Next, the venotomy is made with a small scissors or a No. 11 scalpel blade. Great caution should be taken to incise only the anterior wall of the vein and to avoid transection. The catheter is then inserted with the aid of a small tissue forceps or vein introducer and advanced to the right atrium.

During catheter passage, venospasm may occur, thus obstructing advancement of the catheter. Should this happen, the spasm may be "broken" by withdrawing the catheter 10 cm and then moving it back and forth in short brisk strokes. If this fails, injection of 2 ml of 1% lidocaine via the catheter near its insertion site may relieve the spasm. This method of relieving spasm must be used very cautiously if the patient is already receiving lidocaine as an antiarrhythmic drug, since additional injection may lead to lidocaine intoxication. In many instances, it will be necessary to replace the catheter with one that is one or two French sizes smaller.

The Internal Jugular Approach

The pulmonary artery catheter can also be introduced via the internal jugular vein. There is usually little difficulty in negotiating the catheter into the right atrium, making this route useful when fluoroscopy is not available. However, serious complications may occur at the insertion site, including carotid artery puncture, pneumothorax, and air embolism. In general, we avoid this approach if chronic obstructive pulmonary disease is present, since we feel the likelihood of pneumothorax is increased in this condition. Several different techniques for cannulating the jugular vein may be used. We prefer the posterior approach. The right neck is prepared and draped, and the head is turned to the left. The patient is placed in 15 degree Trendelenburg position, which distends the vessel, making it a bigger target, and decreases the likelihood of air embolism. Next, the posterior head of the sternocleidomastoid muscle is located. The needle will be inserted at the posterior border of this muscle at the junction of its lower and middle thirds. After anesthesia is provided with lidocaine, a 2-inch 16-gauge needle attached to a 5-ml syringe is advanced from the insertion point and is directed caudally toward the suprasternal notch while negative pressure is placed on the syringe. If blood does not appear in the syringe during advancement, the needle is slowly withdrawn while gentle traction is placed on the barrel of the syringe. Frequently, confirmation that one has entered the jugular vein is made only during needle withdrawal. Once free flow of blood returns into the syringe, the syringe is disconnected and a guidewire is inserted into the jugular vein through the needle. The needle is then withdrawn over the wire and a No. 8 French Cordis sheath with a No. 7 French vessel dilator is threaded over the wire with a twisting motion into the vein. The dilator and wire are withdrawn. The Cordis sheath has a one-way valve in its hub, which prevents blood leakage and air embolism. The Swan-Ganz catheter is then passed through this valve and sheath and advanced as previously described.

The Femoral Approach

If other approaches are contraindicated because of previous antecubital cutdowns or chronic obstructive pulmonary disease, the femoral vein may be used for catheter insertion. While this approach is generally successful, we have found greater difficulty in reaching the PCWP position from the femoral vein than from other approaches, particularly is fluoroscopy is not available. Furthermore, after the catheter tip crosses the tricuspid valve, it frequently becomes situated in the right ventricular apex pointed inferiorly instead of superiorly toward the pulmonary artery. Often much manipulation is needed to successfully enter the pulmonary artery from this position.

After the femoral artery is located by palpation, the groin is anesthetized by infiltration with lidocaine. A 0.5 puncture wound is made 1 cm medial to the femoral artery pulsation (Fig. 9-6). A straight hemostat is used to blunt dissect a "tunnel" down to the femoral vein. This facilitates catheter passage and also allows any blood that escapes to come to the surface rather than becoming entrapped as a hematoma. Then, while the femoral artery is palpated, the femoral vein is punctured with an 18-gauge Seldinger needle. The central stylet is removed, and a 5-ml syringe is attached to the needle. The needle is slowly pulled back with one hand, while the other hand gently withdraws on the syringe until there is free flow of blood from the femoral vein into the syringe. The needle is fixed in place with one hand, and the syringe is removed with the other. If the femoral artery has been punctured inadvertently, pulsatile flow from the needle will be noted. In this case, the needle is withdrawn and the bleeding controlled with hand pressure for 5 minutes. Once the vein has been successfully punctured and free flow is noted, a 0.035-inch Teflon-coated J guidewire is advanced

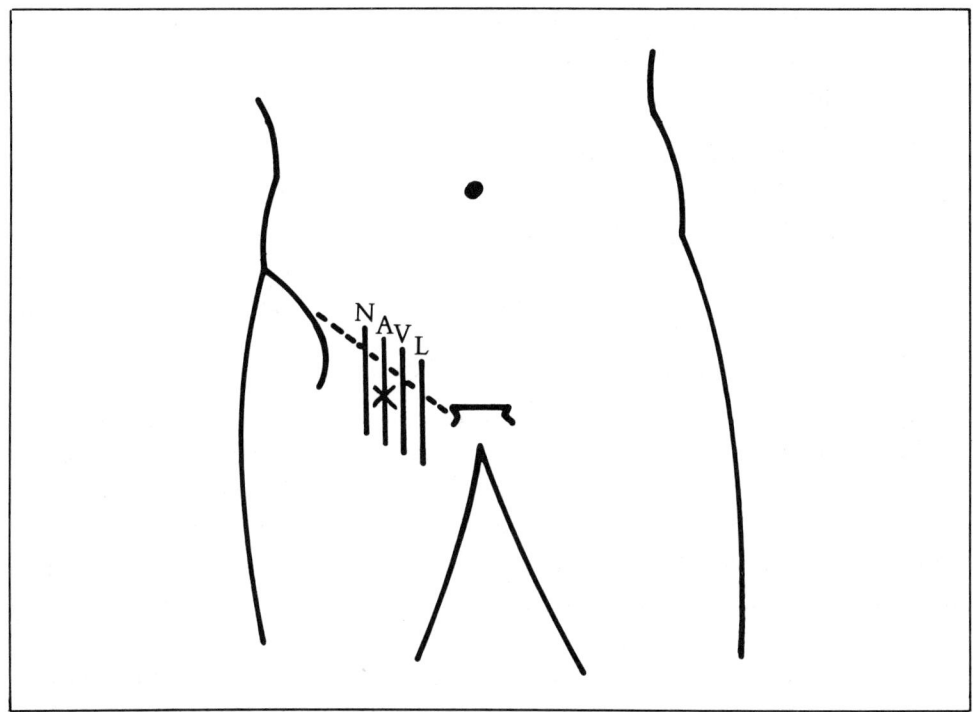

FIGURE 9-6. Diagrammatic representation of the femoral artery (*A*) and vein (*V*) and their relationship to the inguinal ligament (*dotted line*). X marks the point at which the femoral artery pulsation is strongest to palpation, usually near the inguinal skin crease but well below the inguinal ligament. *L* = lymph channel, *N* = femoral nerve. (From CR Conti, DC Levin, W Grossman: *Coronary Angiography.* In W Grossman [ed]: *Cardiac Catheterization and Angiography.* 2nd ed. Philadelphia: Lea & Febiger, 1980, p 54)

through the needle into the femoral vein. The guidewire should pass easily without resistance. If it does not, one withdraws the needle slightly and again attempts to advance the guidewire. The guidewire is advanced approximately 50 cm — under fluoroscopy, if available. The needle is then withdrawn over the guidewire, while one hand is used to control bleeding at the puncture site and to fix the guidewire, guarding against accidental withdrawal. Next, a wet gauze sponge is used to wipe the guidewire free of blood. A No. 7 French vessel dilator inside a No. 8 French venous catheter sheath is then advanced over the guidewire into the femoral vein. The dilator and sheath are advanced together with a brisk twisting motion into the vein with the dilator leading the way. Care should be taken to make sure that enough dilator extends outside the sheath to allow removal of the dilator. Once the sheath is inside the vein, the guidewire and dilator are removed and the sheath flushed with heparinized saline. The Swan-Ganz catheter is then advanced through the sheath into the femoral vein. Preferably, the catheter should be passed into the right atrium under fluoroscopic guidance to avoid its advancing into various inferior vena cava tributaries rather than directly into the right atrium.

Data Acquisition and Interpretation

Implicit in the concept of bedside hemodynamic monitoring is the idea that such monitoring will help in patient management. It is obvious, then, that faulty data acquired by this method or misinterpretation of these data will lead to errors in management. The following suggestions may aid in proper data acquisition and interpretation and in avoiding such misinterpretation.

TRANSDUCERS AND RECORDERS. Miscalibration of transducers and recorders can invalidate data obtained from the most expertly placed catheter. Two major factors that can seriously affect pressure measurement are the zero reference and transducer calibration. We prefer to set the zero reference at the midchest level. If the patient becomes elevated above this level by changes in the bed back position, the pressure recorded will be factitiously high and, conversely, will be factitiously low if the patient is placed below this level. Thus, any change in the patient's position should be accompanied by an adjustment in the zero level.

A second factor leading to inaccurate pressure measurement is improper calibration and balancing of the transducer and recorder. Although most bedside hemodynamic monitors are equipped with accurate internal electronic calibrating circuits, these are not foolproof. Confirmation of accurate calibration can easily be made by placing a mercury manometer in line with the transducer and comparing the pressure recorded by the manometer with that of the transducer-recorder system. This should always be performed when the PCWP recorded is at variance with what one expected clinically.

EVALUATION OF THE PULMONARY CAPILLARY WEDGE PRESSURE TRACING. In most cases, a Swan-Ganz catheter is inserted at the bedside to accurately measure PCWP. However, mere inflation of the catheter balloon does not guarantee that the pressure subsequently noted is a true PCWP. The following are guidelines to help confirm that a true PCWP has been obtained. First, if fluoroscopy is used for initial catheter placement, the balloon should look wedged; it should become fixed in the pulmonary artery without back and forth oscillation. Second, the mean pulmonary capillary wedge pressure should be lower than mean pulmonary artery pressure, since a pressure drop occurs across the resistance imposed by pulmonary vasculature. The absence of a pressure drop suggests that a damped pulmonary artery pressure is still being recorded. Third, since the PCWP is a reflection of left atrial pressure, *a* and *v* waves characteristic of the left atrial pressure tracing should be seen in the PCWP (only a *v* wave will be seen if the patient's rhythm is atrial fibrillation). Fourth, the *v* wave should peak after the T wave of the electrocardiogram. This is important in mitral regurgitation, where large v waves may be mistaken for a pulmonary artery pressure tracing.

Finally, if there is still doubt as to the veracity of the PCWP, blood can be withdrawn from the catheter in the wedge position and measured for oxygen saturation. Highly saturated blood (90–95 percent) confirms that the catheter is in the wedge position. However, failure to obtain highly saturated blood does not necessarily mean the catheter has failed to wedge, since it could be wedged in an area of poorly ventilated lung. If oximetric confirmation of the PCWP is sought, the balloon is inflated, and the distal lumen port of the catheter is disconnected from the transducer and allowed to drip freely until blood appears at the catheter hub. The first blood that returns is frequently pulmonary artery blood flow between the balloon and the capillary bed, and often as much as 5 to 10 ml must be withdrawn before fully oxygenated pulmonary capillary blood is obtained. The hub is then connected to a heparinized 3-ml glass syringe. Blood is sampled by rotating the barrel of the syringe and placing gentle traction on the barrel. If sampling is difficult, one should take care that the balloon not be left inflated for longer than 2 to 3 minutes. Prolonged balloon inflation may lead to pulmonary artery rupture. Only 1 to 2 ml of blood are required for oximetry.

Determination of Cardiac Output

The bedside Swan-Ganz catheter can be equipped with a thermistor to permit quantitation of cardiac output by the thermodilution technique. This relatively accurate, simple way of measuring cardiac output relies on the quantitation of a temperature increase in an injectate bolus of a known colder temperature when it mixes with warmer blood. The injectate enters the circulation in the right atrium, and the temperature is measured by a thermistor in the pulmonary artery. The higher the cardiac output, the less time the injectate has for warming, and the colder the injectate stays. A minicomputer is attached to the thermistor and computes cardiac output (C.O.) according to the formula

$$\text{C.O.} = \frac{V \times (T_B - T_I)}{\int_0^\infty T_B(t)dt}$$

where V = volume of the injectate, T_B = temperature of the blood, T_I = temperature of injectate, and $\int_0^\infty T_B(t)dt$ = area under the thermodilution curve in seconds times degrees Celsius.

Most thermodilution computers are equipped with a temperature probe that detects the temperature of the injectate before injection. The computer can also usually be varied to use 5- or 10-ml injections. It is imperative that exactly 5 or 10 ml be injected for acccurate output determination. The injection should be rapid and steady to produce the desired bolus. Saline or 5% dextrose may be used at room temperature or iced to 0°C. We prefer iced solutions, since this maximizes the difference in temperature between the injectate and blood and theoretically enhances accuracy. When iced solutions are used, we recommend that the sterile injectate be drawn up into 5- or 10-ml syringes and cooled by placement in ice. The injectate temperature probe is then placed into the bath. The assumption that injectate temperature is the same as that recorded by the temperature probe is implicit in this technique. Time must be allowed for the injectate syringes to cool down to the ice bath temperature, and once the syringe is removed from the bath, injection should be performed quickly before the injectate is warmed by the ambient air. Injection of a solution warmer than the temperature sensed by the probe will result in spuriously low cardiac output determinations.

Determination of arteriovenous oxygen difference (a-vO_2) should be obtained on every patient at some point during Swan-Ganz monitoring. According to the Fick principle

$$\text{Cardiac output} = \frac{O_2 \text{ consumption}}{\text{a-}vO_2}$$

Rearranging the terms, O_2 consumption = (cardiac output) × (a-vO_2). If cardiac output falls, a-vO_2 will increase as the tissues are forced to extract more oxygen from each gram of hemoglobin to meet their metabolic needs. Thus, if cardiac output, regardless of its numerical value, is not adequate for a patient's physiologic requirements, a-vO_2 will widen. The normal value for a-vO_2 is 30 to 50 ml/L. Thus, even if the cardiac output is "normal," a high a-vO_2 indicates that the cardiac output is not adequate to deliver adequate oxygen. This principle may be of particular help when double-checking the cardiac output, especially when cardiac output data determined by thermodilution do not seem to fit the clinical situation. A high cardiac output should be associated with a normal or narrow a-vO_2. The finding of a normal or narrow a-vO_2 is reassuring that the cardiac output, regardless of its numerical value, is not adequate for a patient's physiologic increased extraction, regardless of the exact numerical value for cardiac output. Conversely, a high value for a-vO_2 indicates inadequate oxygen delivery.

To determine the a-vO_2, a heparinized sample of blood is withdrawn from a systemic artery and a second sample is withdrawn from the pulmonary artery. These are sent to the blood gas laboratory for determination of oxygen saturation. For increased accuracy, samples should be sent in duplicate. The a-vO_2 = (systemic arterial saturation − pulmonary artery saturation) × patient's hemoglobin × 1.36 ml of O_2/gm Hb × 10. By performing this simple determination, additional and valuable information concerning the adequacy of cardiac output can be easily obtained, enhancing the usefulness of the pulmonary artery catheter.

Complications

Swan and Ganz estimated that between 1 and 2 million balloon-tipped flow-directed pulmonary catheters had been placed as of 1979 [15]. Although the risk of this procedure is thought to be quite low, exact risk has never been defined. Complications include arrhythmia, thromboembolism, damage to tricuspid and pulmonic valves, endocarditis, knotting of the catheter, pulmonary infarction, and pulmonary artery rupture.

Although ventricular tachycardia and/or fibrillation are probably the most common complications, this problem is almost always immediately correctable by withdrawal of the catheter and electrical defibrillation when necessary. Catheter passage without the presence of a defibrillator exposes the patient to a needless risk.

At least one case of tricuspid chordal rupture due to Swan-Ganz catheterization has been reported [16]. Rupture was attributed to withdrawal of the catheter through the tricuspid valve with the balloon inflated. It is obvious that this complication should be completely avoidable with proper catheter use.

Two cases of pulmonary valve injury have recently been reported [17]. In one, the catheter had been in place for 13 days, and the issue of catheter-induced trauma to the valve was raised. In view of the large number of catheters used, this complication must be quite rare.

Ehrie and colleagues found evidence of septic or aseptic tricuspid valve endocarditis in six consecutive burn patients monitored with Swan-Ganz catheters [18]. The use of the catheter in this group of patients should be tempered by the knowledge of this potentially serious and possibly frequent complication.

Complete heart block may be induced by Swan-Ganz catheterization [19]. Since the right bundle lies in close proximity to the right ventricular septum, right bundle branch block may be caused by catheter passage. Right bundle branch block is usually temporary. However, if the patient has preexistent left bundle branch block, damage to the right bundle by catheter passage may induce complete heart block. In the group of patients with left bundle branch block in whom pulmonary artery catheterization is necessary, a prophylactic right ventricular pacemaker insertion should be considered prior to catheter placement. At the very least, all the equipment for pacer insertion including fluoroscopy should be immediately available should pulmonary artery catheter insertion cause complete heart block.

Next to arrhythmia, pulmonary complications of Swan-Ganz catheterization are most common. These include thromboembolism, pulmonary infarction, and pulmonary artery hemorrhage. Goodman et al described two cases in which pulmonary embolism occurred from thrombus formed in the pulmonary artery in close proximity to a Swan-Ganz catheter [20]. This complication is probably quite rare.

Pulmonary infarction was reported in 6 percent of 125 consecutive patients undergoing Swan-Ganz catheterization by Foote and coworkers [21]. This complication was due to unrecognized persistent wedging of the catheter and can be nearly eliminated by careful observation of the pressure tracings obtained from the catheter. When the catheter is thought to be persistently wedged, even with the balloon deflated, it should be withdrawn a few centimeters. If it appears that the catheter is still wedged, fluoroscopy or a chest x-ray should be used to ascertain catheter position. The catheter is withdrawn until it is located in a central pulmonary artery.

A serious complication of pulmonary artery catheterization emphasized recently is pulmonary artery rupture [22, 23]. Again, this complication is avoidable and in general occurs with improper catheter usage. The balloon-tipped catheter was designed to be wedged with the balloon fully inflated which, extending slightly beyond the tip, prevents the tip from contacting the artery wall. Tip contact with the pulmonary artery may lead to eventual perforation. In addition, if wedging occurs only with full inflation, the catheter will be positioned in a relatively large pulmonary artery, which may be stronger than more distal bifurcation sites. Pulmonary artery rupture can best be avoided by careful pressure monitoring during balloon inflation. The balloon should be inflated slowly and inflation should be halted as soon as the wave form changes to that of PCWP. If less than 0.8 ml of air is required to cause wedging, distal migration of the catheter has probably occurred. The catheter should be withdrawn slowly with frequent checks on balloon inflation until the full 0.8 ml of air is required for wedging.

INSERTION OF PERIPHERAL SYSTEMIC ARTERIAL CATHETERS

Placement of a peripheral arterial catheter is a convenient way to monitor blood pressure continuously in shock states and to follow therapy for blood pressure control in hypertensive crisis. In addition, this catheter may be useful in situations in which frequent blood gas determinations must be made to evaluate therapy such as in acute respiratory failure.

The arterial catheter can be placed in the radial, brachial, or femoral artery. Since the major complication of prolonged use of this catheter is thrombosis, we prefer the radial artery for catheter placement. If thrombosis does occur at this site, there is generally adequate collateral circulation to the hand via the ulnar artery to prevent ischemia of the forearm and hand.

Observing sterile technique, the skin over the palpated pulse is infiltrated with lidocaine. A 2-mm puncture wound over the artery is made in the skin with a No. 11 surgical blade. If the femoral artery is employed, a tunnel is blunt-dissected down to the artery with a straight hemostat. Next, while palpating the arterial pulse with one hand, arterial puncture with a Potts-Cournand needle is performed with the other hand. The central stylet is removed and the needle gradually withdrawn until pulsatile blood flow returns through the needle. While steadying the needle with one hand, a 40-cm or 0.032-inch straight guidewire with a flexible tip is advanced through the needle into the artery. No resistance should be encountered during passage of the guidewire. If resistance is encountered, the guidewire should be withdrawn. If pulsatile flow is still present, slight traction on the needle should facilitate guidewire passage. If pulsatile flow has disappeared, the needle may have inadvertently advanced against the posterior wall of the vessel. Again, slight traction on the needle should restore flow. If it does not, the needle is withdrawn slowly until flow returns. If flow cannot be restored, hand compression of the artery for 5 minutes is indicated to provide hemostasis; repeat puncture is then performed. Once the guidewire is successfully negotiated into the artery, the needle is removed while one hand secures the guidewire at the insertion site. A short polyethylene catheter is threaded over the guidewire into the artery. The guidewire is then removed. The catheter is secured and dressed and connected to a pressure transducer. Flushing is performed with a continuous pressurized system such as that used with the Swan-Ganz catheter.

Cardiac Catheterization

General Indications

In general, there are two broad clinical indications for cardiac catheterization. First, cardiac catheterization is indicated to obtain a complete cardiac diagnostic profile of a patient prior to cardiac surgery. Although there are a few exceptions, patients in this category will generally be symptomatic from their heart disease and will show some objective evidence in physical examination or noninvasive cardiologic techniques that cardiac disease is the cause of their symptoms. The possibility of eventual cardiac surgery should always be discussed with the patient prior to referral for catheterization. This will save both the referring and catheterizing physicians from the embarrassing situation of finding out that a patient who is about to be catheterized would refuse surgical intervention no matter what the outcome of the catheterization.

Second, catheterization may establish a firm diagnosis of cardiac disease or rule it out. Even if surgery is not contemplated, the information obtained may be of major importance in guiding medical management and advising the patient of the overall prognosis. A frequent specific indication in this category is that of the patient with chest pain of uncertain etiology in whom noninvasive testing has been inconclusive. Such a patient often is admitted to the coronary care unit several times, causing much anxiety and loss of work days. A positive catheterization will assure the patient's physician that continued therapy for coronary disease is appropriate. A negative catheterization will usually be a relief to the patient; once the patient is no longer petrified that his or her chest pain signifies heart disease, the nature of the symptoms may lessen. In addition, if a search for other causes of the patient's symptoms has not already been undertaken, it may be prompted by negative catheterization results and an alternative source of the pain found, thus leading to appropriate treatment.

Specific Indications

Coronary Artery Disease

The most frequent indication for referral for cardiac catheterization is symptomatic coronary artery disease. In this case, the indications for catheterization are about the same as those for coronary artery bypass surgery. These indications remain controversial. In general, we would recommend catheterization for those patients whose symptoms interfere significantly with their desired lifestyle despite medical antianginal therapy. One exception to this guideline is the young patient (age $\leqslant 50$ years) who has had a myocardial infarction whether or not he or she is symptomatic post infarction. In such a patient, where prognosis is of increased concern because of age, catheterization will help establish prognosis by determining the extent of disease. A second exception is the asymptomatic patient who has a routine stress test performed with markedly positive results and confirmed by a radioisotope study. Such a test result may interfere with a patient's lifestyle, making it difficult for him or her to obtain insurance or forcing him or her to stop working. Catheterization in this case will either confirm that coronary disease does exist, despite the patient's lack of symptoms, or demonstrate that the noninvasive test was a false-positive test, allowing the patient to return to his or her usual activities.

To be sure, many cardiologists will have more liberal indications for catheterization in coronary artery disease and many will have more conservative indications. Until there is more information regarding the utility and long-range effects of coronary bypass surgery, we suggest these guidelines as a "middle-of-the-road" approach.

Aortic Stenosis

When a patient develops symptoms of angina, syncope, or congestive heart failure secondary to aortic stenosis, the risk of death is high [24]. Aortic valve replacement improves the prognosis of this disease and is considered to be the treatment of choice [25]. Once symptoms occur in this disease, surgery should be performed relatively soon thereafter. We believe that nearly every patient suspected of having symptomatic aortic stenosis should be catheterized prior to surgery. The only exception would be an emergency operation in a patient in whom aortic stenosis is strongly suspected clinically and death appears imminent without immediate surgery.

The noninvasive factors suggesting the need for cardiac catheterization and aortic valve replacement in symptomatic patients include (1) a late-peaking ejection murmur, (2) delay in the carotid upstroke, (3) a diminished aortic component of S_2, (4) electrocardiographic evidence of left ventricular hypertrophy, and (5) fluoroscopic evidence of aortic valvular calcification. If at least two of these criteria are present, echocardiography should be performed. Unless at least one valve leaflet is noted to have good excursion at echocardiography, cardiac catheterization should be contemplated in the symptomatic patient to further evaluate the severity of aortic stenosis.

Aortic and Mitral Regurgitation

The proper timing of cardiac surgery for valvular regurgitation is one of the most difficult decisions in cardiology. On the one hand, it is known that patients with regurgitant lesions may tolerate the lesion well for years without decompensation. On the other hand, prolonged regurgitation when neglected may produce irrevocable left ventricular dysfunction. Recent studies indicate that once patients become symptomatic, left ventricular dysfunction is already present [26, 27]. Although we are not advocating valve replacement in asymptomatic patients, we believe that once symptoms do occur, valve replacement should be strongly considered. Noninvasive studies such as chest x-ray and the echocardiogram are helpful in following such patients. An enlarging heart on chest x-ray or a diminution in left ventricular performance on the echocardiogram together with the development of symptoms help to confirm a change in cardiac status and further strengthen the decision to proceed to catheterization and surgery.

Mitral Stenosis

Symptomatic patients with mitral stenosis should undergo valvular commissurotomy or replacement prior to the development of severe pulmonary hypertension, since pulmonary hypertension may adversely affect surgical prognosis [28]. The development of a right ventricular lift and a loud P_2 on physical examination or the presence of right ventricular hypertrophy on the electrocardiogram are clues to the development of pulmonary hypertension.

The echocardiogram is excellent for evaluation of the presence or absence of mitral stenosis. Indeed, with the two-dimensional echocardiogram, even severity can be predicted with relative accuracy [29]. Recently, the need to catheterize patients with pure mitral stenosis has been questioned, since they can be evaluated adequately by echocardiography [30]. Such patients would be young females not apt to have coronary disease, in whom no murmur of valvular regurgitation is heard, and in whom aortic valve motion at echocardiography is normal. Even in this group of patients, catheterization performed at low risk will be useful in quantifying pulmonary hypertension and assessing surgical risk. At the present time, we feel that most patients with mitral stenosis should undergo catheterization prior to surgery (see Chap. 5).

Atrial Septal Defect in the Adult

Often atrial septal defect (ASD) is not detected until a murmur is heard on routine physical examination in adulthood. A systolic ejection murmur heard in the pulmonic area together with fixed splitting of S_2 should raise the suspicion of an ASD. Chest x-ray, echocardiography, and radionuclide angiocardiography will usually confirm the diagnosis. Secundum type ASD is the most common form. This can be corrected with less than a 1 percent operative mortality. Since the occurrence of pulmonary hypertension, which adversely affects prognosis, is unpredictable, it is generally held that in patients with a pulmonary-to-systemic blood flow ratio of 2 : 1 or greater, the defect should be repaired even if the patient is asymptomatic. Although the shunt ratio can usually be quantified by radionuclide techniques, we believe that catheterization is usually indicated in ASD to help evaluate pulmonary vascular resistance, a key prognosticator to surgical outcome. The shunt magnitude will also, of course, be evaluated and confirmed at catheterization. We also would include coronary angiography in the coronary disease-prone population.

Hypertrophic Cardiomyopathy

This cardiomyopathy is suspected by detection of a systolic ejection murmur that increases with the Valsalva maneuver and diminishes with squatting. Echocardiography is almost always diagnostic as long as proper imaging can be performed. Unlike valvular aortic stenosis, mortality is not related to the degree of obstruction as much as to the myopathic disease process itself [31]. In general, medical therapy with beta blocking agents is the treatment of choice. Only if medical therapy fails to control symptoms of chest pain, syncope, and congestion does one usually consider surgery. If surgery is contemplated, prior catheterization is indicated to evaluate the degree of hemodynamic abnormality.

Idiopathic Dilated (Congestive) Cardiomyopathy

This group of diseases is characterized by myocardial systolic dysfunction in the absence of coronary disease, valvular or congenital heart disease, or hypertension; the prognosis is poor. Before one makes the diagnosis of idiopathic dilated cardiomyopathy, one must be sure that no correctable cause of the patient's heart failure can be found. Mitral stenosis, aortic stenosis, left ventricular aneurysm, and constrictive pericarditis may not be suspected clinically and yet are surgically correctable causes of congestive heart failure. Many of these diagnoses can be ruled out by noninvasive means. An adequate echocardiogram should be capable of evaluating the mitral and aortic valves for the presence of stenosis. Radionuclide angiography has been shown reliable in detection of ventricular aneurysms [32]. Constrictive pericarditis, on the other hand, may be difficult to evaluate by any noninvasive means. Despite the utility of noninvasive techniques, we believe that right and left heart catheterization should be performed in most patients with suspected cardiomyopathy. This will allow one to establish a hemodynamic profile that will be helpful in guiding future medical therapy, particularly if the use of vasodilators is planned. If noninvasive imaging is suboptimal or if constrictive pericarditis is suspected, a full catheterization should be planned to rule out correctable causes of congestive heart failure.

Preparation of the Patient

Prior to the actual catheterization, the operator apprises the patient of general and specific risks and discomfort associated with the procedure. Precatheterization orders should include premedication with sedatives or tranquilizers, skin to be prepared and shaved as necessary, and transport orders for the catheterization laboratory. We do not administer antibiotics prophylactically, knowing of no controlled studies to support their use.

Method of Approach

Right heart catheterization is performed by inserting a catheter into a brachial or femoral vein. The techniques are very similar to those described earlier in this chapter for insertion of a Swan-Ganz catheter.

The choice of approach for the arterial catheter — brachial or femoral — is made by the catheterizing physician prior to the procedure on the basis of estimated risk to the patient. The approach considered to be safest and technically easiest will, of course, be chosen.

The direct brachial approach may be preferred in a patient with peripheral vascular disease (involving the abdominal aorta, iliac or femoral arteries), suspected femoral vein or inferior vena caval thrombosis, or coarctation of the aorta. This approach may also be best in the very obese patient, not only because of bleeding problems with the femoral approach, but also because the femoral approach may be technically very difficult in such a patient. Because of the increased hazard of bleeding with the femoral approach in patients with wide pulse pressures (such as in aortic regurgitation) who are receiving anticoagulants, the brachial approach is often used in such instances. However, the percutaneous femoral technique has definite advantages of its own: arteriotomy and artery repair are not required; unlike the brachial approach, the procedure can be performed several times in the same patient at intervals; infection and thrombophlebitis at the catheterization site are rare; and surgical closure of the skin is not necessary. Furthermore, patients with diminished or absent brachial pulsations or with small brachial arteries should be catheterized via the femoral approach. Finally, the operator's experience with each approach must also be entered into the "risk" equation in deciding on technique.

The procedures for insertion of catheters into peripheral arteries have been described earlier. As noted at the beginning of the chapter, a discussion of the techniques for positioning these catheters for left ventriculography and coronary arteriography and for performing the angiographic studies is beyond the scope of this review.

THE CARDIAC CATHETERIZATION PROTOCOL

Every cardiac catheterization should have a sequential plan designed specifically for the patient being studied. In designing such a protocol (which is usually written and posted in the laboratory), certain general principles are followed.

1. An arterial monitor line is present (especially helpful if complications develop).
2. Hemodynamic measurements precede angiographic studies to ensure the basal nature of physiologic pressure and flow measurements.
3. Pressures and oxygen saturations should be measured and recorded in each chamber immediately after entry and before passing on to the next chamber, in case of complications later on.
4. Pressure and cardiac output measurements should be made as simultaneously as possible.

To these general guidelines are added the specific requirements for each patient's study, depending on the diagnosis being entertained. Normal resting values for cardiac catheterization measurements are listed in Table 9-2.

INTERPRETATION OF HEMODYNAMIC AND ANGIOGRAPHIC FINDINGS

Because of its value in Swan-Ganz catheterizations, the evaluation of PCWP tracings has been discussed in detail earlier in this chapter. The interpretation of other right and left heart measurements also depends on their characteristic waveforms (Fig. 9-7). Although marked pressure gradients across the mitral and aortic valves are obviously of prime importance in diagnosing mitral and aortic stenosis, respectively, it is the calculated valve areas that are the most reliable indices of these lesions. If flow across the valve is reduced (low cardiac output), then otherwise unimpressive gradients may actually result in severely reduced valve areas (<0.7 cm^2 for the aortic valve and <1.0 cm^2 for the mitral valve).

The cardiologist evaluates regurgitant lesions in a largely qualitative way, although it is possible to calculate a regurgitant fraction by subtracting the

TABLE 9-2. Range of Normal Resting Hemodynamic Values

	a Wave	v Wave	Mean	Systolic	End-Diastolic	Mean
Pressures						
Right atrium	2–10	2–10	0–8			
Right ventricle				15–30	0–8	
Pulmonary artery				15–30	3–12	9–16
Pulmonary artery wedge and left atrium	3–15	3–12	1–10			
Left ventricle				100–140	3–12	
Systemic arteries				100–140	60–90	70–105
Oxygen consumption index (ml/min/m^2)				110–150		
Arteriovenous oxygen difference (ml/L)				30–50		
Cardiac output index (L/min/m^2)				2.5–4.2		
Resistances (dynes-sec-cm^{-5})						
Pulmonary vascular				22–120		
Systemic vascular				770–1500		

From WH Barry, W Grossman: Cardiac catheterization. In E Braunwald (ed): *Heart Disease*. Philadelphia: WB Saunders, 1980, p 289.

"forward" cardiac output (obtained via the Fick method) from the "total" cardiac output obtained from the left ventriculogram. A grading system has been established for the degree of visualized regurgitation. On a scale of 0 to 4, 1 and 2 are considered mild to moderate and 3 and 4 moderately severe to severe. Recommendations for valve replacement usually require the latter values.

While a detailed discussion of the evaluation of angiographic findings is also beyond the scope of this chapter, several observations are pertinent to the clinician's understanding of the catheterization report. For example, a significant coronary artery stenosis (i.e., one that causes alteration in coronary blood flow) is defined as >70 percent of the vessel diameter. The more proximal the lesion, the greater the area of myocardium at jeopardy with a tight left main coronary artery stenosis being a particularly ominous finding (Fig. 9-8). Areas of myocardium subserved by stenosed coronary arteries often result in areas of abnormal left ventricular wall motion; hence, the value of the ventriculogram. A normal ventriculogram is shown in Figure 9-9; a well-demarcated aneurysm is shown in Figure 11-8C (p. 312). To properly evaluate ventricular function—in both coronary and noncoronary heart diseases—some type of intervention is often necessary. Whether this be exercise, atrial pacing, or the administration of a cardiac drug, the purpose is to compare pressures, flow, and often wall motion changes in the resting (control) state and during or after the intervention. When appropriate,

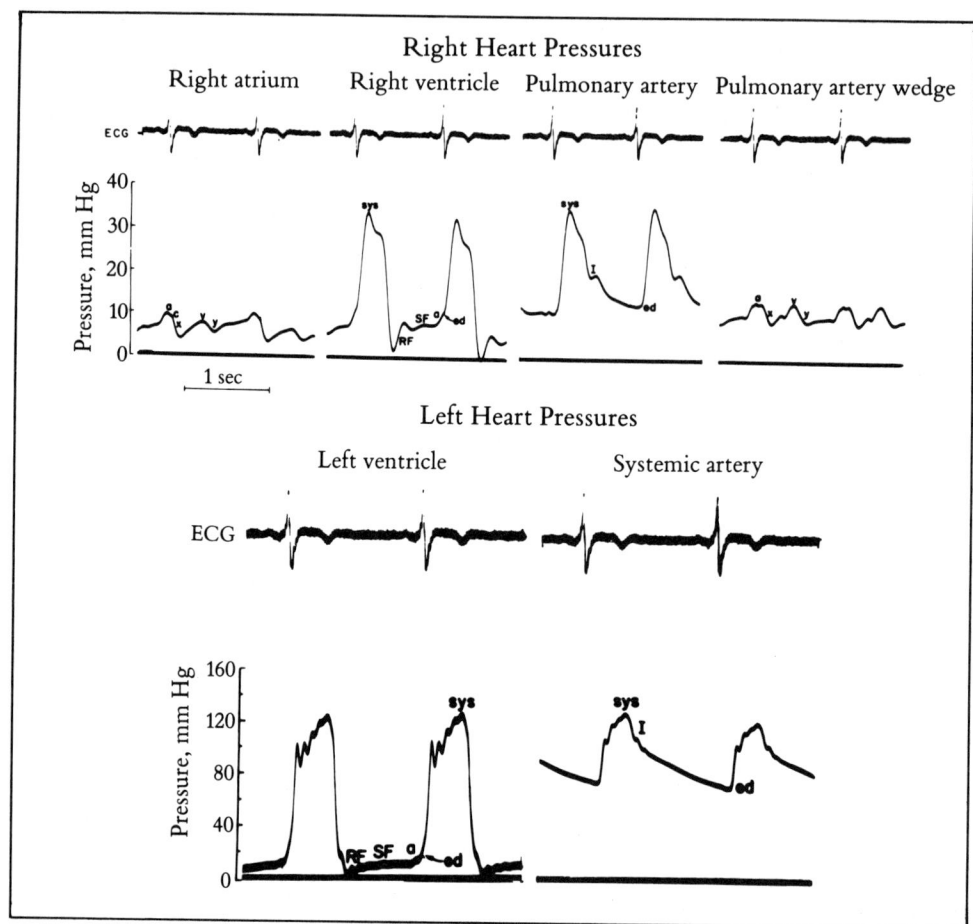

FIGURE 9-7. Intracardiac pressure waveforms recorded with a fluid-filled catheter. Right heart pressures are slightly elevated. a = atrial systolic wave; ed = end-diastolic pressure; I = incisura; RF = rapid filling wave; SF = slow filling wave; Sys = peak systolic pressure. Also shown are a, c, and v waves and x and y descents. (From WH Barry, W Grossman: Cardiac catheterization. In E Braunwald [ed]: *Heart Disease*. Philadelphia: WB Saunders, 1980, p 289)

the results of these interventions should be summarized in the catheterization report along with the standard hemodynamic and angiographic measurements.

POSTCATHETERIZATION CARE

Once the patient is successfully catheterized, he or she will often return to the referring physician for continuing care. We recommend a few simple guidelines to be followed on the first office visit after catheterization.
1. Check the site of catheter insertion for signs of infection. If such signs exist, begin therapy with dry heat and antibiotics.

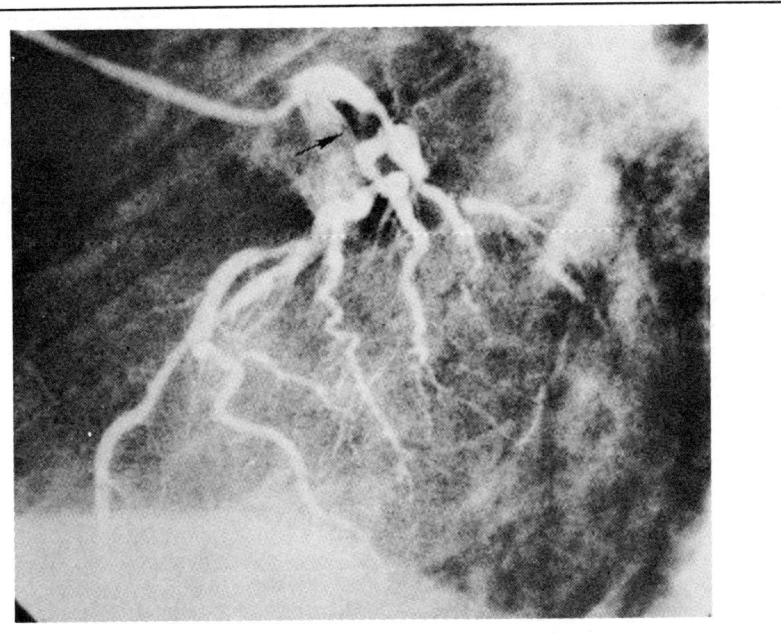

FIGURE 9-8. Left coronary angiogram in the left anterior oblique projection. There is subtotal obstruction at the origin of the main left coronary artery (*arrow*). (From PF Cohn et al: Profiles in coronary artery disease. In W Grossman [ed]: *Cardiac Catheterization and Angiography.* 2nd ed. Philadelphia: Lea & Febiger, 1980, p 328)

2. Check the distal pulses in the limb used for catheterization. Any diminution from previous examinations should be discussed with the catheterizing physician immediately.
3. If the brachial approach has been used, sutures may need to be removed; this should be done 5 to 7 days after catheterization. Many laboratories now use absorbable subcuticular sutures, making suture removal unnecessary.
4. If the femoral approach has been taken, the insertion site should be checked for formation of a pseudoaneurysm of the femoral artery. The palpation of an expansile mass over the femoral artery or the auscultation of a new bruit suggest possible pseudoaneurysm formation. Such findings should be discussed immediately with the catheterizing physician.

COMPLICATIONS
Cardiac catheterization has evolved into a safe, widely used procedure with a relatively low incidence of complications. In a recent cooperative study involving 7553 patients, Davis and associates reported the various complications encountered during coronary angiography [33] (Tables 9-3 and 9-4). Although this study found a higher incidence of complications when the brachial approach was used,

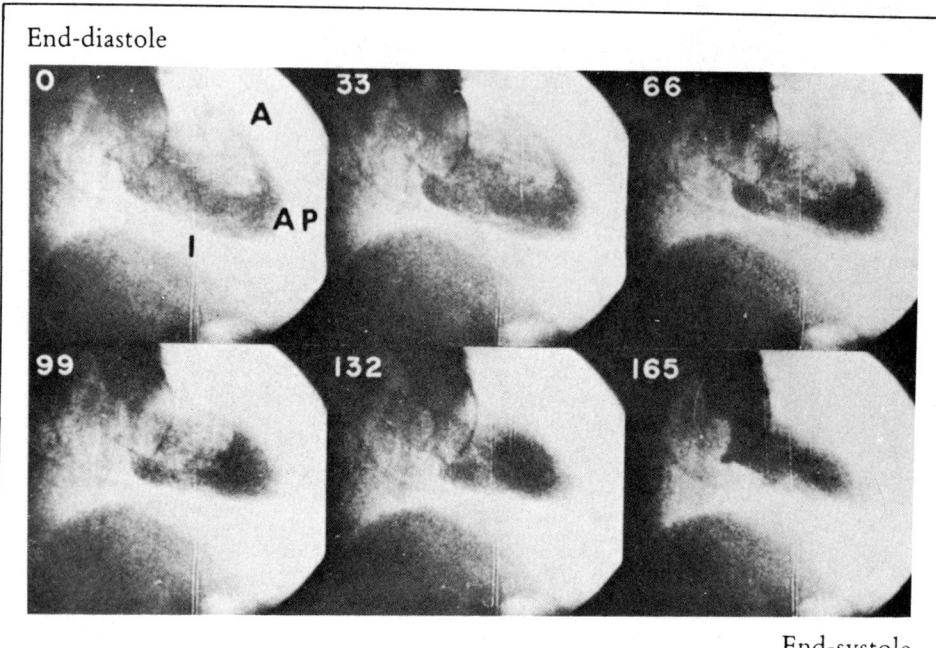

FIGURE 9-9. Left ventriculogram in the right anterior oblique projection. Normal contraction pattern from time zero (0) at end-diastole to end-systole 165 msec later. Three zones are seen in this projection: anterior (A), apical (AP), and inferior (I). (From PF Cohn et al: Profiles in coronary artery disease. In W Grossman [ed]: *Cardiac Catheterization and Angiography.* 2nd ed. Philadelphia: Lea & Febiger, 1980, p 193)

this did not apply in laboratories where that approach was used frequently. In general, we believe that both approaches are safe provided the operator has ample experience.

In addition to these complications, perforation of the heart, pyrogenic reactions, serious arrhythmias, and contrast-induced renal dysfunction also occur rarely. This last complication is most prevalent in diabetic patients with preexisting renal disease [34]. When complications do occur, they usually do so in patients at higher risk because of the disease present. Patients with main left coronary disease, left ventricular dysfunction, unstable angina, or insulin-requiring diabetes fall into our high-risk category. Even in this group, with meticulous care, catheterization can usually be carried out safely.

It should be pointed out that although cardiovascular events occurring within 24 hours after catheterization are usually chalked up as catheterization-related complications, many patients undergoing catheterization are very ill and may have such events as part of the natural history of their disease. Thus, Hildner et al found a similar incidence of cardiovascular events in 48 hours *prior* to catheteriza-

TABLE 9-3. Complications Related to Technique of Coronary Angiography

Complication	Brachial (n = 1187)		Femoral (n = 6328)		Total (n = 7553)
	Day 0 (%)	Day 1 (%)	Day 0 (%)	Day 1 (%)	(%)
Death	0.42	0.08	0.02	0.13	0.20
Myocardial infarction	0.34	0.08	0.17	0.05	0.25
Embolization	0.17		0.08		0.09
Vascular	2.78		0.36		0.74

From K Davis et al: Complications of coronary arteriography from the collaborative study of coronary artery surgery. Circulation 59:1105, 1979, by permission of the American Heart Association, Inc.

TABLE 9-4. Comparison of Mortality for Brachial and Femoral Procedures

	Femoral Procedures (%)	Brachial Procedures (%)	p Value
Clinics using			
Majority ($\geq$ 80%) brachial procedures	0.00 (0/105)	0.00 (0/654)	NS
Minority (1–43%) brachial procedures	0.05 (2/3770)	1.13 (6/533)	0.0002*
No brachial procedures	0.29 (7/2453)		

*Fisher's exact test of significant difference in mortality between brachial and femoral technique.
From K Davis et al: Complications of coronary arteriography from the collaborative study of coronary artery surgery. Circulation 59:1105, 1979, by permission of the American Heart Association, Inc.

tion as in the 24 hours *following* catheterization [35]. This underlines the fact that not every cardiovascular event following catheterization is necessarily a direct consequence of the procedure.

Pulmonary Angiography

INDICATIONS

By far the most frequent indication for pulmonary angiography is to document the presence of clinically suspected pulmonary embolism. In this regard, pulmonary angiography is considered to be the most accurate diagnostic modality. However, it should be clear that not every patient suspected of having a pulmonary embolism can or should undergo pulmonary angiography. Prior to consideration of pulmonary angiography, a chest x-ray and lung scan should be obtained. A perfusion lung scan will be abnormal in any area of almost any lung pathology, since perfusion is altered readily by any lung abnormality. Thus, the mere presence of a defect on lung scan is not specific for pulmonary embolism. However, a normal scan indicates that a pulmonary embolism is not present, and the need for angiography is obviated [36]. Since vascular obstruction by pulmonary embolism usually produces lobar hypoperfusion, a lobar defect on lung scan is likely to indicate pulmonary embolism. Pulmonary embolism is present in 80 percent of patients with such a defect, and it is termed a high probability scan. Segmental defects are intermediate in their likelihood of indicating pulmonary embolism, while subsegmental defects usually do not indicate embolism. The addition of the ventilation scan to detect areas that are ventilated but not perfused increases the specificity of the test. A schema for the use of chest x-ray, lung scan, and pulmonary angiography is presented in Table 9-5.

In addition to diagnosing pulmonary embolism, pulmonary angiography can also be used to evaluate pulmonary arteriovenous malformations, peripheral pulmonary artery stenosis, and anomalous pulmonary venous drainage.

TECHNIQUES

The brachial approach is the preferable site of venous entry. First, these patients are usually anticoagulated, which increases the morbidity of the percutaneous femoral approach. Second, entry of the catheter into the femoral and iliac veins could dislodge thrombi and cause additional pulmonary emboli. A variety of catheters with multiple sideholes can be used. The method of insertion is similar to that described earlier in the chapter for the Swan-Ganz catheters. When the catheter has been placed in the main pulmonary artery, the patient is ready for the injection of contrast medium. When mainstream injections are equivocal, selective injections may be made. (If primary pulmonary hypertension is present, mainstream injections are contraindicated.) For completeness — in addition to filming the passage of the contrast medium — hemodynamic measurements should also be obtained in the right heart.

INTERPRETATION OF ANGIOGRAPHIC FINDINGS

While the normal pulmonary angiogram is easily recognized, angiographic recognition of pulmonary embolism is not as simple as would first appear. In addition to classic filling defects and abrupt arterial cutoff (Fig. 9-10), there may be more subtle variations. Thus, the presence of nonspecific angiographic abnormalities (asymmetry of flow and/or oligemia) may be helpful in borderline cases, though the latter by themselves do not confirm the diagnosis of pulmonary embolism. By contrast, a normal angiogram effectively rules out this diagnosis.

CONTRAINDICATIONS AND RISKS

Recent myocardial infarction, severe systemic illness, and pulmonary hypertension are relative contraindications to pulmonary angiography. When these conditions

TABLE 9-5. The Role of Scintigraphy in Pulmonary Embolism

Largest Perfusion Defect	X-Ray	Ventilation	Interpretation	Strategy
Normal			No pulmonary embolism within past 48 hours	No pulmonary angiography
Subsegmental		Indicated only if large subsegmental deficit; then interpretation same as segmental lobar below	Low probability of PE (10%)	Pulmonary angiography only if clinical suspicion is high
Segmental or lobar	Normal in region of defect	Perfusion-ventilation match	Low probability of PE	Pulmonary angiography only if clinical suspicion is high
Segmental or lobar	Abnormal density in region of defect	Not Indicated	Indeterminate	Pulmonary angiography recommended
Segmental or lobar	Normal in region of defect	Perfusion-ventilation mismatch	High probability of PE (PE > 90%)	Treat
Segmental or lobar	Normal in refion of defect	Cannot be performed	Moderate probability of PE (25% in segmental and 80% in lobar defects	Pulmonary angiography recommended

PE = pulmonary embolism.
From BL Holman: Radioisotopic examination of the cardiovascular system. In E Braunwald (ed): *Heart Disease.* Philadelphia: Saunders, 1980, p 363.

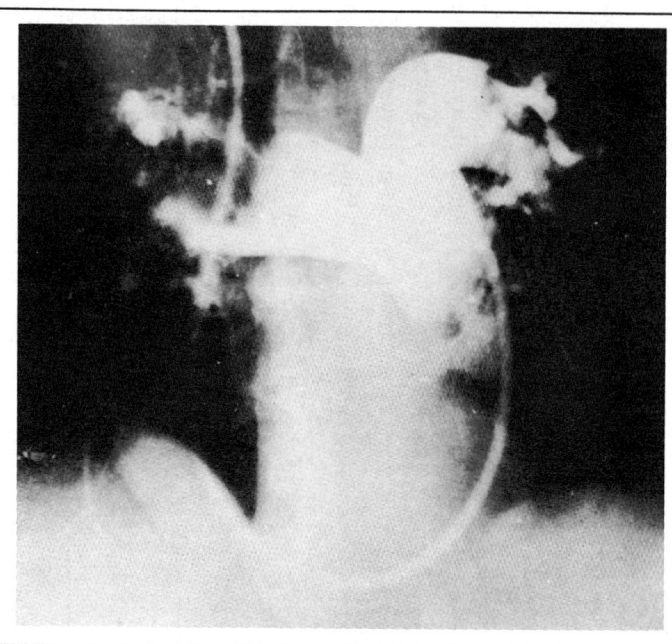

FIGURE 9-10. Pulmonary angiogram in a patient with massive pulmonary emboli. Intraluminal filling defects are present in the main right and left pulmonary arteries. There are also cutoffs of the right and left lower lobar arteries. (From JE Dalen, W Grossman: Pulmonary angiography. In W Grossman [ed]: *Cardiac Catheterization and Angiography.* 2nd ed. Philadelphia: Lea & Febiger, 1980, p 193)

TABLE 9-6. Complications of Pulmonary Angiography (544 Consecutive Studies, 1964–1973), Peter Bent Brigham Hospital

Complications	Number	Fatal
RELATED TO CARDIAC CATHETERIZATION		
Cardiac perforation	3	0
Pyrogen reaction	7	0
Arrhythmia	5	0
RELATED TO ANGIOGRAPHY		
Bronchospasm	3	0
Pulmonary edema	1	0
Hypotension	1	0
Angioneurotic edema	1	0
Anaphylaxis	1	0
Cardiogenic shock	2	2
Total	24 (4%)	2 (0.4%)

From W Grossman: Pulmonary angiography. In W Grossman (ed): *Cardiac Catheterization and Angiography.* 2nd ed. Philadelphia: Lea & Febiger, 1980, p 191.

are present, the risk of therapy for pulmonary embolism, i.e., heparinization, must be weighed against the risk of the procedure. If there is no contraindication to anticoagulation, it is probably safer to assume that the patient has had a pulmonary embolism and proceed with anticoagulation. Conversely, if the patient also has a contraindication to heparinization, such as gastrointestinal hemorrhage, and the suspicion of pulmonary embolism is high, then angiography should be performed. If positive, inferior vena caval interruption is indicated.

The risk of pulmonary angiography as performed at the Peter Bent Brigham Hospital is depicted in Table 9-6. As with any procedure, this risk is related to the experience of the operator and may be higher in institutions where the study is performed infrequently.

References

1. Swan HJC, Ganz W, Forrester JS, Marcus H, Diamond G, Chonette D: Catheterization of the heart in man with the use of a flow-directed balloon tipped catheter. *N Engl J Med* 283:447, 1970
2. Russell RO Jr, Rackley CE, Pombo J, Hunt D, Potanin C, Dodge HT: Effect of increasing left ventricular filling pressure in patients with acute myocardial infarction. *J Clin Invest* 48:1539, 1970
3. Crexells C, Chatterjee K, Forrester JS, Dikshit K, Swan HJC: Optimal level of filling pressure in the left side of the heart in acute myocardial infarction. *N Engl J Med* 289:1263, 1973
4. Carabello BA, Cohn PF, Alpert JS: Hemodynamic monitoring in patients with hypotension after myocardial infarction. *Chest* 74:5, 1978
5. Forrester JS, Diamond G, Swan HJC: Correlative classification of clinical and hemodynamic function after acute myocardial infarction. *Am J Cardiol* 39:137, 1977
6. Rotman M, Chen JTT, Seningen RP, Hawley J, Wagner GS, Davidson RM, Gilbert MR: Pulmonary artery diastolic pressure in acute myocardial infarction. *Am J Cardiol* 33:357, 1974
7. McHugh TJ, Forrester JS, Adler L, Zion D, Swan HJC: Pulmonary vascular congestion in acute myocardial infarction: Hemodynamic and radiologic correlations. *Ann Intern Med* 76:29, 1972
8. Rahimtoola SH, Loeb HS, Ehsani A: Relationship of pulmonary artery to left ventricular diastolic pressures in acute myocardial infarction. *Circulation* 46:283, 1972
9. Forrester JS, Diamond G, McHugh TJ, Swan HJC: Filling pressures in the right and left sides of the heart in acute myocardial infarction: A reappraisal of central venous pressure monitoring. *N Engl J Med* 285:190, 1971
10. Saunder RH, Kern WH, Blount SG Jr: Perforation of the interventricular septum complicating myocardial infarction. *Am Heart J* 51:736, 1956
11. Johnson RA, Daggett WM Jr: Heart failure resulting from coronary artery disease: Acute myocardial infarction complicated by ventricular septal rupture. In Johnson RA,

Haber E, Austen WG (eds): *The Practice of Cardiology.* Boston: Little, Brown, 1980, p 355

12. Antman EM, Marsh JD, Green LH, Grossman W: Blood oxygen measurements in the assessment of intracardiac left to right shunts: A critical appraisal of methodology. *Am J Cardiol* 46:265, 1980
13. Robin ED, Cross CE, Zelis R: Pulmonary edema. *N Engl J Med* 288:239, 280, 1973
14. Cohn JN, Franciosa JA: Vasodilator therapy of cardiac failure. *N Engl J Med* 297:27, 254, 1977
15. Swan HJC, Ganz W: Complications with flow-directed balloon-tipped catheters. *Ann Intern Med* 91:494, 1979
16. Smith WR, Glaser FL, Jemison P: Ruptured chordae of the tricuspid valve: A consequence of flow-directed Swan-Ganz catheterization. *Chest* 70:790, 1976
17. O'Toole JD, Wuhzbacher JJ, Wearner NE, Jain AC: Pulmonary-valve injury and insufficiency during pulmonary artery catheterization. *N Engl J Med* 301:1167, 1979
18. Ehrie M, Morgan AP, Moore RD, O'Connor NE: Endocarditis with indwelling balloon-tipped pulmonary artery catheter in burn patients. *J Trauma* 18:664, 1978
19. Abernathy WS: Complete heart block caused by Swan-Ganz catheter. *Chest* 65:349, 1974
20. Goodman DJ, Rider AK, Billingham ME, Schroeder JS: Thromboembolic complications with the indwelling balloon-tipped pulmonary arterial catheter. *N Engl J Med* 291:777, 1974
21. Foote GA, Schabel SI, Hodges M: Pulmonary complications of flow-directed balloon-tipped catheter. *N Engl J Med* 290:927, 1974
22. Pape LA, Haffajee CI, Markis JE, Ockene IS, Paraskos JA, Dalen JE, Alpert JS: Fatal pulmonary hemorrhage after use of the flow-directed balloon-tipped catheter. *Ann Intern Med* 90:344, 1979
23. Paulson DM, Scott SM, Sethi GK: Pulmonary hemorrhage with balloon flotation catheters: Report of a case and review of the literature. *J Thorac Cardiovasc Surg* 80:453, 1980
24. Rapaport E: Natural history of aortic and mitral valve disease. *Am J Cardiol* 35:221, 1975
25. Cohn LH, Koster JK, Mee RB, Collins JJ Jr: Long term follow-up of the Hancock bioprosthetic heart valve. *Circulation* 60(Suppl I):87, 1979
26. Carabello BA, Nolan SP, McGuire LB: Assessment of preoperative left ventricular function in patients with mitral regurgitaion: Value of the end systolic wall stress–end systolic volume ratio. *Circulation* 64:1212, 1981
27. Osbakken M, Boue AA, Spann JF: Left ventricular function in chronic aortic regurgitation with reference to end systolic pressure, volume and stress relations. *Am J Cardiol* 47:193, 1981
28. Ward C, Hancock BW: Extreme pulmonary hypertension caused by mitral valve disease. *Br Heart J* 37:74, 1975
29. Martin RP, Rakowski H, Kleiman JH: Reliability and reproducibility of two dimensional echocardiographic measurement of the stenotic mitral valve orifice area. *Am J Cardiol* 43:560, 1979

30. Montro M, Neufeld HN: Should patients with pure mitral stenosis undergo cardiac catheterization. *Am J Cardiol* 46:515, 1980
31. Frank S, Braunwald E: Idiopathic hypertrophic subaortic stenosis. Clinical analysis of 126 patients with emphasis on natural history. *Circulation* 37:759, 1968
32. Rigo P, Murray M, Strauss HW, Pitt B: Scintiphotographic evaluation of patients with suspected left ventricular aneurysm. *Circulation* 50:985, 1974
33. Davis K, Kennedy JW, Kemp HG Jr, Judkins M, Gosselin AJ, Killip T: Complications of coronary arteriography from the collaborative study of coronary artery surgery. *Circulation* 59:1105, 1979
34. Weinrauch LA, Healy RW, Leland OS Jr, Goldstein HH, Kassissieh SD, Libertino JA, Takacs FJ, D'Elia JA: Coronary angiography and acute renal failure in diabetic azotemic nephropathy. *Ann Intern Med* 86:56, 1977
35. Hildner FJ, Javier RP, Ramaswamy K: Pseudocomplications of cardiac catheterization. *Chest* 63:15, 1973
36. Humphries JD, Bell WR, White RI: Criteria for the recognition of pulmonary emboli. *JAMA* 235:2011, 1976

Chapter 10

Electrophysiologic Studies

Stephen C. Vlay and Peter F. Cohn

In reviewing the subject of cardiac electrophysiologic studies, we will consider indications for the procedures; the measurements, definitions, and mechanisms that form the basis for cardiac electrophysiology; and the equipment used in these studies. We will then consider specifically the three disease entities that these procedures are most helpful in evaluating: conduction disturbances, supraventricular arrhythmias, and ventricular arrhythmias.

Indications

The ability to record intracardiac electrograms and stimulate extra beats facilitates evaluation of conduction abnormalities and arrhythmias. Presently, there are three major indications for cardiac electrophysiologic testing: (1) evaluation of symptoms of syncope or dizziness, (2) evaluation of supraventricular tachycardia, and (3) evaluation of ventricular tachycardia. Not every patient with these diagnoses requires study, however, and careful selection of appropriate patients for testing is necessary to avoid unnecessary utilization of resources as well as potential morbidity. Two types of asymptomatic patients do not require study. *Asymptomatic patients with sinus bradycardia* will not benefit from the study, since there are no data that assess the prognostic importance of normal or abnormal sinus node function [1]. *Asymptomatic patients with chronic bifascicular disease* similarly do not benefit from measurement of the His bundle-to-ventricle (HV) interval, since the rate of progession to complete heart block is unclear [2]. Prophylactic transvenous pacing in patients with chronic bifascicular disease has produced no clear advantage in terms of survival. The underlying cardiac disease in this population is usually advanced organic heart disease, primarily coronary artery disease. Congestive heart failure is common [3]. Morbidity and mortality is usually due to progression of intrinsic disease and failure. In addition, these patients have a high incidence of sudden death due to malignant ventricular arrhythmias [4, 5].

SYNCOPE OR DIZZINESS
These patients deserve a careful medical evaluation and neurologic assessment. Very often, noncardiac etiologies, such as endocrine imbalance (including hypo-

glycemia, hypothyroidism), electrolyte imbalance, renal failure, hypoxia, drug toxicity or overdose, and a vast variety of neurologic disorders, to name only a few, will explain the patient's syncope or dizziness. Should this evaluation fail to determine the cause of the symptoms, 24- to 36-hour electrocardiographic monitoring is recommended [6] (see Chap. 3). This allows the patient to go about his or her normal activities while constant recording of the rhythm proceeds. Patients are instructed to keep a diary and to press an event marker on their recorder if they are symptomatic. In this manner, correlation between rhythm and symptoms is made. If the patient is symptomatic when the rhythm is normal sinus, medical and neurologic reevaluation is indicated. Morganroth et al [7] feel that at least 72 hours of electrocardiographic monitoring should be obtained before the Holter tape is considered nondiagnostic. Shorter periods of monitoring fail to account for the day-to-day variability of arrhythmias. Conduction disorders can similarly be intermittent.

If the patient is asymptomatic during normal sinus rhythm and has a history of medically and neurologically unexplained syncope or dizziness, he or she becomes a candidate for cardiac electrophysiologic evaluation. During the study, assessment is made of sinus node function, atrioventricular (AV) conduction and inducibility of supraventricular and ventricular arrhythmias. If all of these are normal, the patient is referred back for further medical and neurologic reevaluation. Patients with abnormally slow sinus node recovery time or prolonged sinoatrial conduction may have the sick sinus or tachycardia/bradycardia syndrome. It is important to note that long periods of asystole following cessation of sinus activity implies disease of the distal conduction system. Pacemakers situated lower in the patient's conducting system should provide an escape rhythm if the sinus mechanism fails but because this may not always occur, these patients should be candidates for permanently implanted pacemakers.

Should the electrophysiologic study reveal evidence of significant distal conduction disease by demonstrating block below the His bundle or document high degrees of AV block (even if intermittent), the patient similarly becomes a candidate for a pacemaker. If the Holter recording reveals advanced AV block in a symptomatic patient, electrophysiologic testing is unnecessary. One caveat regarding pacemakers should be mentioned. Some patients with conduction disease may continue to display symptoms of dizziness or syncope despite the fact that their pacemaker is functioning properly, since their symptoms were, and still are, noncardiac in origin.

Supraventricular or Ventricular Arrhythmias

These arrhythmias may be manifest on the Holter recording or be induced by programmed electrical stimulation. Supraventricular (more often than ventricular) arrhythmias may be managed by antiarrhythmic drugs alone and do not always require study. Patients with severely symptomatic recurrent supraventricular arrhythmias deserve a study for diagnostic purposes and assessment of drug efficacy. In some cases, electrophysiologic evaluation is necessary to distinguish supraventricular from ventricular tachycardia. Patients with the Wolff-Parkinson-White (WPW) or Lown-Ganong-Levine (LGL) preexcitation syndrome are prone to paroxysmal supraventricular tachycardias. Although the rhythm originates in the atrium, the rapid 1:1 conduction that may occur and result in ventricular responses of 300 beats/min creates a de facto ventricular tachycardia. The patient's hemodynamic response and predisposition to ventricular fibrillation depends on the state of the ventricle and the amount of coronary artery disease present. Certainly any patient with a preexcitation syndrome who ever has been even mildly symptomatic deserves an electrophysiologic study to test the efficacy of his or her drug regimen.

Patients with symptomatic ventricular tachycardia (VT) require treatment. Suspected but undocumented cases of ventricular arrhythmias merit study to determine whether VT can be induced. The initial study should be performed, if possible, in the absence of any antiarrhythmic drug, since many of these may, in fact, be arrhythmogenic. Drug efficacy may be assessed either by acute intravenous drug challenge or by testing after oral loading [8, 9]. Care must be taken to test only one drug at a time, allowing for washout of previously used agents. Electrophysiologic testing has, in fact, provided the impetus for the development of electropharmacology. Certain antiarrhythmic agents produce changes in the rate and morphology of the induced ventricular tachycardia (which most often resembles the spontaneous variety). Some drugs may slow the rate of the VT, avoiding hypotension and allowing the patient to seek medical attention. Some drugs speed the rate of the tachycardia, allowing appropriate sensing by devices such as the automatic internal defibrillator [10].

Refinement in techniques of programmed stimulation and recording has allowed location of the site of an irritable focus. Mapping [11] of the ventricle and identification of the site of origin of the ventricular tachycardia has allowed surgical extirpation of the focus by endocardial resection [12]. Presently, candidates for electrophysiologic evaluation include individuals with symptomatic ventricular tachycardia and survivors of sudden death/ventricular fibrillation, unless either of these events was associated with the early state of acute myocardial infarction. At this time, study is not recommended for survivors of myocardial infarction unless they are symptomatic with dizziness or syncope in the convalescent stage.

Electrophysiologic Measurements, Definitions, and Mechanisms

The purpose of this section is to acquaint the reader with some of the basic terms and mechanisms of electrophysiology. For further details, the reader is referred to more specialized texts [13].

Basic Intervals

A-H interval measures the conduction time from the low right atrium through the AV node to the His bundle (Fig. 10-1). The range of normal values in adults is 60 to 125 msec.*

H-V interval measures the conduction time from the proximal His bundle to ventricular myocardium and is measured from the His deflection on the intracardiac electrogram to the earliest activation on the surface tracing of the QRS complex. The range of normal values in adults is 35 to 55 msec.*

Refractory Periods

The refractory period measures the response of cardiac tissue to premature stimuli. In practical electrophysiology, the most valuable of these measurements is the effective refractory period (ERP). The ERP is dependent on both cycle length and stimulus strength. Therefore, when measuring this interval, constant pacing at a fixed basic cycle length for 8 to 10 beats is followed by premature stimuli. By convention, the stimulus strength is set at twice diastolic threshold.

In atrial, His-Purkinje, and ventricular tissue, the refractory periods decrease as the basic cycle length shortens. In the AV node, however, the opposite is seen with an increased refractory period at shorter basic cycle lengths.

Effective refractory period (ERP) refers to the longest coupling interval between the basic drive and the premature beat that fails to propagate through that tissue.

Relative refractory period (RRP) refers to the longest coupling interval of a premature beat that results in prolonged conduction of that beat relative to that of the basic drive.

Functional refractory period (FRP) refers to the minimum interval between two consecutively conducted impulses.

Sinus Node Assessment

Sinus node function is assessed by measurement of sinus node recovery time (SNRT) and sinoatrial conduction time (SACT). SNRT is dependent on automaticity, SACT, and the presence of acetylcholine and norepinephrine as well as the stimulation site of the exploring atrial electrode. It is considered the best test of

*These ranges may vary from laboratory to laboratory.

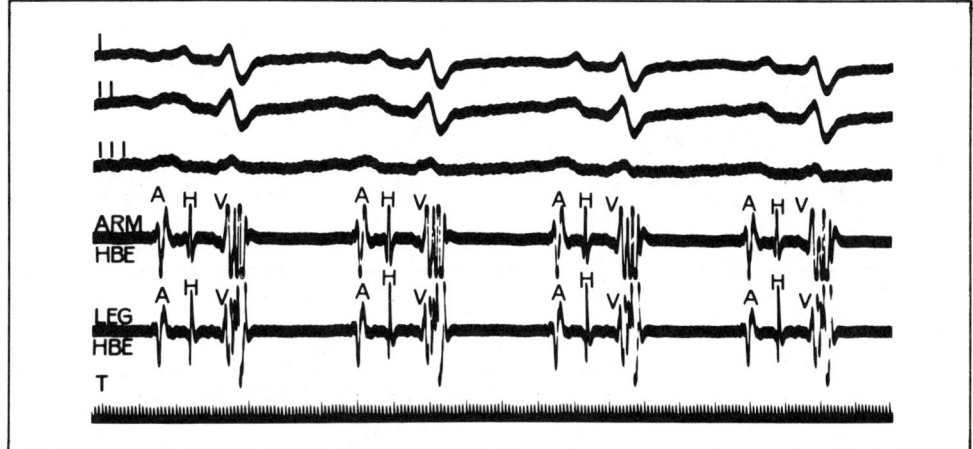

FIGURE 10-1. Simultaneous recording of the His bundle electrogram (*HBE*) from catheters advanced from the upper and lower extremities. From top to bottom, Standard leads I, II, and III; His bundle electrograms obtained from the arm via the antecubital vein and from the leg by the standard femoral technique; and time lines at 10 and 100 msec. Note that His bundle electrograms obtained from the upper and lower extremities are nearly identical. (From JJ Gallagher, AN Damato: Technique of recording His bundle activity in man. In W Grossman (ed): *Cardiac Catheterization and Angiography.* Philadelphia: Lea & Febiger, 1980, p 283. Reprinted with permission.)

sinus node automaticity and function currently available. SACT is not considered a sensitive indicator of sinus node dysfunction.

Corrected sinus node recovery time (CSNRT) measures the longest pause from the last paced atrial deflection to the first sinus recovery beat with the subtraction of the sinus cycle length. The normal value should be less than 550 msec.

Sinoatrial conduction time (SACT) measures the return cycle length after atrial pacing with premature atrial beats with the subtraction of half the basic atrial cycle length.

MECHANISMS OF ARRHYTHMIAS: REENTRY VS. AUTOMATICITY

Both reentry and automaticity are postulated mechanisms of action for both supraventricular and ventricular arrhythmias [14–18]. Automaticity involves the spontaneous diastolic depolarization of cells. An automatic tachycardia results from enhanced spontaneous depolarization and usually cannot be initiated nor terminated by programmed stimulation. Reentry theoretically involves the combination of dual pathways, unidirectional block, and slowed conduction (Fig. 10-2). The ability to reproducibly induce or terminate a tachycardia by programmed stimulation is characteristic of a reentrant mechanism.

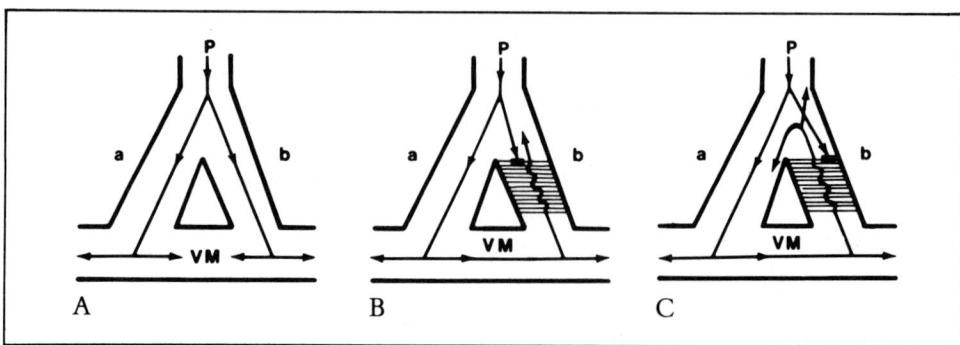

FIGURE 10-2. Schematic representation of reentry in the Purkinje system. The Purkinje fiber (P) in the distal ventricular conducting system divides into two branches (a and b) before making contact with ventricular muscle (VM) to form a loop. A shows the sequence of activation under normal conditions; the sinus impulse descends via the main Purkinje bundle leading to the loop, conducts through both branches (a and b) into ventricular muscle, collides, and terminates. B shows the pattern of activation when an area of unidirectional conduction block is present (shaded area in branch b). Conduction is blocked in the antegrade direction in b but not in the retrograde direction (from VM to b). The impulse in limb a conducts slowly around the loop and returns to the site of antegrade block in limb b. Because of slowed conduction, this impulse arrives at the site of antegrade block in b after the refractory period has passed and is able to conduct in a retrograde manner. In C, the impulse traveling retrograde past the site of antegrade block into b conducts into P, activating the ventricle, and gives rise to a reciprocal beat. It may also continue its movement via limb a, producing repetitive reciprocal beats. The rate of this reciprocal beating will be determined by the total conduction time around the loop. (From A Vera, DT Mason: Reentry versus automaticity: Role in tachyarrhythmia genesis and antiarrhythmic therapy. *Am Heart J* 101:329, 1981.)

Most ventricular tachycardias are thought to be due to reentry. Occasionally, after ventricular pacing, a repetitive response will be observed that is preceded by a His deflection. This response is physiologic rather than pathologic and is thought to represent macroreentry in the His-Purkinje system [19, 20]. Also called bundle branch reentry (BBR), the postulated explanation involves retrograde conduction block in the right bundle, conduction through myocardium to the left bundle, retrograde activation to the His bundle, and propagation back down the right bundle. In contrast, pathologic microreentry or intraventricular reentry (IVR) is caused by a microcircuit near the site of stimulation. Distinction between IVR and BBR is important if management decisions are to be made on the basis of nonsustained repetitive ventricular responses after ventricular pacing. Some laboratories, however, would recommend treatment of only induced sustained tachycardia.

Equipment and Techniques

EQUIPMENT

The basic equipment required for electrophysiologic testing includes a stimulator, amplifier, oscilloscope, and recording device. The stimulator must have the ability to pace, induce multiple extrastimuli, and have a dropout switch to allow for observation of the response to stimulation. The amplifier processes the signals and has an oscilloscope to provide constant monitoring of the surface and intracardiac potentials as well as display the arterial pressure tracing. The recording device may be an ink jet, photographic, or tape recorder. Z-fold paper facilitates interpretation of the studies.

Various electrode catheters may be employed. We routinely use No. 5 or 6 French quadripolar pacing electrodes, which enable us to record from two sets of bipoles or to pace from one and record from the other. The interelectrode distance is 1 cm. Some catheters contain a movable core that permits fashioning of curves.

TECHNIQUES

Our usual approach is percutaneous, through the femoral veins. Although the type of catheter is different, techniques for insertion are similar to those described in Chapter 9. We usually limit the number of entry sites to two per vein. For example, two electrodes will be placed in the right and one in the left femoral vein. These electrodes will be advanced to positions in the high right atrium, His position, and right ventricle. An additional venous catheter will be placed into the coronary sinus if required (e.g., in the evaluation of WPW syndrome). Pressure is recorded via an 18-gauge catheter inserted, again percutaneously, into the femoral artery. Should stimulation of the left ventricle be required, this catheter is replaced with a sheath that allows pressure monitoring through a side arm as well as electrode access. Occasionally, if necessary, the basilic vein is used as access, either percutaneously or by cutdown. In some cases, one electrode is inserted via the subclavian vein and retained, under sterile conditions, for repeated studies.

COMPLICATIONS

Complications of electrophysiologic studies should be minimal. Nationwide experience has shown only rare deaths, myocardial infarctions, or cerebrovascular accidents as a result of the studies. The major risk that the patient faces, particularly during ventricular stimulation, is the induction of sustained ventricular tachycardia and possible ventricular fibrillation. It must be recalled, however, that the purpose of the study is to determine inducibility of arrhythmia, either on or off drugs. Approximately half of the patients with sustained ventricular tachycardia will have the rhythm restored to sinus by overdrive pacing. Some individuals are able to maintain their blood pressure and consciousness by coughing during ventricular tachycardia [21]. This allows additional time for attempts at overdrive pacing. Failure to restore sinus rhythm requires cardioversion (or defibrillation) in the other half of cases. When doing ventricular tachycardia studies, it is recommended that two defibrillators be available, one as a backup unit.

Minor risks include phlebitis and thromboembolism. All patients are routinely anticoagulated with heparin during the study (100 U/kg intravenously) and receive a similar amount of protamine at the end of the study for reversal. Significant hemorrhage is rarely a problem if the entry sites are compressed for suitable periods of time (at least 15 minutes for an artery) after removal of the catheters and the patient is confined to bed rest for at least 12 hours post study.

A rare but serious complication involves perforation of the heart by the pacing electrode, which may result in pericardial effusion or tamponade. Other serious complications may occur during retrograde catheterization of the left heart, particularly with the relatively stiff pacing electrode. A skilled operator can minimize these risks by caution and meticulous technique.

Infection is not common, and our patients do not receive prophylactic antibiotics. Chronic indwelling catheters provide a focus for infection and deserve careful monitoring.

STIMULATION PROTOCOLS

Atrial pacing is accomplished via the pacing electrode in the high right atrium. Commonly, the protocol begins with eight atrially paced beats (A_1) at a constant basic cycle length followed by a premature atrial stimulus (A_2). After a dropout of 2 to 5 seconds, the cycle is repeated with A_2 more premature (i.e., closer to the prior A_1). The cycle is repeated until the refractory period of first the AV node (failure to conduct to the His) and then the atrium (failure to produce atrial deflection) is achieved. This is performed with at least two different pacing cycle lengths. After this is completed, incremental pacing is performed (for 30–60 seconds at constant cycle lengths) to measure SNRT.

Ventricular pacing is accomplished via the exploring electrode in the right or the left ventricle. Four protocols are available with the $V_1V_2V_3$ and V_{burst} modes reported to have the highest predictive accuracy [22–24]. The first protocol, now used infrequently, is termed A_1V_1 [25] and involves eight atrially paced beats followed by one premature ventricular beat. Diastole is scanned until the refractory period of the ventricle is achieved. A positive response (i.e., a repetitive ventricular response) is defined as a repetitive beat following V_1. If it is preceded by a His deflection, it is classified as BBR, if not as IVR. The phenomenon must be reproducible. The number of responses is noted.

The second protocol, termed V_1V_2, involves eight ventricularly paced beats (with eight simultaneous atrially paced beats to avoid atrial premature beats and competition) followed by a premature ventricular beat. Again, diastole is scanned for repetitive responses until the ERP is reached. The third protocol, termed $V_1V_2V_3$, involves eight ventricularly paced beats (again with eight simultaneous atrially paced beats) followed by a premature ventricular couplet (Fig. 10-3). To arrive at the coupling intervals, 50 msec is added to the ventricular ERP determined by V_1V_2 for V_2 and V_3 is brought in at twice the cycle length of V_2. For example, if the ventricular ERP is 280 msec, V_2 is entered at 330 msec and V_3 at 660 msec. V_3 is brought in by 10 msec decrements until V_3 becomes refractory; then V_2 is brought in by 10 msec decrements until V_3 is again able to depolarize the ventricle. This continues until the refractory period of V_2 is reached. A similar recording of repetitive responses is tabulated as for the other protocols.

V_{burst}, the final protocol, involves a series of 10 ventricular beats at a constant cycle length and observation of response. The paced cycle length is decreased by 50 to 100 msec until within 50 msec of the predicted ERP (by V_1V_2), then the decrement proceeds by 10 msec intervals until ERP is achieved by V_{burst}.

Noninvasive Electrophysiology

Efforts are under way to develop a noninvasive His bundle electrogram [26]. Although this method may not be applicable to various stimulation techniques, it has the potential to eliminate one diagnostic step for the symptomatic patient who requires a pacemaker. The technique is based on high gain amplification of external signals, use of filters to eliminate random noise, and averaging of amplified signals over several hundred cardiac cycles. Recent advances may make averaging unnecessary. Thus the initial work appears promising that this is a reproducible means to obtain measurement of the HV interval.

Evaluation of Intracardiac Conduction Disturbances

The indications for cardiac electrophysiologic study in patients with conduction disturbance have already been considered. This section will correlate the measurements on the surface ECG with specific sites of intracardiac conduction delay [27, 28].

The P-R interval on the ECG describes AV conduction but not the location of the block. First-degree heart block may represent delay in the AV node, the bundle of His, the bundle branch–Purkinje system, or in multiple sites. If first-degree block occurs on the ECG with a QRS of normal duration, the delay will be in the AV node in the vast majority of cases. Electrophysiologically, the A–H interval is prolonged, but the HV interval is normal. The reasons for the delay include increased vagal tone, inferior wall infarction, myocarditis, drug effect (digitalis, beta blockade, calcium antagonists), and degenerative disease. Delay in

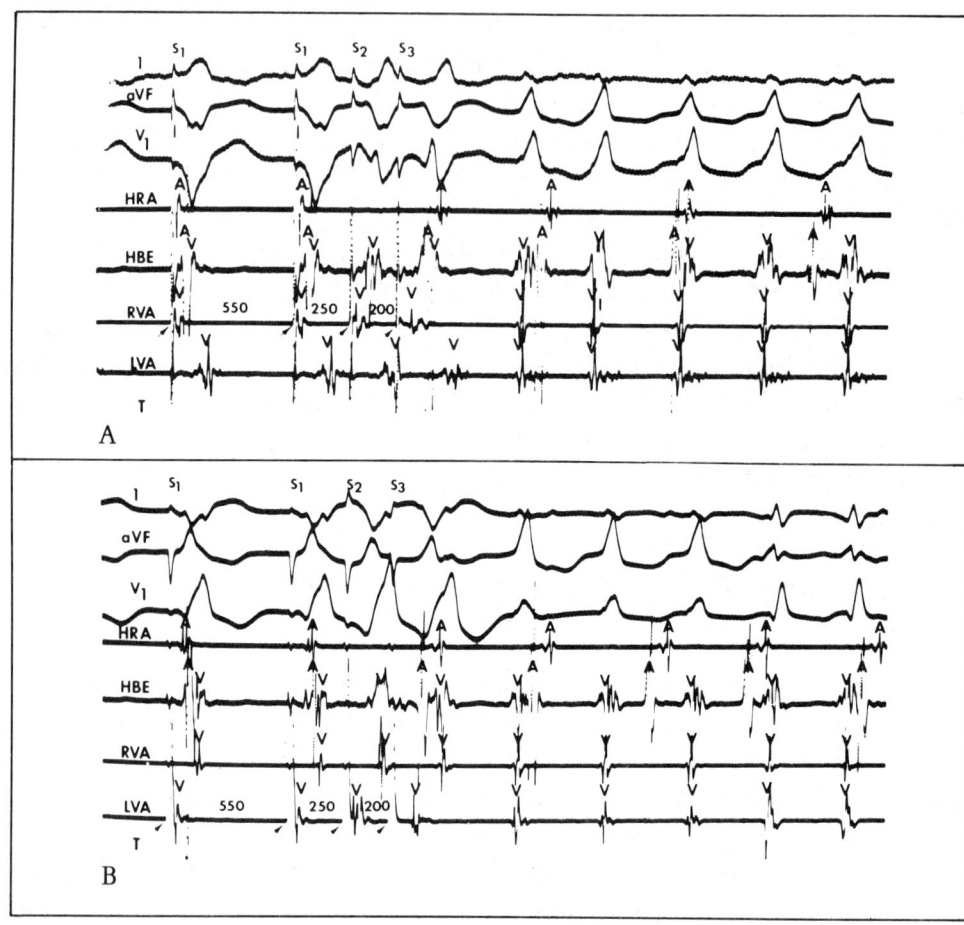

FIGURE 10-3. Initiation of ventricular tachycardia by right or left ventricular stimulation. Both panels are organized from top to bottom: ECG leads I, aVF, V1, and electrograms from the high right atrium (*HRA*), His bundle (*HBE*), right ventricular apex (*RVA*), left ventricular apex (*LVA*). In A, two right ventricular premature stimuli (S_2, S_3) are introduced after the eighth RV paced complex (S_1), resulting in ventricular tachycardia. In panel B, two left ventricular stimuli (S_2, S_3) are delivered after the eighth LV paced complex (S_1), resulting in ventricular tachycardia. Note that the coupling intervals of the premature stimuli are identical. Stimulus artifacts are indicated by small arrows. (From ME Josephson, et al: *Circulation* 57:431, 1978, by permission of the American Heart Association, Inc.)

the His or distal conduction system is manifest by split His potentials indicating impaired intra-His conduction or by a prolonged HV interval consistent with disease in the bundle branch–Purkinje system.

Second-degree heart block of the Wenckebach (Mobitz type I) variety generally represents impaired conduction at the AV node, less commonly in the distal conduction system, and uncommonly in the His bundle. The prolonged intracardiac intervals are the same as for first-degree block. If the block occurs at the AV node, atrial pacing with atrial premature beats will first result in a prolonged A–H interval as the relative refractory period (latency) is approached. When the effective refractory period of the AV node is reached, atrial depolarization will be seen, but this His deflection will be absent. If the block occurs in the distal conduction system, the HV interval will be prolonged. As the atrial premature beats (APBs) become more premature, block will eventually occur below the His, i.e., a His deflection will be observed without conduction to the ventricle and therefore no ventricular electrogram.

Second-degree block of Mobitz type II is associated with block below the His bundle and is recognized as described above. Third-degree or complete heart block may also occur at each level in the conduction system, but most commonly is infra-His, and only occasionally in the AV node or His bundle. If the patient is asymptomatic and the third-degree block is at the AV node level, permanent pacing may not be mandatory.

Patients with bundle branch block of the various varieties and combinations may still have normal HV intervals if some portion(s) of the fascicular conduction system remains intact. Although the vast majority of patients with bundle branch block who develop complete heart block have prolonged HV intervals, the incidence of HV prolongation is high and the incidence of complete heart block low. If atrial pacing studies produce infra-His block, permanent pacing should be considered. In the evaluation of the distal conduction system, attention must be paid to the patient's antiarrhythmic drug regimen. Certain drugs may impair conduction and cause infra-His block.

Evaluation of Supraventricular Tachycardias

The etiology of supraventricular tachycardia may be divided into two major categories [29, 30]. By far the most common is AV nodal reentry, accounting for 60 percent of cases in some series, followed by AV reentry due to a concealed bypass tract (30 percent). Sinoatrial nodal reentry, intraatrial reentry, and automatic atrial tachycardias constitute the remaining 10 percent. Programmed electrical stimulation identifies these arrhythmias by characterizing the response to atrial premature beats and incremental pacing of the ventricle as well as the atrium.

Preexcitation syndromes (e.g., WPW, LGL) are described by activation of the ventricles by the atrium before the impulse has time to pass through the AV node [31, 32]. Conduction therefore occurs through a bypass tract (Fig. 10-4). Connections may occur between the atrium and ventricle, AV node and ventricle, atrium and His bundle, and finally fascicular branches of the His-Purkinje system and ventricle. Electrophysiologic testing is performed as described earlier. The goals include localization of the bypass tract and determination of the ability to conduct antegrade and/or retrograde as well as the selection of an appropriate antiarrhythmic drug regimen. At the close of the study, atrial fibrillation is induced to determine the risk for a rapid ventricular response. Certain antiarrhythmic agents increase the refractory period of the accessory pathway and may prevent life-threatening rapid rates during atrial fibrillation. Other modalities of treatment for accessory pathway syndromes include pacemakers and surgery to interrupt the bypass tract.

Evaluation of Ventricular Tachycardia

Electrophysiologic (EP) testing of patients with ventricular arrhythmias has facilitated understanding of the mechanism of ventricular tachycardia and permitted laboratory assessment of antiarrhythmic therapy. Management of this life-threatening rhythm disturbance may also be accomplished by repeated 24-hour ambulatory recordings [33, 34] and attention to drug levels [35, 36]. Programmed electrical stimulation allows immediate therapeutic decision-making without the necessity of waiting for Holter reports or long-term follow-up. If a drug regimen is ineffective, it is likely to be exposed during the EP study, while it may otherwise become apparent only after discharge from the hospital. Interpretation of the results of the EP study still fails to meet universal agreement [37]. Some laboratories consider the induction of sustained ventricular tachycardia (VT) to be the only significant result, with nonsustained self-terminating VT of lesser importance. The goal is to prevent induction of sustained VT. Other laboratories consider three or more repetitive ventricular responses due to intraventricular reentry to be a significant predictor of recurrent symptomatic ventricular tachycardia. Both the absence of any repetitive response and the presence of nonsustained responses due to bundle branch reentry are considered to be normal responses. Therefore, the management of patients with nonsustained ventricular tachycardia on the electrophysiologic study will depend upon the bias of the investigator until more data are available.

In addition to the stimulation protocols described in the techniques section, some laboratories include isoproterenol infusions and short pacing cycle lengths as part of the provocative protocol. In the majority of cases, the VT reproduced in the laboratory has been demonstrated to be identical to the VT occurring in the clinical setting, no matter what the stimulation protocol. One criticism of the electrophysiologic study is that it may be a more potent stimulus than may occur in life. However, the evidence has suggested that 80 to 90 percent of patients with inducible VT will have out-of-hospital recurrences. Some drugs, however, may possibly provide protection even though VT can be induced in the laboratory.

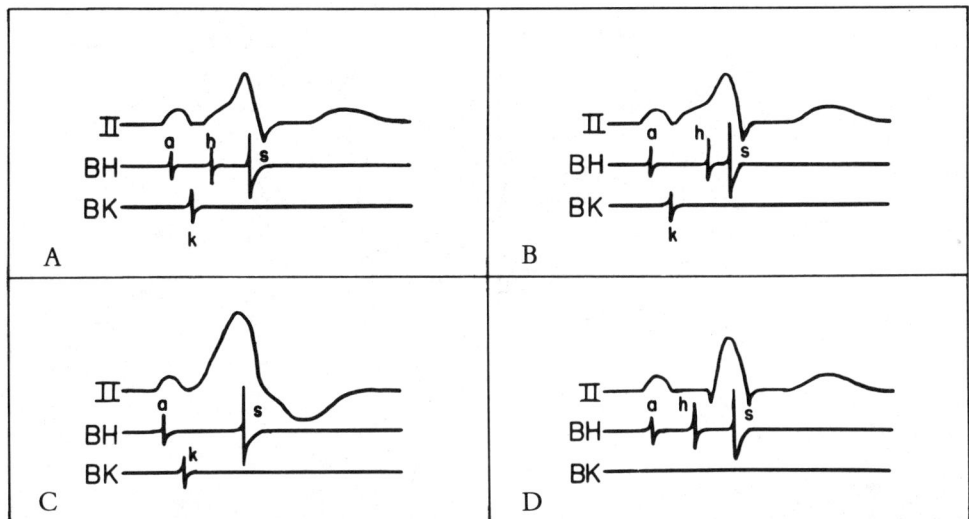

FIGURE 10-4. Simultaneously recorded electrocardiograms (lead II), bundle of His electrograms (BH) and bundle of Kent electrograms (BK) during normal preexcitation (A), preexcitation with delayed conduction within the atrioventricular node (B), preexcitation with blocked conduction through the atrioventricular node (C), and blocked conduction over the anomalous bundle of Kent (D). a = atrial, h = His bundle, k = bundle of Kent as recorded by epicardial (but not endocardial) mapping, s = ventricular septal activation. (Reprinted with permission from EN Moore, et al: *N Engl J Med* 289:956, 1973.)

Although the EP study has improved understanding of the mechanism of VT, it is not absolute. It provides evidence for either reentry or automaticity by the ability to initiate and terminate the tachycardia by programmed stimulation. The tachycardia, however, may be influenced by the basic cycle length, the location and size of the tachycardia circuit, electrophysiologic properties of the tissue, and the effect of pharmacologic therapy.

Endocardial mapping techniques [11] (Fig. 10-5) have added new dimension to the EP study. The actual site of origin of the tachycardia is determined by recordings at multiple sites (Fig. 10-6). The morphology of the VT on the surface electrocardiogram represents epicardial activation, but does not necessarily correspond to endocardial activation [38]. Therefore, different morphologies of VT may result from the same site. Of course, multiple irritable foci certainly are possible in patients with diffuse disease.

Preferably, all drugs should be discontinued for the first EP study. Once the response is observed, acute drug testing may be performed to test the ability of an agent to prevent induction of VT. Before a second drug can be evaluated, however, washout of the first drug (at least five half-lives) should occur; otherwise, the individual drug effects cannot be interpreted. Occasionally combinations of drugs are useful, and in this case acute administration of a second drug would be

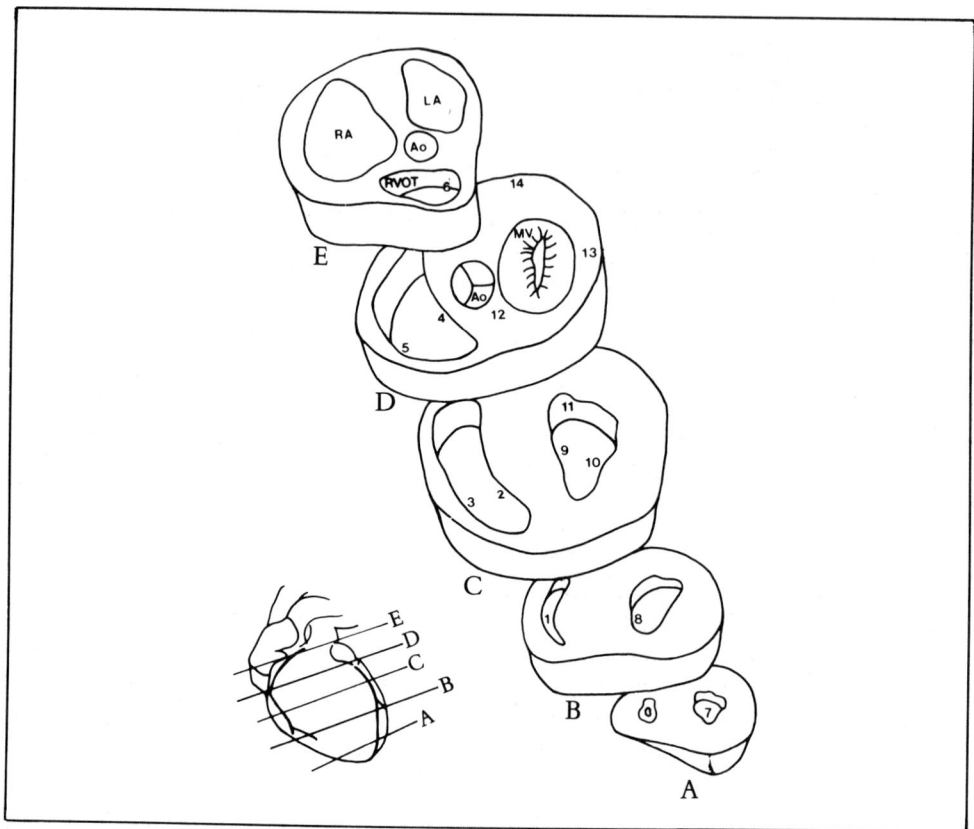

FIGURE 10-5. Schematic view of the heart in serial sections indicating the endocardial mapping sites. The inset shows the level of transection for each section. The sites are (1) right ventricular (*RV*) apex; (2) RV midseptum; (3) RV free anterior wall; (4) AV junction; (5) RV inflow tract; (6) RV outflow tract; (7) left ventricular (*LV*) apex; (8) LV low septum; (9) LV midseptum; (10) LV anterior free wall; (11) LV inferoposterior wall; (12) LV high septum (under aortic valve); (13) LV lateral wall (under mitral valve), and (14) posterobasilar LV (recorded from coronary sinus). *Ao* = aorta, *LA* = left atrium, *MV* = mitral valve, *RA* = right atrium, *RVOT* = right ventricular outflow tract. (From ME Josephson, et al: Recurrent sustained ventricular tachycardia. 2. Endocardial mapping. *Circulation* 57:440, 1978, by permission of the American Heart Association, Inc.)

acceptable. Serial testing with a number of agents allows a choice of the most optimal regimen. If the patient is electrically unstable off medications, it is acceptable to perform the study on the intended discharge regimen.

For patients with VT refractory to all drugs, endocardial mapping will allow consideration of a surgical procedure to eradicate the irritable focus. Subendocardial resection [12] has proven to be successful in preventing recurrence of the

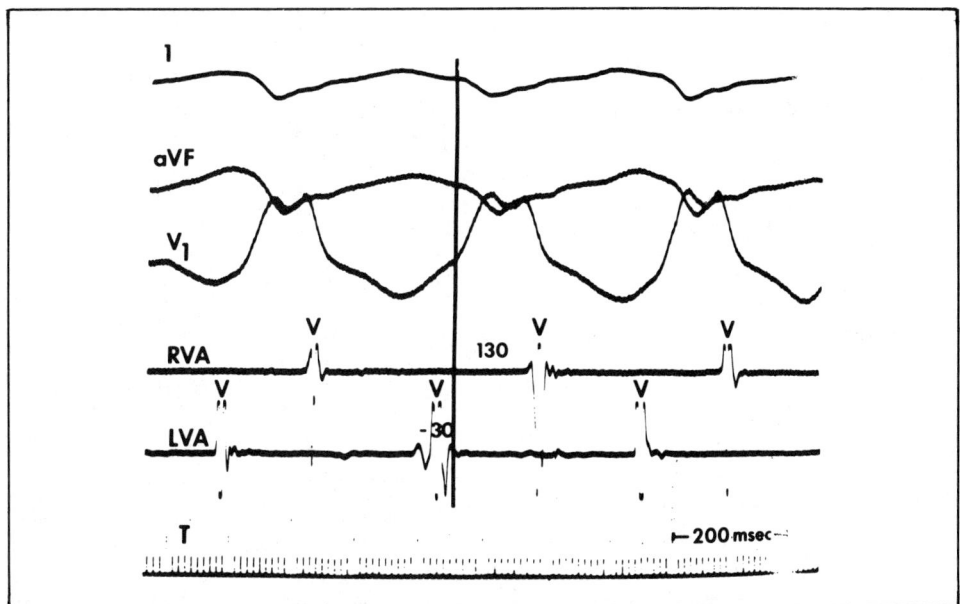

FIGURE 10-6. Earliest endocardial site of activation at left ventricular apex in a ventricular tachycardia with right bundle branch block morphology and wide QRS. ECG leads I, aVF, and V1 and electrograms at the right ventricular (*RVA*) and left ventricular apex (*LVA*). Of all sites mapped, the LVA was the earliest site of activation, occurring 30 msec prior to the inscription of the QRS. (From ME Josephson, et al: Recurrent sustained ventricular tachycardia. 2. Endocardial mapping. *Circulation* 57:440, 1978, by permission of the American Heart Association, Inc.)

arrhythmia. In this procedure, stripping of the endocardium has been performed in the areas identified at the EP study. The EP study has compared favorably with intraoperative mapping [39]. Intraoperative endocardial mapping occasionally may fail to induce VT owing to technical problems and therefore may not allow definition of the tachycardia zone. In the initial report of the subendocardial stripping, repeat electrophysiologic studies in 10 of 12 survivors revealed failure to induce VT. These patients remained free of sustained VT over the next 9 to 20 months, with one late nonarrhythmic death [12].

Electrophysiologic testing is also indicated for the patient in whom a manually activated overdrive pacemaker for refractory VT is considered. The potential hazard in this type of device is that the rapid bursts of ventricular pacing [40] may accelerate the VT in some patients. The role of the EP study is not only to determine inducibility but also the response to overdrive pacing.

Refractory patients may be considered for the automatic internal defibrillator (AID), a device that recognizes ventricular fibrillation and/or ventricular tachy-

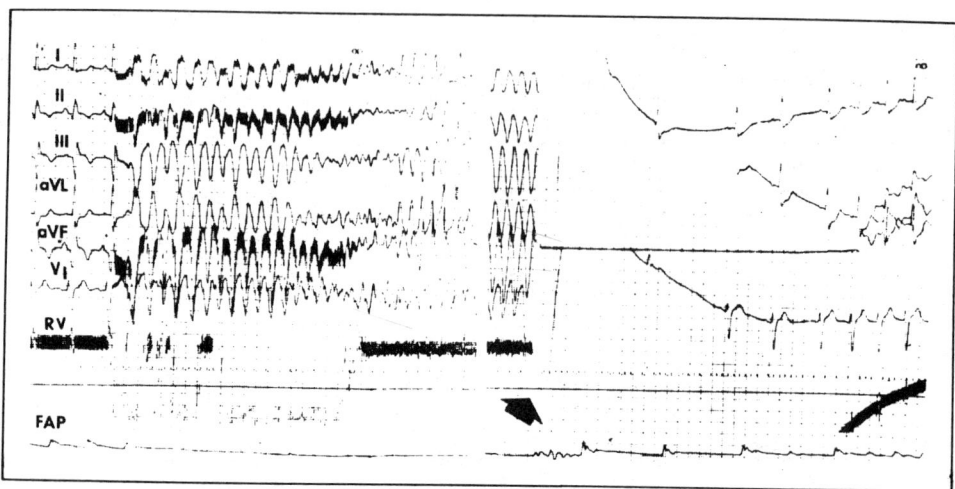

FIGURE 10-7. *Left,* Initiation of ventricular flutter-fibrillation by a burst of rapid ventricular pacing. *Right,* Automatic reversion of the arrhythmia to normal sinus rhythm by the implanted defibrillator (*arrow*). FAP = femoral artery pressure, RV = right ventricular electrogram. (From M Mirowski, et al: The automatic implantable defibrillator. *Am Heart J* 100:1089, 1980.)

cardia and then discharges, delivering 30 joules through internal electrodes to restore sinus rhythm. After implantation, these patients undergo repeat EP study to test the efficacy of the AID [41] (Fig. 10-7).

With increased awareness of the magnitude of the problem of sudden cardiac death (400,000–600,000 cases/year), electrophysiologic evaluation of ventricular arrhythmias will become a more widely utilized technique. It involves considerable time and expense on the part of the physician and patient alike and therefore must not be utilized indiscriminately. Certain situations are definite indications for study. The patient with recurrent ventricular tachycardia deserves evaluation of the final discharge drug regimen. Patients with subendocardial resection or implanted devices (pacemakers or defibrillators) require testing for efficacy. Other cases for EP testing are not as clear. If there is doubt as to the necessity for therapy, such as in the patient with underlying heart disease and high-grade ventricular arrhythmias (Lown class 3 or 4A, as depicted in Table 3-2) at rest or on Holter tapes, EP study may be considered. One caveat must be mentioned. The prognostic value of EP studies is valid as long as the underlying heart disease remains unchanged. If the substrate changes, such as worsening heart failure or ischemia, reevaluation may become necessary. At present, electrophysiologic testing remains an important procedure for uncovering electrical instability and assessing the therapeutic regimen.

References

1. Narula OS, Shantha N, Narula LK, Alboni P: Clinical and electrophysiologic evaluation of sinus node function. In Narula OS (ed): *Cardiac Arrhythmias: Electrophysiology, Diagnosis, and Management.* Baltimore: Williams & Wilkins, 1979, p 176
2. Fisch GR, Zipes DP, Fisch C: Bundle branch block and sudden death. *Prog Cardiovasc Dis* 23:187, 1980
3. Denes P, Dhingra RC, Wu D, Chuquimia R, Amat-y-Leon F, Wyndham C, Rosen KM: HV interval in patients with bifascicular block (RBB + LAHB). Clinical, electrocardiographic, and electrophysiologic correlations. *Am J Cardiol* 35:23, 1975
4. Lie KI, Liem KL, Schuilenburg RM, David GK, Durrer D: Early identification of patients developing late in-hospital ventricular fibrillation after discharge from the coronary care unit. A 5 1/2 year retrospective and prospective study with 1897 patients. *Am J Cardiol* 41:674, 1978
5. Denes P, Dhingra RC, Wu D, Wyndham C, Amat-y-Leon F, Rosen KM: Sudden death in patients with bifascicular block. *Arch Intern Med* 137:1005, 1977
6. Kennedy HL, Chandra V, Sayther KL, Caralis DG: Effectiveness of increasing hours of continuous ambulatory electrocardiography in detecting maximal ventricular ectopy. *Am J Cardiol* 42:925, 1978
7. Morganroth J, Michelson EL, Horowitz LN, Josephson ME, Pearlman AS, Punkman WB: Limitations of routine long-term electrocardiographic monitoring to assess ventricular ectopy frequency. *Circulation* 58:408, 1978
8. Winkle RA, Alderman EL, Fitzgerald JW, Harrison DC: Treatment of recurrent symptomatic ventricular tachycardia. *Ann Intern Med* 85:1, 1976
9. Horowitz LN, Josephson ME, Farshidi A, Spielman SR, Michelson EL, Greenspan AM: Recurrent sustained ventricular tachycardia. 3. Role of the electrophysiologic study in selection of antiarrhythmic regimens. *Circulation* 58:986, 1978
10. Mirowski M, Reid PR, Mower MM, Watkins L, Gott VL, Schauble JF, Langer A, Heilman MS, Kolenik SA, Fischell RE, Weisfeldt ML: Termination of malignant ventricular arrhythmias with an implanted automatic defibrillator in human beings. *N Engl J Med* 303:322, 1980
11. Josephson ME, Horowitz LN, Farshidi A, Spear JF, Kastor JA, Moore EN: Recurrent sustained ventricular tachycardia. 2. Endocardial mapping. *Circulation* 57:440, 1978
12. Josephson ME, Harken AH, Horowitz LN: Endocardial excision: A new technique for the treatment of recurrent ventricular tachycardia. *Circulation* 60:1430, 1979
13. Josephson ME, Seides SF: *Clinical Cardiac Electrophysiology.* Philadelphia: Lea & Febiger, 1979
14. Wellens HJJ, Schuilenburg RM, Durrer D: Electrical stimulation of the heart in patients with ventricular tachycardia. *Circulation* 46:216, 1972
15. Wellens HJJ, Lie KI, Durrer D: Further observations on ventricular tachycardia studied by electrical stimulation of the heart. Chronic recurrent ventricular tachy-

cardia and ventricular tachycardia during acute myocardial infarction. *Circulation* 49:647, 1974
16. Wellens HJJ: Observations on the pathophysiology of ventricular tachycardia in man. *Arch Intern Med* 135:473, 1975
17. Wellens HJJ, Duren DR, Lie KI: Observations on mechanisms of ventricular tachycardia in man. *Circulation* 54:237, 1976
18. Josephson ME, Horowitz LN, Farshidi A, Kastor JA: Recurrent sustained ventricular tachycardia. 1. Mechanisms. *Circulation* 57:431, 1978
19. Akhtar M: Re-entry within the His-Purkinje system. In Narula OS (ed): *Cardiac Arrhythmias: Electrophysiology, Diagnosis and Management.* Baltimore: Williams & Wilkins, 1979, p 397
20. Castellanos A, Sung RJ, Ghahramani A, Myerburg RJ: The retrograde His bundle deflection: Its recognition and value in the analysis of tachyarrhythmias induced by stimulation of the T wave. *Eur J Cardiol* 4:295, 1976
21. Wei JY, Greene HL, Weisfeldt ML: Cough facilitated conversion of ventricular tachycardia. *Am J Cardiol* 45:174, 1980
22. Mason JW: Repetitive beating after single ventricular extrastimuli: Incidence and prognostic significance in patients with recurrent ventricular tachycardia. *Am J Cardiol* 45:1126, 1980
23. Kent KM: Assessing the electric stability of the heart in human beings. *Am J Cardiol* 45:1305, 1980
24. Platia EV, Vlay SC, Reid PR: Predictive value of programmed electrical stimulation in patients with sudden death or recurrent ventricular tachycardia (Abstract). *Am J Cardiol* 47:397, 1981
25. Greene HL, Reid PR, Schaeffer AH: The repetitive ventricular response in man. *N Engl J Med* 299:729, 1978
26. Flowers NC, Shvartsman V, Kennelly BM, Sohi GS, Horan LG: Surface recording of His-Purkinje activity on an every beat basis without digital averaging. *Circulation* 63:948, 1981
27. Rosen KM: The contribution of His-bundle recording to the understanding of cardiac conduction in man. *Circulation* 43:961, 1971
28. Gomes JAC, El-Sherif N: His bundle recordings: Contributions to clinical electrophysiology. In Samet P, El-Sherif N (eds): *Cardiac Pacing.* 2nd ed. New York: Grune & Stratton, 1980, p 375
29. Josephson ME, Kastor JA: Supraventricular tachycardia: Mechanisms and management. *Ann Intern Med* 87:346, 1977
30. Wu D, Denes P, Amat-y-Leon F, Dhingra R, Wyndham CRC, Bauernfeind R, Latif P, Rosen KM: Clinical electrocardiographic and electrophysiologic observations in patients with paroxysmal supraventricular tachycardia. *Am J Cardiol* 41:1045, 1978
31. Wellens HJJ: Contribution of cardiac pacing to our understanding of the Wolff-Parkinson-White syndrome. *Br Heart J* 37:231, 1975
32. Gallagher JJ, Pritchett ELC, Sealy WC, Kasell J, Wallace AG: The pre-excitation syndromes. *Prog Cardiovasc Dis* 20:285, 1978

33. Lown B: Sudden cardiac death: The major challenge confronting contemporary cardiology. *Am J Cardiol* 43:313–328, 1979
34. Vlay SC, Kallman CH, Reid PR: Identification by Holter of patients at risk for recurrent sudden death or syncope despite abolition of hypotensive ventricular tachycardia (Abstract). *Circulation* 62(Suppl III):84, 1980
35. Myerburg RJ, Conde C, Sheps DS, Appel RA, Kiem I, Sung RJ, Castellanos A: Antiarrhythmic drug therapy in survivors of prehospital cardiac arrest: Comparison of effects on chronic ventricular arrhythmias and recurrent cardiac arrest. *Circulation* 59:855, 1979
36. Vlay SC, Kallman CH, Reid PR: Improved survival in sudden death/ventricular tachycardia patients with therapeutic antiarrhythmic drug levels (Abstract). *Am J Cardiol* 47:438, 1981
37. Wellens HJ: Value and limitations of programmed electrical stimulation of the heart in the study and treatment of tachycardias. *Circulation* 57:845, 1978
38. Josephson ME, Horowitz LN, Farshidi A, Spielman SR, Michelson EL, Greenspan AM: Recurrent sustained ventricular tachycardia. 4. Pleomorphism. *Circulation* 59:459, 1979
39. Josephson ME, Horowitz LN, Spielman SR, Greenspan AM, VandePol C, Harken AH: Comparison of endocardial catheter mapping with intraoperative mapping of ventricular tachycardia. *Circulation* 61:395, 1980
40. Ruskin JN, Garan H, Poulin F, Harthorne JW: Permanent radiofrequency ventricular pacing for management of drug resistant ventricular tachycardia. *Am J Cardiol* 46:317, 1980
41. Reid PR, Mirowski M, Mower M, Vlay SC, Platia EV, Weisfeldt ML: Electrophysiologic studies before and after implantation of the automatic defibrillator (Abstract). *Am J Cardiol* 47:397, 1981

Part V

Additional Diagnostic Procedures

Chapter 11

Nonangiographic Radiologic Examination of the Heart

Donald P. Harrington and J. Daniel Garnic

Fluoroscopy of the heart, performed on November 8, 1895, was the first cardiac application of Wilhelm Konrad Roentgen's newly discovered x-rays. In the United States, the first comprehensive report of medical radiography of the heart and lungs dates to the 1897 notation of Francis H. Williams in the *Medical and Surgical Reports of the Boston City Hospital* [1]. The fluoroscopic and subsequent radiographic technique was quickly incorporated into the diagnostic evaluation of cardiac patients; it soon took its place with the medical history, physical examination, and electrocardiogram as one of the basic elements in the work-up of such patients. For many years after the introduction of x-rays, there were few substantial modifications in methods or in technology. However, in the last several decades, remarkable technical developments in nonradiographic cardiac diagnostic procedures (such as echocardiography) have called into question the value of the previously established procedures. The first four sections of this chapter will attempt to evaluate the present usefulness of established radiographic and fluoroscopic studies. The final section will be concerned with newer diagnostic procedures (such as computed tomography).

Cardiac Diagnostic Procedures: A Comparison

In order to put into perspective the well-established radiographic procedures, it is important to review some of the newer diagnostic modalities: modern cardiac catheterization, echocardiography, and cardiac nuclear medicine.

The modern practice of cardiac catheterization has changed profoundly the way in which we approach the analysis of the chest radiograph. At first glance, the chest x-ray might seem obsolete in light of the precise intracardiac and pulmonary measurements and the exquisite anatomic detail that are available with modern angiocardiography; such factors tend to overshadow the admittedly less precise evaluation afforded by radiographic techniques. Nonetheless, the older methods provide unique anatomic, physiologic, and prognostic information on a wide variety of cardiac diseases at a considerably lower risk and financial expense than the more sophisticated and complex diagnostic procedures. Cardiac catheterization has indeed had a beneficial effect upon plain film analysis, in that it has provoked a reassessment of the way in which the anatomic information contained in the radiograph is interpreted. Prior to wide use of cardiac catheterization the radiographic picture was correlated to the pathologic specimen. The newer method of diagnostic evaluation enables the physician to correlate the radiograph with a broad range of physiologic information. First fruits of this type of correlation can be seen in the physiologic explanation in the 1960s for some manifestations of Kerley's patterns of interstitial edema that were first described in the 1930s [2, 3]. A more balanced interpretation of the radiograph enhances the value of the radiographic examination.

Cardiac ultrasound and radionuclide studies — including myocardial perfusion scanning and the radionuclide ventriculogram — offer new noninvasive approaches to cardiac diagnosis, and these too must be compared to previously established examinations. In general, radionuclide studies complement simple radiography, since, although they provide direct physiologic information, their anatomic detail is relatively poor in comparison to the highly resolved anatomic data offered by the radiograph. The physiologic information provided by the radiographic examination, while not as direct, can be quite useful. Left ventricular function is estimated radiographically by alterations in cardiac size and changes in pulmonary venous circulation. These estimates can be provided on a broader scale more efficiently and less expensively than with radionuclide methods. In most cases, however, evaluation of extent of myocardial infarction and ischemia is far beyond the scope of simple radiographic and fluoroscopic techniques but can be assessed with other radiographic methods. Computed tomography (CT) scanning and intravenous angiography may have a substantial future role in these areas.

Echocardiography, on the other hand, competes directly with the anatomic imaging advantages of the radiograph. In the evaluation of cardiac chamber enlargement and valve motion, echocardiography is superior to the radiographic method, although overall cardiac size is best determined by chest roentgenogram. Both methods have their place in evaluating the presence and extent of cardiac calcification. Cardiac ultrasound can detect valve leaflet calcification earlier than can radiography, but fluoroscopy provides superior definition of coronary artery calcification. Newell and his colleagues maintain that these two procedures are complementary, and a brief description of this comparison will be discussed in a later section [4].

Cardiac Radiography and Fluoroscopy
FRONTAL AND LATERAL CHEST RADIOGRAPHY
The upright frontal and lateral chest films, which constitute the standard roent-

genographic survey for cardiac and pulmonary disorders, provide a unique view of the heart and pulmonary vascularity. A substantial body of literature has developed over the years to describe the radiographic features of various cardiac diseases; extensive reviews may be found in several major texts of both cardiac medicine and radiology [5, 6]. A brief discussion of basic precepts is necessary in order to assess both the older and the newer radiologic methods.

Roentgenographic visualization of the heart is possible because of the contrast differences provided by air in the surrounding lung and by the tissue densities of muscle and blood within the heart itself. The image provides an outline of the heart from which a precise measurement of overall cardiac size is available. Enlargement of specific chambers, such as the left atrium, can be detected because of changes in cardiac contour. Further contrast differences are provided by the fat around the heart; these serve to identify pericardial effusions and to outline cardiac chambers, such as the left ventricle. Calcification within the heart provides the greatest degree of contrast. Its presence is considered pathologic in virtually all cases, indicating destruction or degeneration of valves, pericardium, or heart muscle; in many instances its recognition leads to a specific diagnosis, such as previous pericarditis (Fig. 11-1) or valvular heart disease (Fig. 11-2). The frontal and lateral chest films, in addition, permit analysis of the arterial and venous components of the pulmonary vascular tree, thus providing supplemental anatomic and physiologic information. Such data include, for example, a reliable estimate of capillary wedge pressure and pulmonary artery pressure and flow. The most diagnostically useful information comes from integrating knowledge of overall cardiac size with the physiologic state of the pulmonary vasculature and with pathologic calcifications within the heart.

Estimates of Cardiac Size

A wide variety of formulas have been used to assess cardiac size. The simplest and probably most useful is the cardiothoracic ratio. Volume measurements, on the other hand, provide a more precise evaluation of cardiac size but involve more complicated calculations. The cardiothoracic ratio, first described in 1919 by Danzer, is the ratio of the transverse diameter of the heart to the transverse inner diameter of the rib cage [7]. This is calculated by first establishing a vertical line through the spinous processes and then measuring the transverse length from this point to the furthest point of the right heart border added to the length from the vertical line to the left heart border. In measuring the left heart border, it is important not to include the cardiac fat pad. The denominator in this ratio is obtained by measuring the longest transverse diameter between the inner aspects of the rib cage (Fig. 11-3). While the cardiothoracic ratio represents the most widely used evaluation of overall cardiac size, it has some disadvantages, in that the thoracic diameter does not adequately correct for body habitus. Its accuracy

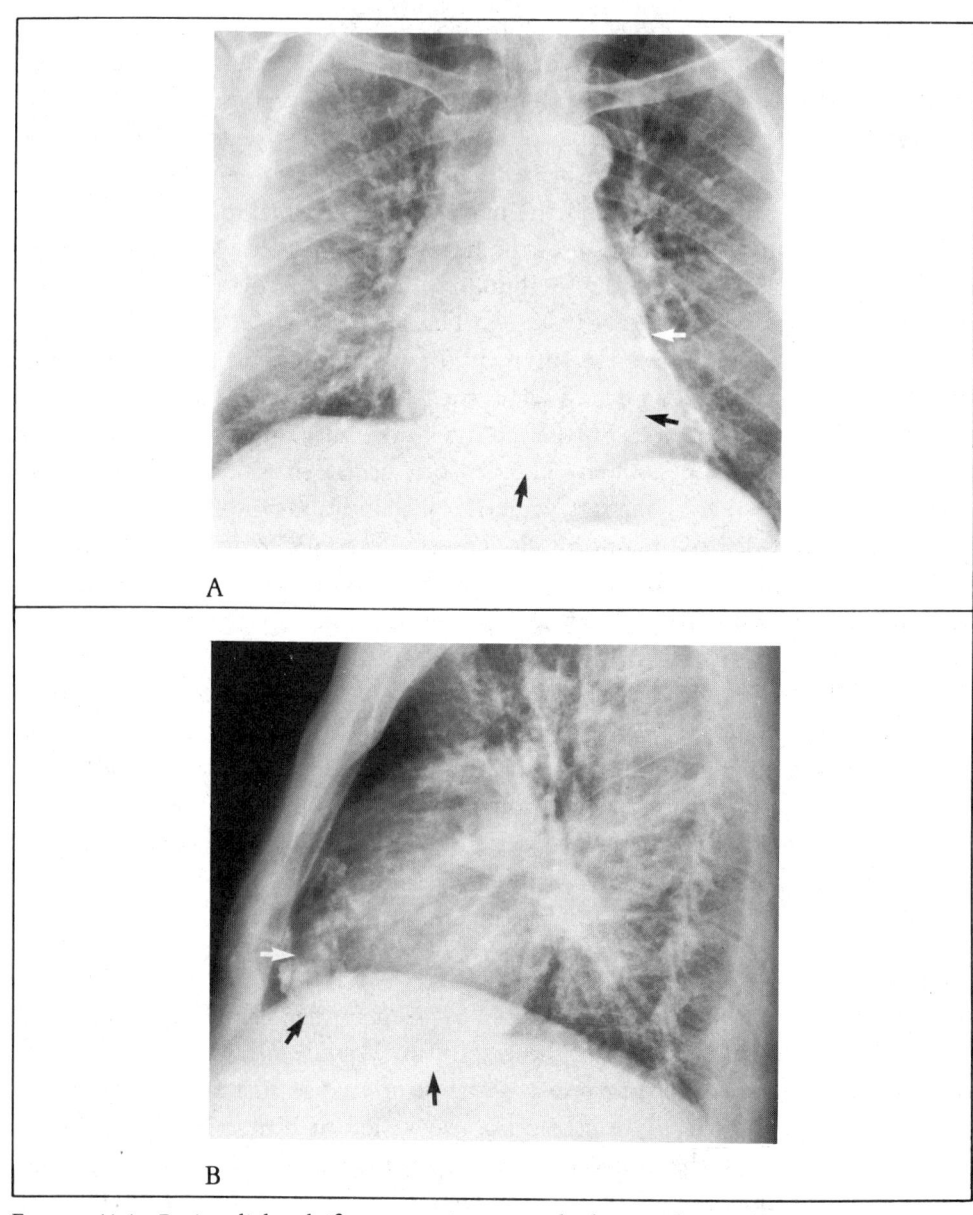

FIGURE 11-1. Pericardial calcification. (A) Frontal chest radiograph. Arrows indicate extensive pericardial calcification involving the right and left ventricles. The extensive nature and location of the calcification distinguishes the pericardial process from calcification in an old myocardial infarction. (B) Lateral chest radiograph. The extent of the pericardial calcification (*arrows*) is confirmed by the lateral projection. A specific etiologic agent could not be determined in this particular patient, although tubercular pericarditis is the most common cause of pericardial calcification. Rotation and a slight scoliosis make the right heart border somewhat more prominent than normal.

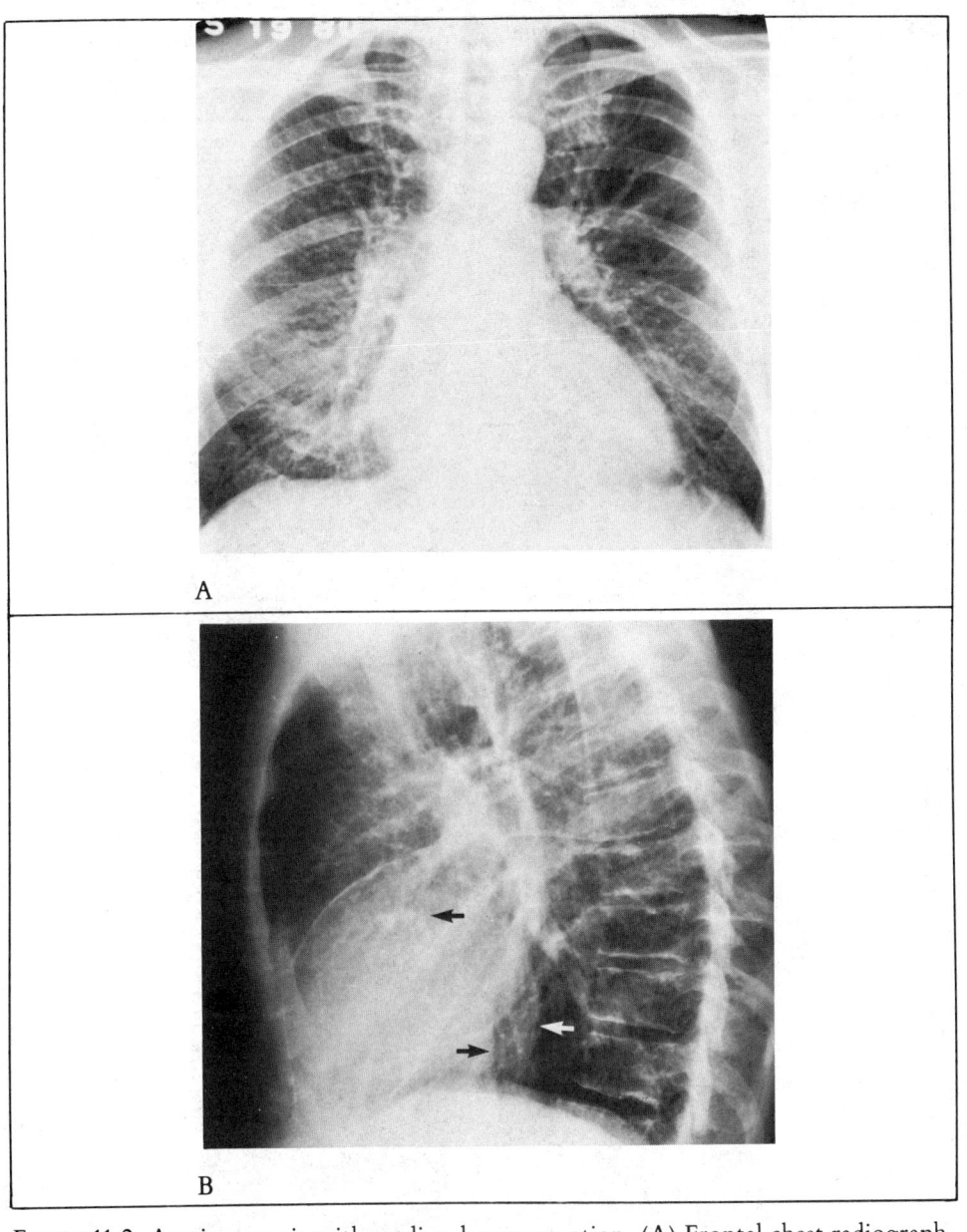

FIGURE 11-2. Aortic stenosis with cardiac decompensation. (A) Frontal chest radiograph. Cardiomegaly is present with prominence of ascending aorta and normal aortic knob. Prominence of upper lobe veins coupled with loss of hilar angle, haziness of both hila, diffuse interstitial pattern, and suggestion of alveolar edema indicate congestive heart failure. (B) Lateral chest radiograph. Left ventricular enlargement is suggested by the extension of the left ventricle (*white arrow*) behind the inferior vena cava (*lower black arrow*). Right ventricular enlargement cannot be completely ruled out because retrosternal space is not clearly seen. Aortic valve calcification is clearly visualized (*upper black arrow*). The chest radiograph provides the most specific information when only one cardiac lesion is present. In this example, cardiac catheterization and coronary angiography indicated that cardiac decompensation was probably caused by a combination of aortic stenosis and coronary artery disease. The chest radiograph can frequently identify early congestive heart failure prior to clear-cut clinical signs and symptoms.

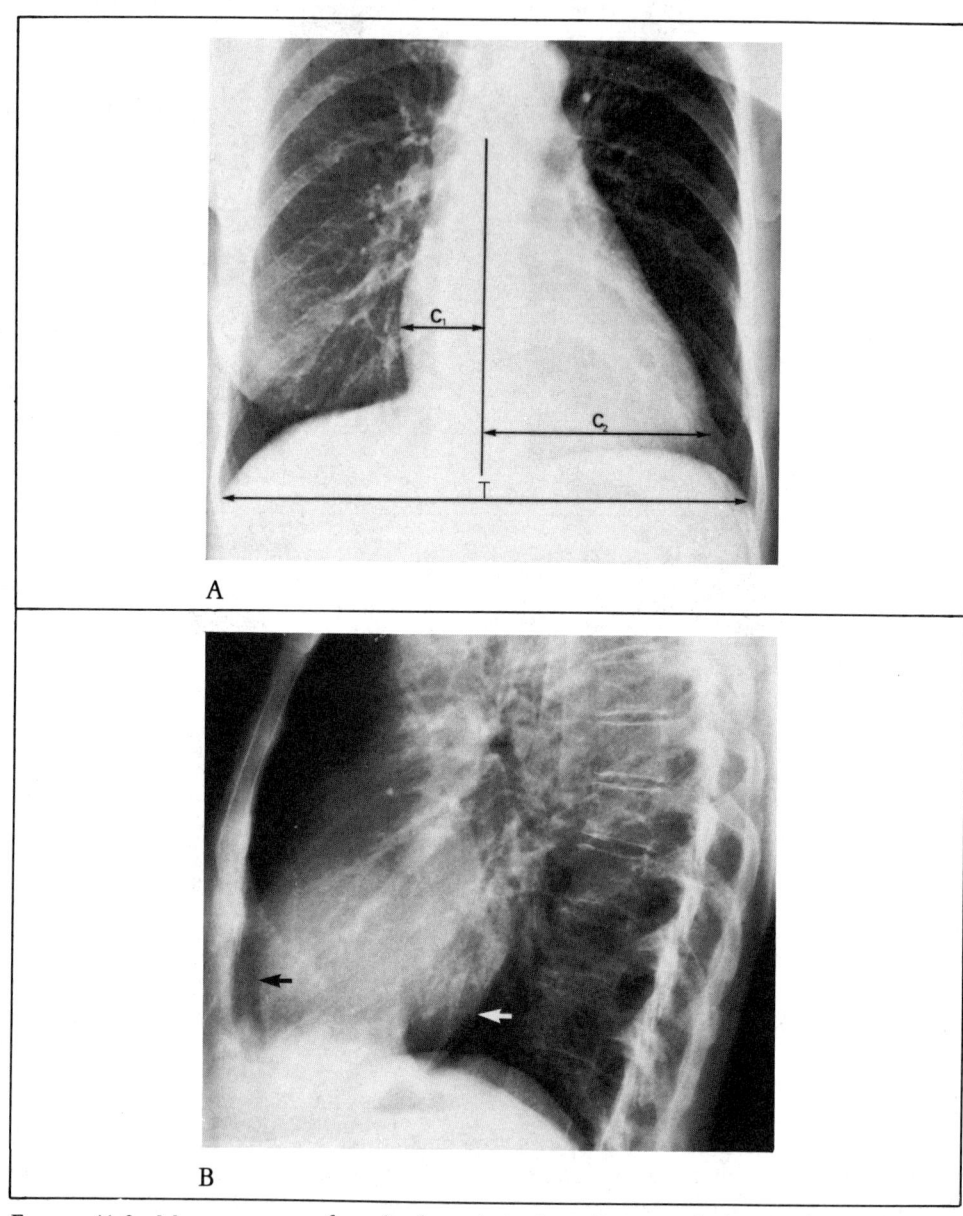

FIGURE 11-3. Measurement of cardiothoracic ratio. (A) Frontal chest radiograph. The cardiothoracic ratio is established using $C_1 + C_2/T$. In this patient with aortic insufficiency the ratio was 59 percent. The values used to determine cardiomegaly vary from 50 to 60 percent depending on the author (see text). (B) Lateral chest radiograph. The left ventricle (*white arrow*) extends well beyond the inferior vena cava, indicating left ventricular enlargement. The pericardial fat pad is well seen (*black arrow*) in the normal position just posterior to the retrosternal clear space.

can be enhanced using a correction factor for height and weight [8]. The generally accepted value for the normal cardiothoracic ratio is 50 percent, but Glover and colleagues suggest use of 60 percent for the normal value in order to reduce the false-positive rates [9], whereas Newell et al use a 55 percent cutoff point [4].

A more precise but also more complex estimate of cardiac size is derived from cardiac volume [10] (Fig. 11-4). This measurement is established by determining the long axis of the heart (L) in the frontal view, an axis that extends to the apex from the junction of the superior vena cava and the right atrium. The short axis, S, which is perpendicular to L, is measured from the right cardiophrenic angle to the junction of the left atrium and pulmonary arteries on the upper left heart border. The third dimension, D, is obtained from the lateral chest roentgenogram and consists of the widest anterior-posterior diameter of the cardiac shadow, extending from the anterior margin of the heart, behind the sternum, to the posterior margin, which is most easily identified as the anterior portion of the barium-filled esophagus. Relative cardiac volume (RCV) is calculated as follows:

$$RCV = \frac{L \times S \times D \times K}{BSA}$$

K is a correcting factor for the focal-film distance and is 0.42 for the standard six-foot chest x-ray. The number finally obtained must then be indexed to body surface area (BSA), using the DuBois standards. The results are expressed in ml/m^2; the average range for females is 450 to 490 ml/m^2 and 500 to 540 ml/m^2 for males. As might be imagined from the complexity of the calculations, cardiac volume is not routinely used in most institutions, although it is the most accurate measurement of overall heart size. The cardiothoracic ratio is more commonly employed in ordinary practice, and its results hold up well in comparison to those derived from cardiac volume. Both techniques are reproducible, although they are susceptible to technical errors. The radiographic technique must be standardized, as it is impossible to rely upon comparisons between upright and supine chest films or between different phases of respiration.

Cardiac size measurements are optimally used in conjunction with estimates of pulmonary vascular changes and of other factors, such as abnormal calcifications. Cardiac size alone, however, provides considerable information concerning left ventricular function and serves as a prognostic indicator in many cardiac diseases regardless of how it is derived [11]. The question can be asked as to what we are really measuring in our estimates of cardiac size or volume. In patients with aortic valve disease, Chikos et al showed good correlation between total heart volume and the sum of angiographically determined left ventricular end-diastolic volumes, mass, and wall thickness [12]. Glover et al studied 254 adult patients

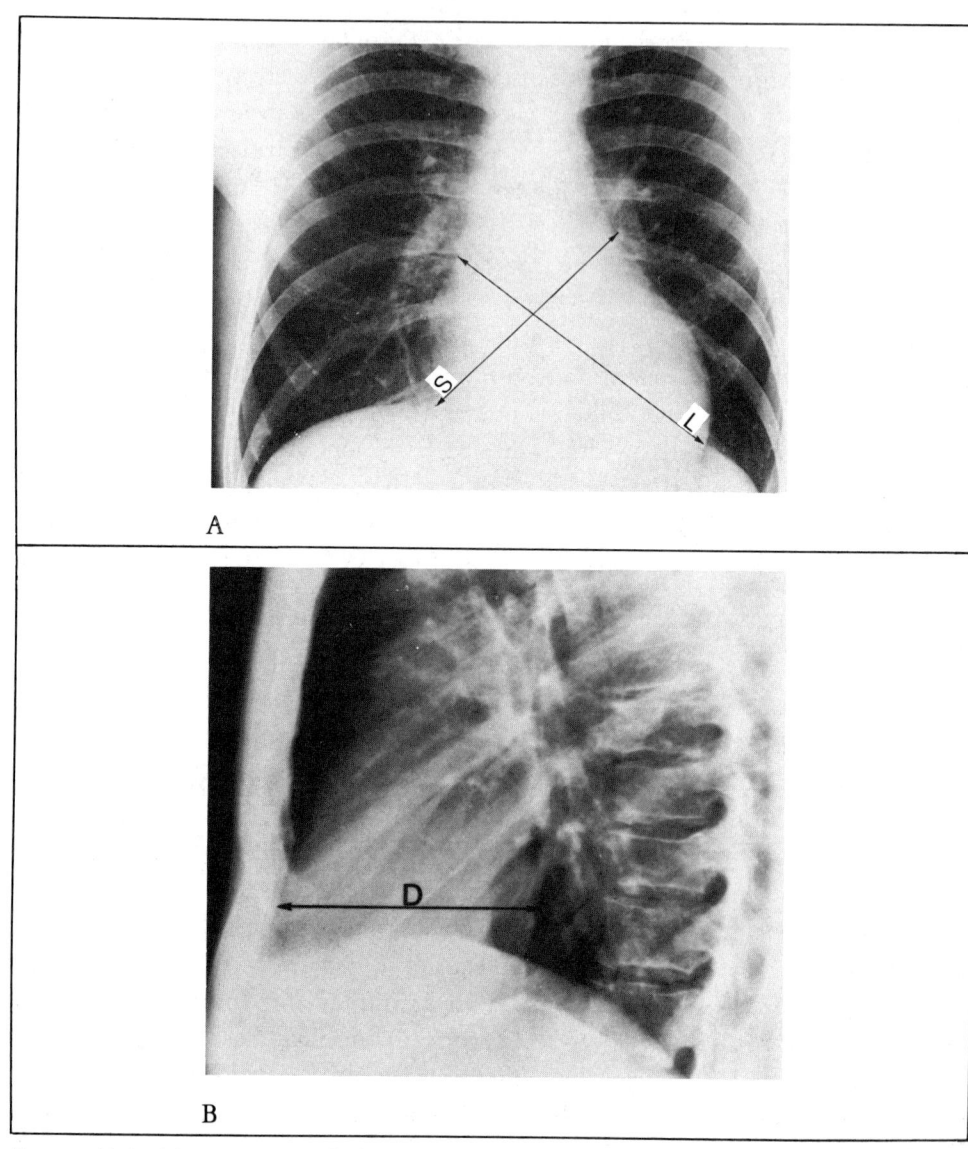

FIGURE 11-4. Measurement of cardiac volume. (A) Frontal chest radiograph. Relative cardiac volume is calculated from the formula L × S × D × K/BSA (see text). The values of L and S are measured from the frontal chest as marked. K is a constant that equals 0.42 for routine 6-foot chest films. BSA is the body surface area obtained from the DuBois Standards. D is obtained from the lateral film. (B) Lateral chest radiograph. D is obtained from the lateral chest radiograph as indicated. Left ventricular enlargement is indicated by the posterior extension of the left ventricle behind the inferior vena cava in this patient with aortic insufficiency.

with a variety of heart diseases and correlated heart volume on plain film with the sum of left ventricular volume, diastolic volume, mass, and left atrial volume [9]. When heart volume based on cardiothoracic ratio was compared to quantitative estimates based on angiography alone, the correlations were significant but scattered. Correlation increased as other left heart components — such as volume, mass, and left atrial volume — were added to the assessment; it was accurate in 79 percent of patients when heart volume was compared to the left heart mass, and in 70 percent of patients when a simple cardiothoracic ratio was compared to left heart mass. Factors that are uncontrolled in this type of assessment include the upright position for the x-ray and the supine position for the angiographic measurement. In addition, enlargement of the right heart cannot be calculated accurately. However, accuracy can be improved at the time of film interpretation if the limitations of the method are taken into consideration. The value of cardiac size measurements is greatest when serial films are available and when clinical information can contribute to the final analysis.

For detection of cardiac abnormalities, radiographic measurements of cardiac size provide information comparable to that of other modalities, such as the electrocardiogram (ECG). Glover et al noted heart volume calculations to have been 70 percent accurate and cardiothoracic ratios 67 percent accurate in assessing cardiac enlargement in a group of patients with angiography-proven left heart enlargement. This compares to a study by Baxley et al, who were able to identify two-thirds of patients with angiography-proven increases in left ventricular mass by standard ECG criteria of left ventricular hypertrophy [13].

The usefulness of the cardiothoracic ratio as a measure of heart volume on plain film was assessed by Hammermeister and coworkers, who found that these measurements were highly sensitive but not specific indicators of abnormal left ventricular end-diastolic volume and ejection fraction [11]. Sensitivity refers to the number of times that each technique detected left ventricular enlargement or reduced ejection fraction when these were present; expressed as a percentage of total cases, this was 88 percent for the cardiothoracic ratio and 86 percent for heart volume on plain film. Specificity refers to the ability to identify normal rather than abnormal patients. In this regard, both the cardiothoracic ratio and heart volume on plain film were less accurate — 41 percent and 51 percent of times, respectively — indicating that the volume of the heart may appear to be increased despite a normal end-diastolic volume or ejection fraction. However, Hammermeister's findings do support the view that abnormal volume results by these methods are an accurate indicator of the presence of a disease process.

The chest radiograph was shown to be a key source of information by Sherman and associates, who used this test as a screening method for a large employee population [8]. Chest radiographs were performed on 22,394 asymptomatic subjects over 40 years of age whose electrocardiograms were normal. Eighty-two employees were found to have cardiac enlargement based on an abnormal cardiothoracic ratio corrected for the patient's height and weight. This evidence of cardiomegaly was considered to be the only indicator of an underlying disease process. Sherman's work gives credence to this technique as an important indicator of disease when other clinical and laboratory factors are normal. It must be noted, parenthetically, that the cost-benefit ratio in this population may not justify the use of the chest x-ray as a survey technique for asymptomatic cardiac disease but clearly indicates its capacity to identify cardiac disease.

Pulmonary Vascularity

The chest radiograph provides a unique view of the pulmonary venous and arterial vascularity. The pulmonary capillary wedge pressure measurement is a very sensitive indicator of a variety of left-sided abnormalities ranging from left ventricular failure — with causes as diverse as cardiomyopathy and myocardial infarction — to mitral valve disease. This physiologic measurement is reflected in the plain chest film by variations in the distribution of the pulmonary venous blood flow and fluid shifts within the lung [3, 14–16]. In patients with a normally compliant left ventricle and without obstruction to the left heart, the frontal upright chest film demonstrates pulmonary veins in the lower lung fields. There is relatively little venous vascularity in the upper lung fields, indicating selective flow to the lower lung field (Figs. 11-3 and 11-4). Equal filling of the upper and lower pulmonary veins is present if the chest radiograph is taken in the supine position, demonstrating that this phenomenon is in part a gravitational effect on pulmonary venous blood flow. The pattern of lower lobe venous prominence is present when the pulmonary capillary wedge pressure is in the normal range of 6 to 15 mm Hg. Elevation of capillary wedge pressure above 18 mm Hg can be roughly correlated with a progressive prominence of the pulmonary venous vascularity and flow to the upper lung fields (Fig. 11-5). In the first stage of pulmonary venous hypertension, there is equalization of vascularity in the upper and lower lung fields; in the second stage the chest film demonstrates relative oligemia of the lower lung fields and plethora of the upper lung fields. As the wedge pressure increases to the range of 20 to 25 mm Hg, interstitial edema is added to the radiographic picture, characterized by a loss of hilar angle, clouding of the overall lung fields, the lo of distinction of the lung markings, and the appearance of interstitial Kerley B lines (see Fig. 11-2). Frank alveolar edema is noted to occur at or above 25 mm Hg. The correlation between radiographic findings and capillary wedge pressure is, as previously noted, a rough correlation and is subject to errors such as in the case of rapid onset of pulmonary edema. In this situation there can be a diagnostic lag of hours before the radiographic appearance is comparable to the elevated wedge pressure as outlined. Alternatively, a therapeutic lag can last up to days after the capillary wedge pressure has returned to normal with treatment (Fig. 11-6). The residual interstitial and pleural fluid is evidence of the therapeutic lag in an assessment of the frontal and lateral chest x-ray. In this situation the value of serial films cannot be overstated. Serial films allow for identification of physiologic and pathophysiologic changes that may not be discernible on a single film.

Pulmonary vascular changes associated with mitral stenosis or left ventricular failure initially affect the pulmonary *venous* bed. However, long-standing left-sided disease processes will lead to precapillary pulmonary *arterial* hypertension as opposed to pulmonary venous hypertension. Precapillary pulmonary hypertension is a primary process in pulmonary embolization or in the pathophysiologic changes associated with Eisenmenger's syndrome. In the early stages of precapillary pulmonary hypertension, the chest radiograph will usually be normal or will reflect changes of the inducing process such as the pulmonary parenchymal changes of pulmonary infarction. If the pulmonary pressure remains elevated over a period of time, chest radiography demonstrates enlargement of the main pulmonary artery segment with pruning of distal vessels and an increased radiolucency of the peripheral lung fields (Fig. 11-7). These findings are reliable indicators of pulmonary arterial hypertension. Increased pulmonary arterial flow from a left-to-right shunt and poststenotic dilatation of the pulmonary artery will enlarge the main pulmonary artery but will not result in pruning of the pulmonary arterial tree.

FLUOROSCOPY OF THE HEART

Fluoroscopy of the heart and chest was the earliest application of roentgen diagnosis of cardiac disease. It was considered an integral part of the cardiac evaluation, especially in patients with congenital and valvular heart disease. The utilization of this technique was reduced considerably with the introduction of cardiac catheterization. Many believed that any useful data derived from fluoroscopy could either be obtained by the more sophisticated hemodynamic and angiographic examination or could be gained at the time of catheterization without the necessity of separate radiation exposures. Consequently, when fluoroscopy of the heart is performed in conjunction with cardiac catheterization, the fluoroscopic examination of the heart is frequently accomplished in a very superficial manner or totally overlooked for the angiographic and hemodynamic findings. However, a cursory fluoroscopic examination of the heart can result in the loss of important diagnostic and prognostic information that is available with an adequate study. Margolis and associates, after assessing 800 patients at cardiac fluoroscopy or at the time of cardiac catheterization, found 250 patients with coronary artery calci-

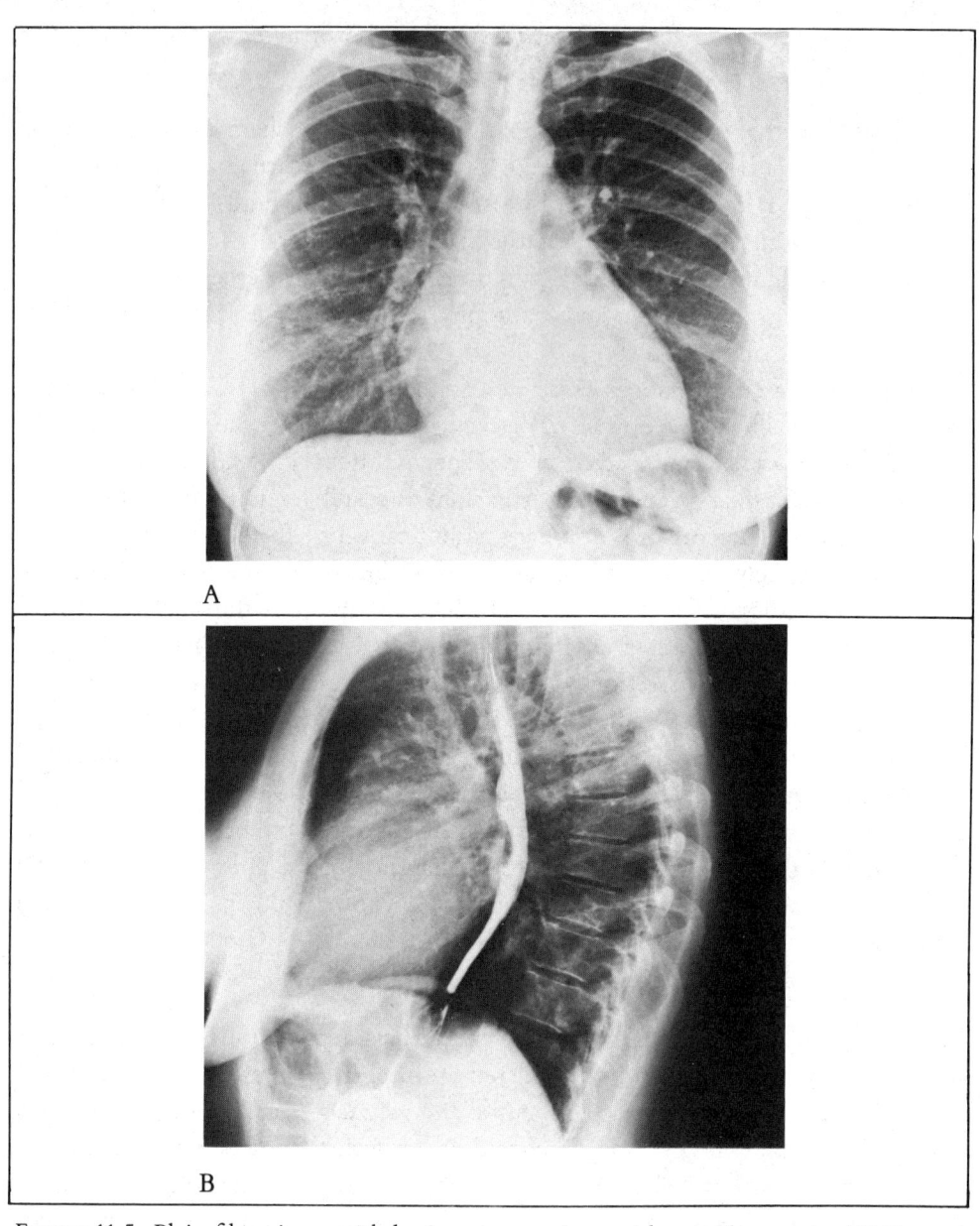

FIGURE 11-5. Plain film views with barium in a patient with mitral stenosis. (A) Frontal chest radiograph. The cardiothoracic ratio is 54 percent, which is borderline for cardiomegaly. The double density of the enlarged left atrium is present as is slight prominence of the left atrial appendage. There is prominence of the upper lobe pulmonary venous vascularity indicating pulmonary venous hypertension. (B) Lateral chest film. There is posterior deviation of the barium-filled esophagus by the enlarged left atrium. The left and right ventricles are normal in size. (C) Right anterior oblique film. Minimal devia-

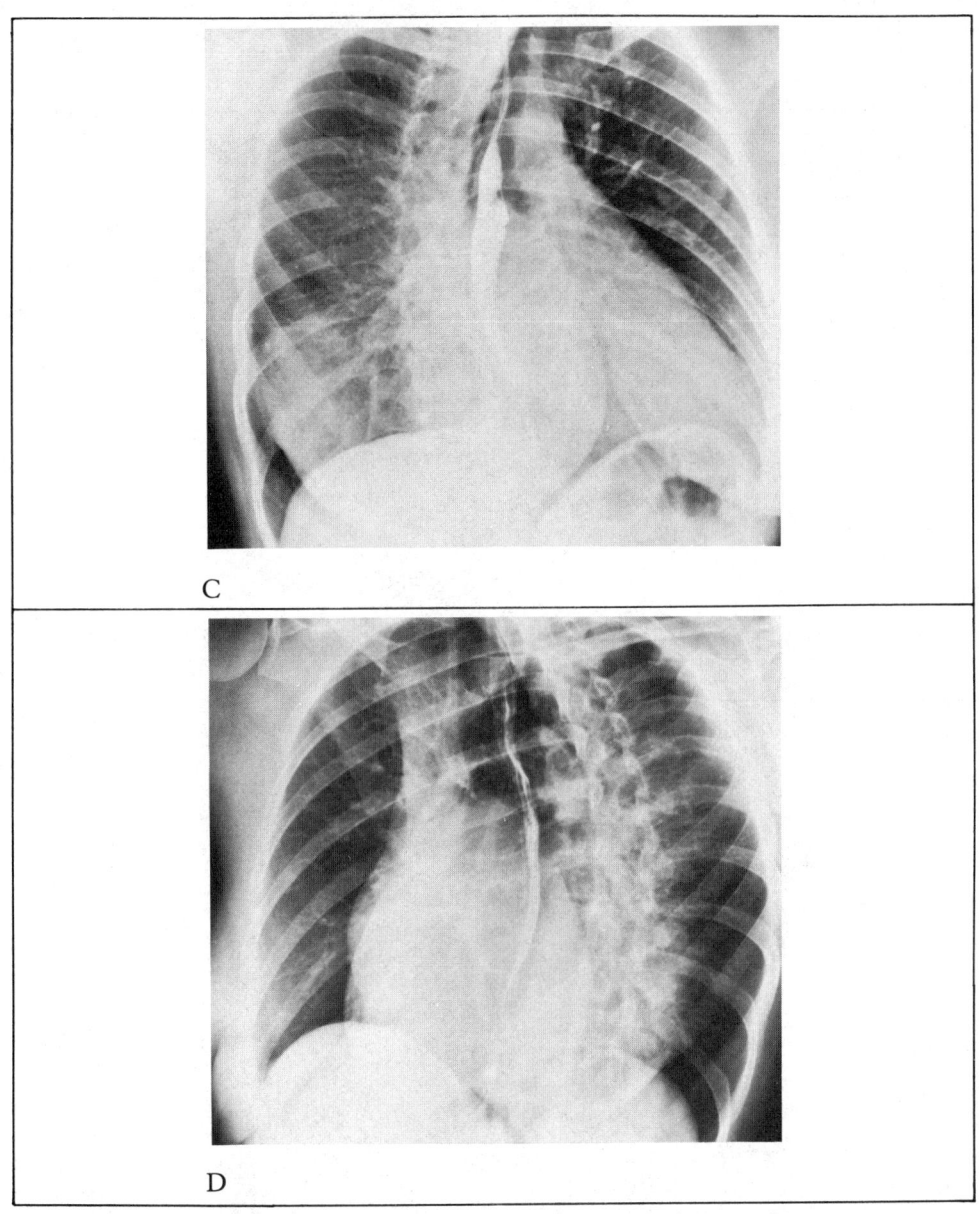

tion of the barium column is caused by the enlarged left atrium. This is the least helpful of the four views. (D) Left anterior oblique film. The normal clear space between the left atrium and left mainstem bronchus is lost with mild elevation of the left mainstem bronchus. The left ventricle is normal. There is minimal prominence of the right atrium, but overall the right side of the heart is normal. There is no calcification of the mitral valve. The findings are consistent with mild to moderate mitral stenosis. The pulmonary capillary wedge pressure was 23 mm Hg.

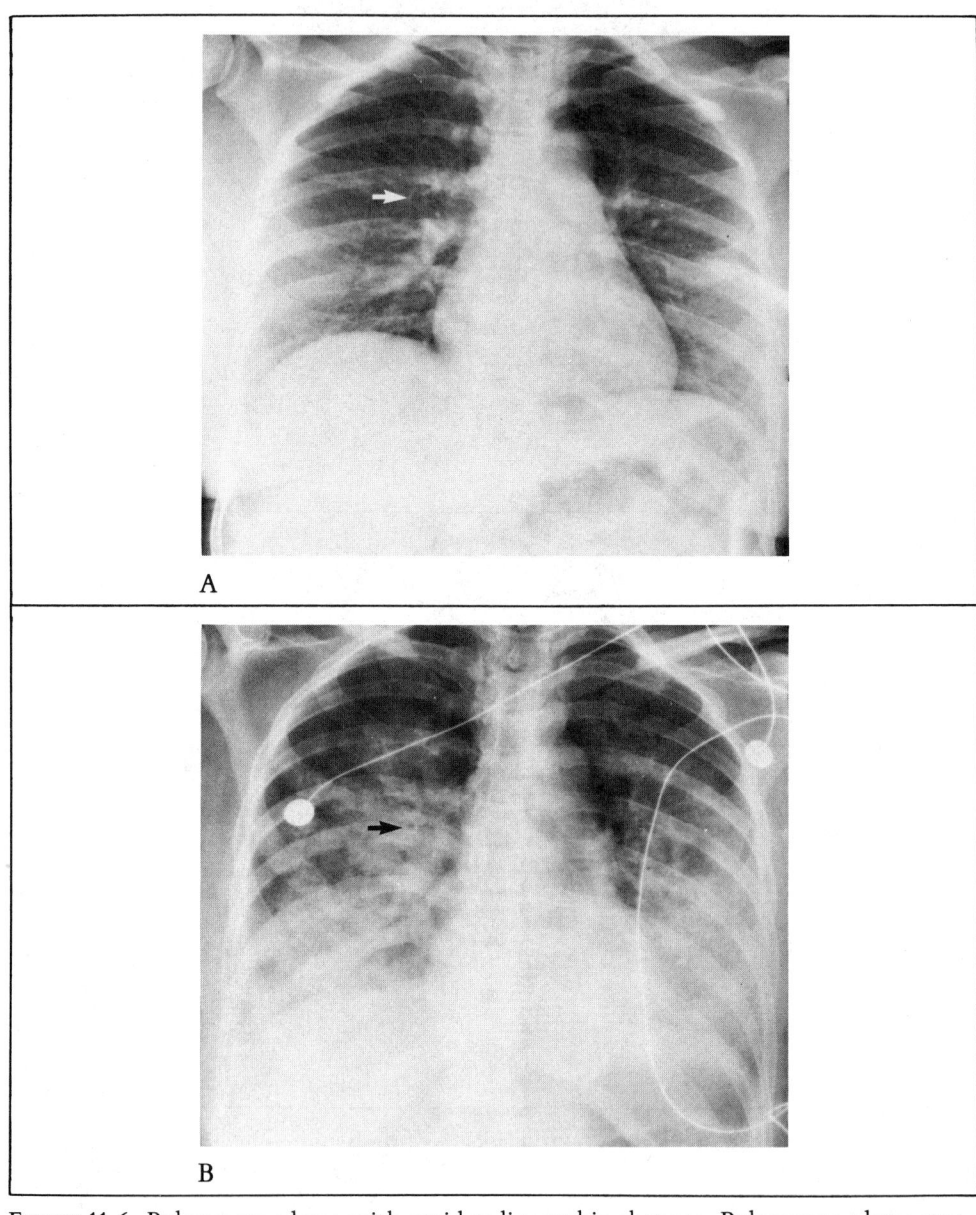

FIGURE 11-6. Pulmonary edema with rapid radiographic changes. Pulmonary edema was induced by fluid overload in this otherwise healthy young woman with ectopic pregnancy. (A) Supine preoperative chest radiograph demonstrates normal heart size and no evidence of pulmonary edema. A bronchus on end (*arrow*) shows normal wall thickness. (B) Supine chest radiograph performed 1-1/2 hours later, just after surgery, shows frank alveolar edema without significant change in heart size. Peribronchial cuffing is clearly illustrated (*arrow*). (C) Supine chest radiograph performed 6 hours after (B). Clinical signs of pulmonary edema had subsided but not cleared. Some clearing of edema is evident radio-

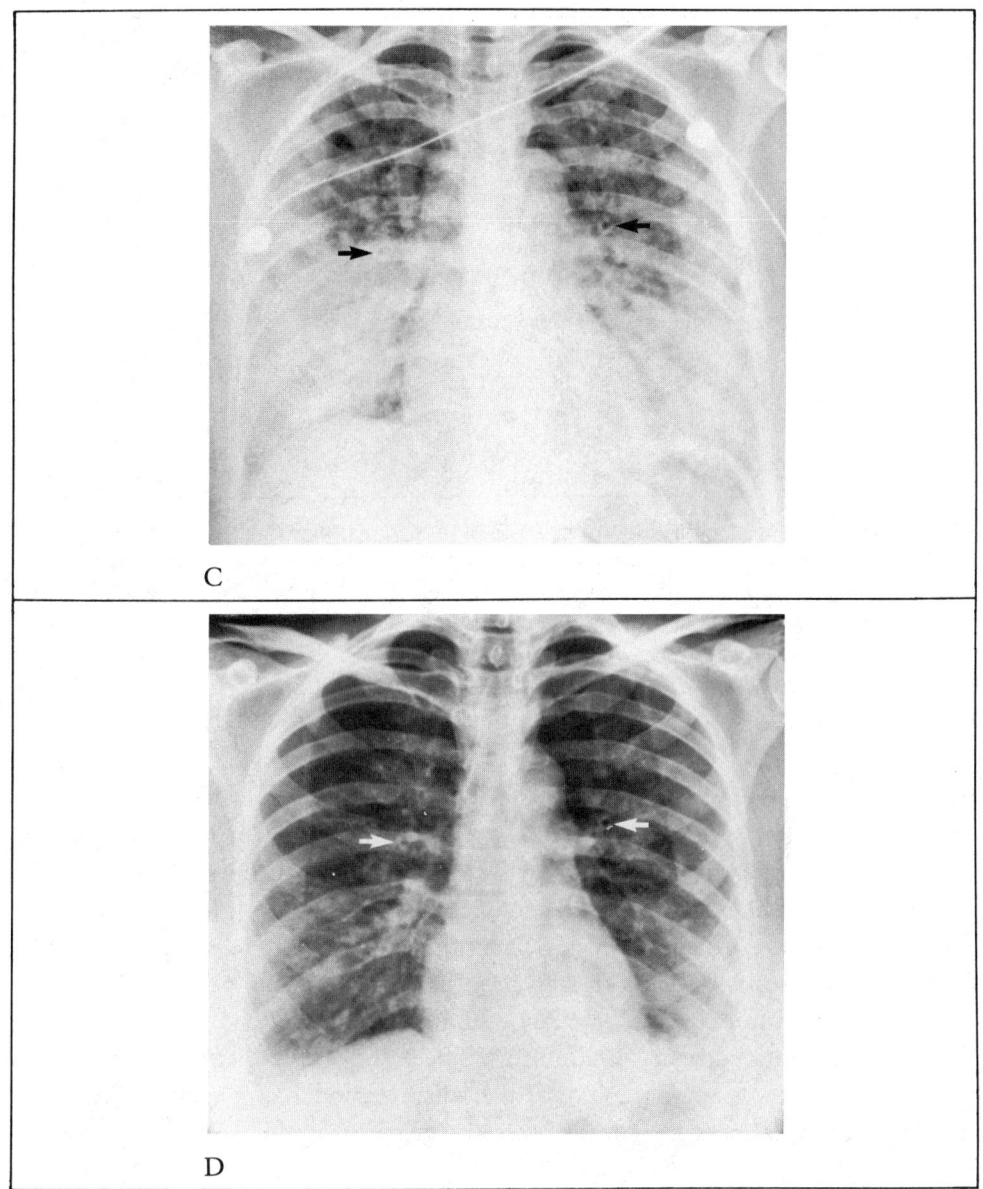

graphically but peribronchial edema remains (*arrows*). (D) Upright frontal chest radiograph 24 hours after (C). There is complete clearing of alveolar edema, but bilateral pleural effusions persist. Peribronchial cuffing is reduced but not to normal dimensions (*arrows*). Cardiac size remains normal. This case illustrates minimal lag in the radiographic detection of onset of pulmonary edema. A therapeutic lag of hours is noted in the clearing of edema. Serial chest films are very useful in following pathophysiologic changes of both pulmonary and cardiac origin.

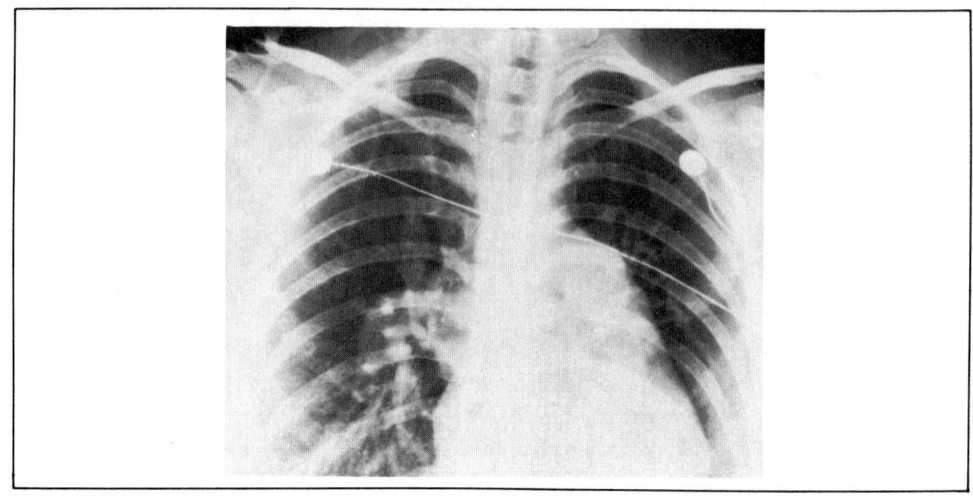

FIGURE 11-7. Pulmonary hypertension in a patient with atrial septal defect. Frontal chest radiograph shows a greatly enlarged main pulmonary artery segment with corresponding enlargement of right pulmonary artery. The left pulmonary artery is obscured by the main pulmonary artery. The most important finding is the lack of peripheral pulmonary vessels in contrast to large proximal arteries. The result is the "pruned tree" effect with increased radiolucency of the peripheral lung fields. The shunt at the atrial level was converted to a right-to-left shunt by the pulmonary hypertension.

fication [17]. Of that group 236 (94 percent) had angiographic evidence of significant coronary artery obstruction equal to or greater than 75 percent of one or more coronary arteries. By reversing the equation, the authors found that 236 patients (40 percent) from a group of 585 patients with significant coronary artery disease had coronary artery calcification. In follow-up of the patients with and without coronary calcification (6 months to 5 years), 87 percent of patients without calcification survived 5 years, while 58 percent survival was noted in those patients with coronary calcification. The authors note that the survival data are independent of angiographic and cardiac hemodynamic data. The false-negative rate of 60 percent reduces the value of the study for identifying patients in a screening situation.

A study by Langou and coworkers evaluating the predictive accuracy of coronary artery calcification detected by fluoroscopy (coupled with an abnormal exercise test) for coronary artery disease detection in asymptomatic males indicates its possible value as a screening test [18]. They found 13 males in a population of 129 subjects who had coronary calcification and a positive exercise test. These 13 patients went on to coronary angiography, which revealed greater than 50 percent stenosis in one or more coronary arteries in 12 of 13 patients and coronary arteriosclerosis of some degree in all 13. Follow-up evaluation of the 129 patients to determine the presence or absence of angina pectoris was carried out over 36 months. Three patients (23 percent) of those with positive exercise test and coronary calcification developed angina pectoris. Of 24 patients with coronary artery calcification and normal stress test, one (4 percent) developed angina, and one (1.5 percent) of the remaining patients developed angina pectoris. Thus the combination of fluoroscopic identification of calcification and stress testing seems to have reduced the false-positive rate. Coronary angiography would have to be performed on all the normal subjects in Langou's series in order to compare these findings to those of Margolis et al, but further clinical evaluation seems justified.

Cardiac fluoroscopy coupled with cineradiography has proven to be of great value in assessing function of prosthetic heart valves. Bream and Elliott assessed disk opening and valve tilt in Bjork-Shiley valves; they found that those valves tilt up to 9 degrees in the immediate and postoperative period both in the mitral and aortic position [19]. The authors demonstrated that serial evaluation of these prosthetic valves can predict changes in valve tilt, which could be used to identify abnormal valve function prior to gross failure of the valve. The authors recommend baseline studies after valve placement in order to evaluate future deleterious changes.

Four Views of the Heart with Barium

Four views of the heart — with barium in the esophagus — is a long established supplement to the standard frontal and lateral chest film. In the past this procedure was routinely performed in conjunction with fluoroscopy of the heart, but in present practice the study functions as a separate examination. The examination consists of the standard frontal and lateral chest films coupled with a right anterior oblique (RAO) and a left anterior oblique (LAO) projection (see Fig. 11-5). The RAO projection provides better visualization of the outflow tract of the right ventricle and is very important fluoroscopically because it allows the best views of the mitral valve; however, because this is the least productive view in plain films of the heart, RAO projections are not widely utilized. On the other hand, the left anterior oblique view offers optimum visualization of the left atrium and its relationship to the left mainstem bronchus and the esophagus. This view also offers good visualization of the right side of the heart, which at times allows separation of the right atrium from the ventricle and provides a reliable indication of enlargement of the right heart. Visualization of aortic valve calcification is excellent in this projection. The posterior and lateral aspects of the left ventricle are also clearly seen, and criteria for left ventricular enlargement that relates the extension of the left ventricle to the left of the spine in the LAO projection have been defined. Unfortunately, small changes in angulation can result in extension of the ventricle beyond the spine in normal subjects. As a result, this criterion for left ventricular enlargement is considered unreliable. The oblique positioning does allow for a second view of possible valvular calcification not afforded by the frontal view. In general, four views of the heart may be helpful in the evaluation of patients with valvular disease or in those suspected of adult congenital heart lesions but should not be used routinely in other cardiac abnormalities.

Portable Chest Radiographs

Sometimes overlooked in any assessment of noninvasive radiographic evaluation of the heart is the portable supine chest x-ray. This method is limited by a number of technical factors, including the usually severe illness of the patient in the postoperative and intensive care situation, which frequently precludes optimum positioning. The use of portable x-ray equipment also has inherent limitations for optimum technical factors. These limitations in a sense define the usefulness of the method: on serial examinations easily identifiable changes such as heart size and the status of the pulmonary vascular bed can be used as major indicators of disease or of a changing physiologic status. As in standard x-ray examinations, attention to the technical details of the examination are important. For instance, knowledge of the patient's exact position at the time of examination is critical to accurate interpretation, since the upright position, although preferable, is not always obtainable. In addition, radiographic factors must be consistent at each examination for comparisons to be meaningful.

In those patients who do not require continuous pulmonary capillary wedge pressure measurements, the daily chest x-ray or portable chest x-ray can give indirect but accurate assessment of capillary wedge pressure. This assessment is based on changes in cardiac size as well as changes in the pulmonary venous vascular bed and pulmonary parenchyma. These changes are frequently seen prior to the clinical evidence afforded by auscultation. Portable chest films are also ideally suited for the postoperative cardiac or thoracic surgical patient where both postsurgical complications and rapidly changing physiologic states can be monitored by frequent radiographic examination. Some limitations of the radiographic method include the relative lag period of some hours from the onset of ventricular failure to the presence of fluid or an interstitial parenchymal pattern. This same lag in a reverse fashion can be seen after therapeutic intervention, where ventricular function as measured by capillary wedge pressure returns to normal but residual fluid within the pleural space or interstitial lung tissue takes some time to be totally resolved. In the post-therapeutic stages this can be measured sometimes in days. Figure 11-6 illustrates rapid changes in fluid accumulation with clearing and reaccumulation, indicating that a period of days is not always necessary for radiographic identification of change.

Radiographic Examination of Specific Disease Processes

CORONARY ARTERY DISEASE

In the majority of patients with ischemic coronary artery disease, the chest x-ray is normal. In patients with angina alone, 7 to 21 percent show cardiomegaly [20]. Even with extensive myocardial ischemia or fibrous scarring, the myocardial reserve is often sufficient for normal cardiac compensation. However, in patients with acute myocardial infarction, 50 percent will have abnormal chest x-rays [20]. In these patients, roentgenographic abnormalities usually include an increase in cardiac size and/or evidence of pulmonary venous hypertension. One-third to one-half of patients with radiographic abnormalities will demonstrate some degree of pulmonary venous hypertension within 24 hours of the acute event [21]. This change may occur without evidence of obvious cardiomegaly and probably reflects the rapid decrease in left ventricular compliance of the ischemic left ventricle. Roentgenographic abnormalities appearing within 24 hours of acute myocardial infarction provide prognostic as well as physiologic information. Battler and associates reported mortality in excess of 80 percent in 30 days and 100 percent in one year in patients with generalized alveolar edema in contrast to less than 10 percent mortality in patients with normal chest x-rays and 30 percent mortality in patients with any lesser signs of pulmonary venous hypertension, such as shift of flow to the upper lobes [21]. Persistence of cardiomegaly after the acute phase of the infarction is indicative of a combined early and late mortality of 50 percent as compared to a 25 percent mortality for patients whose cardiomegaly returns to normal after the acute phase [21].

The chest radiograph may be very useful in evaluation of the complications of myocardial infarction. True aneurysms of the left ventricle can be heralded by abnormal configurations in the cardiac contour (Fig. 11-8). The usual location of such aneurysms is the apex and anterolateral portions of the left ventricle. These aneurysms can result in localized bulgings at the lower left heart border in the frontal projection or anteriorly in the lateral projection. Small aneurysms will not be visualized routinely. False aneurysms usually extend posteriorly and can be seen as retrocardiac masses. These aneurysms can at times be calcified, which facilitates diagnosis. False aneurysms with or without impending rupture tend to be larger in size as compared to true aneurysms, which are usually more localized. Ventricular septal rupture usually occurs in the muscular portion of the septum and reveals dramatic evidence of a left-to-right shunt associated with signs of severe pulmonary venous congestion and pulmonary edema. Rupture of a papillary muscle is marked by the rapid onset of pulmonary edema without change in cardiac size.

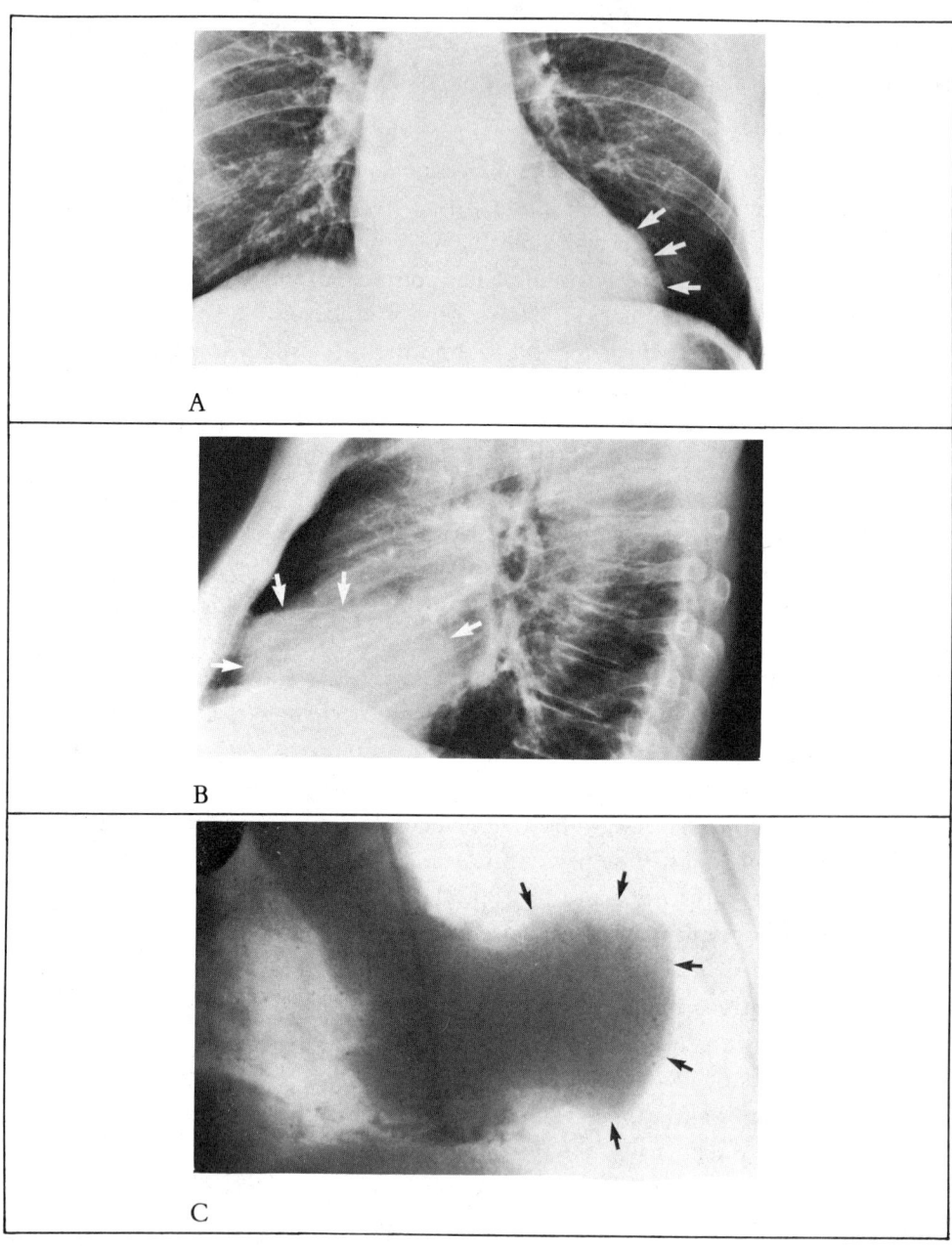

FIGURE 11-8. Left ventricular aneurysm. (A) Frontal chest radiograph shows slight bulging along the lower left heart border (*arrows*). (B) Lateral chest radiograph demonstrates the full extent of the left ventricular aneurysm above the diaphragm (*arrows*). The extension of the lower aspect of the aneurysm is obscured by the diaphragm. (C) Single frame from a cine left ventriculogram performed in the RAO projection shows a smooth-walled, well circumscribed aneurysm (*arrows*) of the apex of the left ventricle with extension to anterior and inferior walls of the left ventricle.

Cardiogenic shock can also present as pulmonary edema. Cascade and coworkers used the chest roentgenogram in the evaluation of patients in cardiogenic shock and concluded that (1) the roentgenographic estimate of hemodynamic factors was less reliable when patients were in cardiogenic shock, and (2) that those patients in whom the radiographic evidence of cardiac decompensation showed rapid clearing within 24 hours of heart failure had a significantly higher rate of survival than those without clearing or in whom the radiographic evidence of failure worsened [22].

Valvular Heart Disease

Mitral Valve Disease

The pathophysiology of mitral stenosis reflects obstruction at the mitral valve level, with anatomic and physiologic changes that are radiographically well documented. In the early stages of mitral stenosis, pulmonary congestion is not a factor, and enlargement of the left atrium is the first radiologic finding. Left atrial enlargement is identified in the frontal chest x-ray by the double density of the left atrium as it expands posteriorly, and straightening or bulging out of the left heart border by the enlarging left atrial appendage (see Fig. 11-5). If barium is used to outline the esophagus, this organ is seen to be deflected posteriorly. Late findings include elevation of the left mainstem bronchus as the left atrium continues to enlarge. Massive enlargements of the left atrium are generally associated with regurgitation as opposed to stenosis, but this does not hold in all cases. Calcification within the mitral valve is not as common as in aortic stenosis, but the amount of calcification within the valve is related to the degree of stenosis [23]. Calcification within the mitral annulus, as opposed to the valve leaflets, is considered a reflection of the aging process and does not routinely produce detectable pathologic changes. Annular calcification has a typical C- or J-shaped configuration as opposed to the smaller, more irregular-shaped calcifications of the mitral valve leaflets. Identification of mitral valve calcification in mitral stenosis is an important consideration for surgical therapy. The presence of calcification precludes commissurotomy and dictates valve replacement. In isolated mitral stenosis without heart failure, the overall heart size is normal. In contrast, mitral regurgitation, as an isolated lesion or in conjunction with stenosis, is identifiable by dilatation of the left ventricle as a result of the volume overload (Fig. 11-9).

Physiologic consequences of mitral stenosis on the pulmonary circulation, and ultimately on the right side of the heart, are well demonstrated roentgenographically (see Fig. 11-5). Mitral stenosis was the model in the correlation of radiographic changes of pulmonary venous hypertension and pulmonary capillary wedge pressure measurements [3]. Because the pathophysiologic changes in mitral stenosis are slow and persistent, they allow for good correlation between

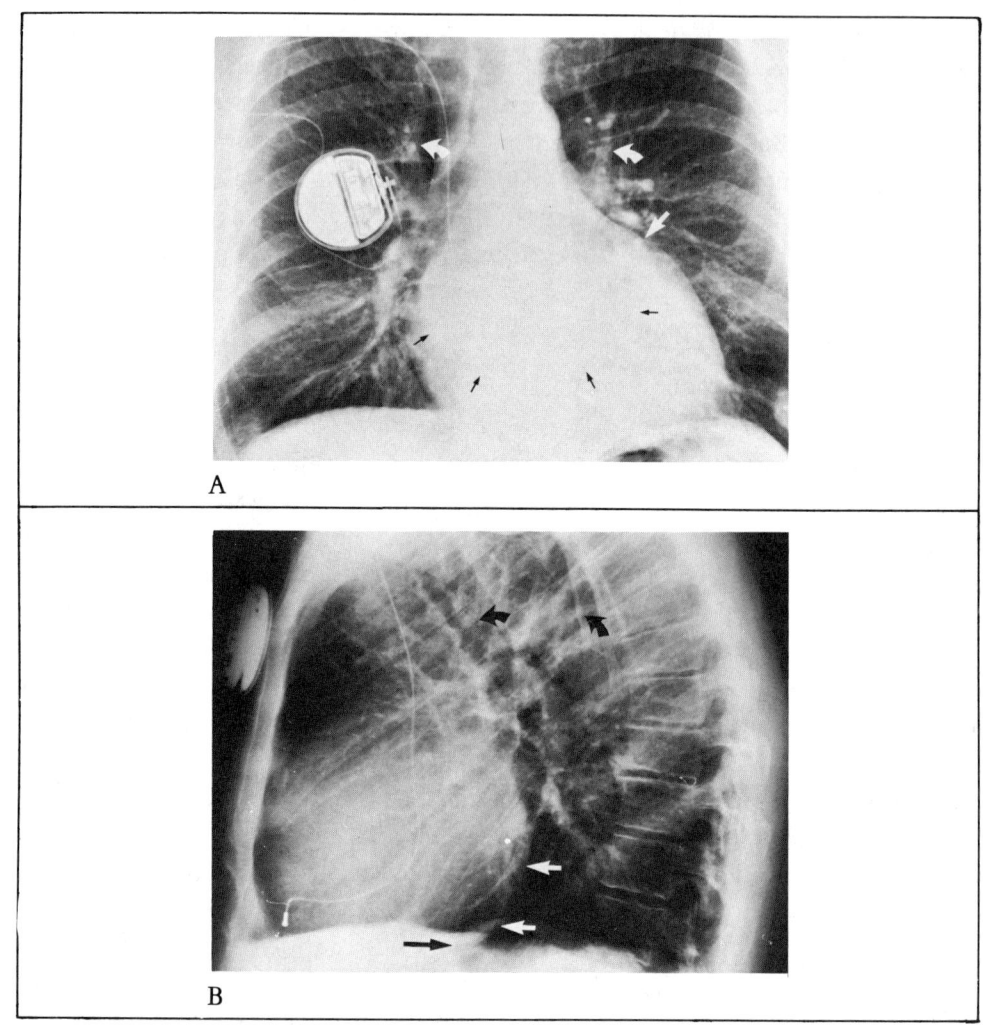

FIGURE 11-9. Combined mitral stenosis and regurgitation. (A) Frontal chest radiograph. Cardiomegaly is present. The double density of the enlarged left atrium (*black arrows*) is well demonstrated. The enlarged left atrial appendage (*straight white arrow*) is somewhat obscured by the expansion and rounding off of the left heart border caused by the left ventricular dilatation in response to mitral regurgitation. The upper lobe veins are very prominent (*curved white arrows*), while the normal lower lobe vessels are not seen, all in response to pulmonary venous hypertension. The pacemaker was necessary because of arrhythmias induced by the enlarged left atrium. (B) Lateral chest radiograph. The enlarged left ventricle (*white arrows*) extends far posterior to the inferior vena cava (*straight black arrow*). Note that the retrosternal clear space is preserved, suggesting that the right ventricle is not enlarged. The upper lobe venous vascularity is also well seen in this view (*curved arrows*). The presence of mitral regurgitation as the predominant lesion is suggested by the left ventricular dilatation. Of all valvular lesions, mitral valve disease is the easiest to diagnose radiographically.

the capillary wedge pressure measurement and the radiographic changes in the lung and pulmonary vascularity. (As noted earlier in the chapter, the accuracy of the radiographic method for wedge pressure estimates is diminished by rapidly changing hemodynamic factors.) The earliest radiographic changes are the shift of pulmonary venous flow to the upper lung fields, which results in equalization of the venous pattern in the upper and lower lung fields, followed by a diminution of the caliber of veins in the lower lung fields and a preponderance of flow in the upper lung fields. When the pulmonary capillary wedge pressure rises into the 20 to 25 mm Hg range, interstitial edema is noted; above 25 mm Hg, frank pulmonary edema is present. Prolonged elevation of pressure in the pulmonary bed leads to increased pulmonary artery pressure. Right heart involvement is indicated by right ventricular enlargement and finally right heart failure. The latter is manifested by right atrial enlargement and appearance of the azygos vein in conjunction with peripheral edema. Tricuspid regurgitation will cause similar enlargement of the right heart chambers (Fig. 11-10).

Aortic Valve Disease
Aortic valve disease presents less clear-cut roentgenographic changes than those associated with mitral valve disease. The first radiographic change consists of dilatation of the ascending aorta as a result of poststenotic dilatation. The dilatation may be absent with subaortic stenosis. Valvular calcification is more common in aortic valve stenosis than with mitral stenosis, but there is little correlation with the amount of valve calcification and degree of stenosis. Obstruction at the level of the aortic valve leads to hypertrophy of the left ventricle, but unless failure supervenes there is no clear-cut cardiac enlargement as measured by cardiothoracic ratios or heart volumes. Aortic regurgitation is differentiated from aortic stenosis on the basis of enlargement of the left ventricle due to volume overload as opposed to pressure overload of the left ventricle (see Figs. 11-3 and 11-4). The final stages of aortic valve stenosis and/or regurgitation include left-sided heart failure with cardiomegaly and redistribution of pulmonary flow, pulmonary venous hypertension, interstitial edema, and frank alveolar edema (see Fig. 11-2).

Myocardial Disease
There may be little evidence of roentgenographic abnormality in the early stages of congestive or restrictive cardiomyopathy. Hypertrophic changes are well visualized by echocardiography but generally are not reflected in the overall cardiac size or cardiothoracic ratio. Late manifestations of this process have been well documented with changes in the pulmonary venous bed, indicative of elevations in end-diastolic pressure. These are similar to the changes of mitral valve obstructive disease and progress from evidence of pulmonary venous hypertension to interstitial edema and frank alveolar edema.

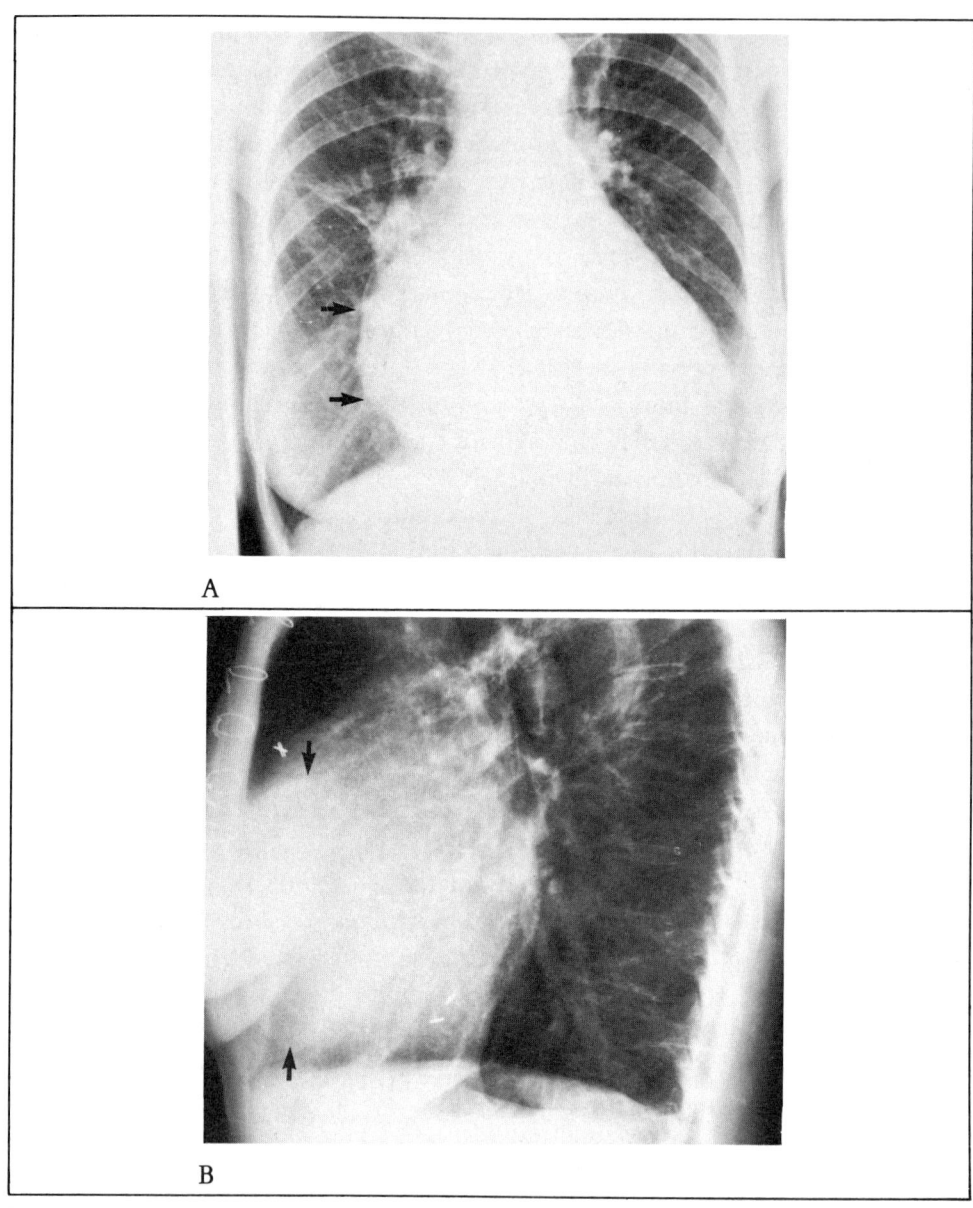

FIGURE 11-10. Tricuspid regurgitation. (A) Frontal chest radiograph reveals massive enlargement of the right heart (*arrows*) with overall cardiomegaly. Pulmonary venous hypertension is reflected in the prominence of upper lobe veins. (B) Lateral chest radiograph. The enlarged right heart is seen anteriorly in this view (*arrows*). Right heart enlargement cannot usually be as easily identified, especially with combined disease.

PERICARDIAL DISEASE

Pericardial disease produces few radiographic changes, yet pericardial calcification associated with constrictive pericarditis can be quite specific. The changes associated with a large pericardial effusion are also striking. The diagnostic value of the chest radiograph in acute uncomplicated pericarditis is limited, although it is useful for the evaluation and particularly the follow-up of patients with pericardial effusion in excess of 250 ml. Echocardiography is a more precise and reliable indicator of effusions and can identify even very small amounts of pericardial effusion. Despite the echocardiographic diagnosis of effusion, the plain chest film is often obtained prior to echocardiography and can represent an early warning for the possible presence of pericardial effusion.

Pericardial effusion presents on plain film as a generalized enlargement of the heart and a smoothing out of normal cardiac contours, which results in a "water-bottle" configuration. While this configuration alone cannot always be used to distinguish pericardial effusion from cardiac enlargement of any origin, an evaluation of the pulmonary vascularity will provide the added diagnostic clues. With pericardial effusion, the pericardium expands in all directions. The superior expansion of the pericardium tends to partially obscure the pulmonary arteries, whereas in congestive heart failure the pulmonary vasculature is enlarged and well seen, although there may be some haziness in the hilum due to fluid accumulations (Fig. 11-11). A second sign, best seen at fluoroscopy but also present on some 40 percent of lateral chest x-rays, is the epicardial fat pad, located just behind the sternum (see Fig. 11-3). The epicardial and pericardial portions are separated by effusion as pericardial fluid accumulates. This is evident radiographically as the fat pad moves away from the sternum and into the cardiac shadow (Fig. 11-11). While the fat pad sign is reliable when seen, absence of this sign has no clinical significance.

Pericarditis usually has no roentgenographic evidence of its presence, although pericardial calcification is suggestive of constrictive pericarditis usually as a result of tuburculous infection; the absence of calcification does not exclude the process (see Fig. 11-11).

Complementary Role of Chest Radiograph and Cardiac Ultrasound

The introduction of newer methods of study in any field frequently results in a polarization between proponents of the new method versus those of the old method. In reality, newer diagnostic methods infrequently replace older techniques; generally, an accommodation between the techniques is established based on the best attributes of each. Newell and associates use a system for assessing acquired heart disease that is facilitated by the complementary role of M-mode

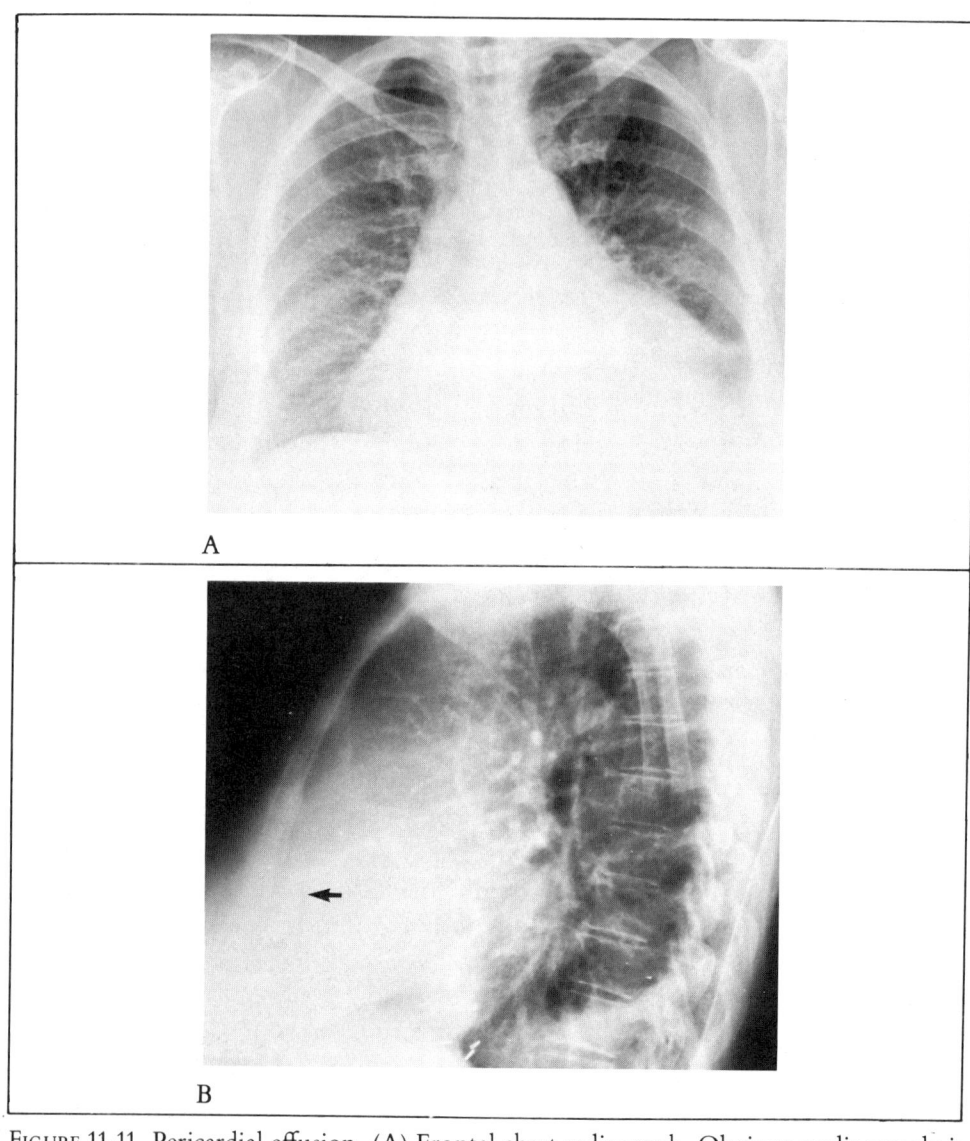

FIGURE 11-11. Pericardial effusion. (A) Frontal chest radiograph. Obvious cardiomegaly is present; in addition, pleural effusion on the left and atelectasis in the left lower lobe obscures the left hemidiaphragm. The overall cardiac shape is smooth, giving a symmetric appearance to the heart that has been termed the "water-bottle" configuration. Also characteristic for pericardial effusion is the overlap of the cardiac outline with the right and left pulmonary arteries, totally obscuring these vessels. The pulmonary vessels seen outside the cardiac outline are somewhat prominent but with normal distribution, usual with pericardial effusion. (B) Lateral chest radiograph. The pericardial fat pad (*arrow*) is seen to be displaced into the cardiac outline and away from the normal retrosternal location (see Fig. 11-3).

TABLE 11-1. Cardiac Lesions and Cardiomegaly

Cardiac lesions associated with normal heart size or mild cardiomegaly (in compensated states)
  Aortic stenosis
  Systemic hypertension
  Mitral stenosis
  Acute myocardial infarction
  Hypertrophic cardiomyopathy
  Restrictive cardiomyopathy
  Constrictive pericarditis
Cardiac lesions associated with moderate or marked cardiomegaly
  Aortic regurgitation
  Mitral regurgitation
  Tricuspid regurgitation
  Dilated (congestive) cardiomyopathy
  Pericardial effusion

From JD Newell et al [4].

echocardiography and plain chest radiography [4]. The radiographic assessment of pulmonary vascularity and cardiac size is used as a guide to the pathophysiology of the predominant cardiac pathology. The M-mode echocardiogram provides specific information about dilatation and hypertrophy of individual chambers and precise information on the functional capacities of normal and abnormal cardiac valves.

In this approach, two broad categories of acquired heart disease are defined based on overall cardiac size (Table 11-1). The first group consists of patients with mild or no cardiomegaly who present with lesions of pressure overload (aortic stenosis) or reduced myocardial compliance (myocardial infarction) but who are in a state of cardiac compensation. The second group comprises patients with cardiomegaly defined by a cardiothoracic ratio in excess of 55 percent, which is related to lesions causing volume overload, myocardial failure, or fluid distension of the pericardium but will also result from cardiac decompensation from all causes. The radiographic method for defining the presence and severity of diverse acquired heart disease has been discussed previously. Table 11-2 summarizes the findings on radiograph and M-mode echocardiography used by Newell and his colleagues.

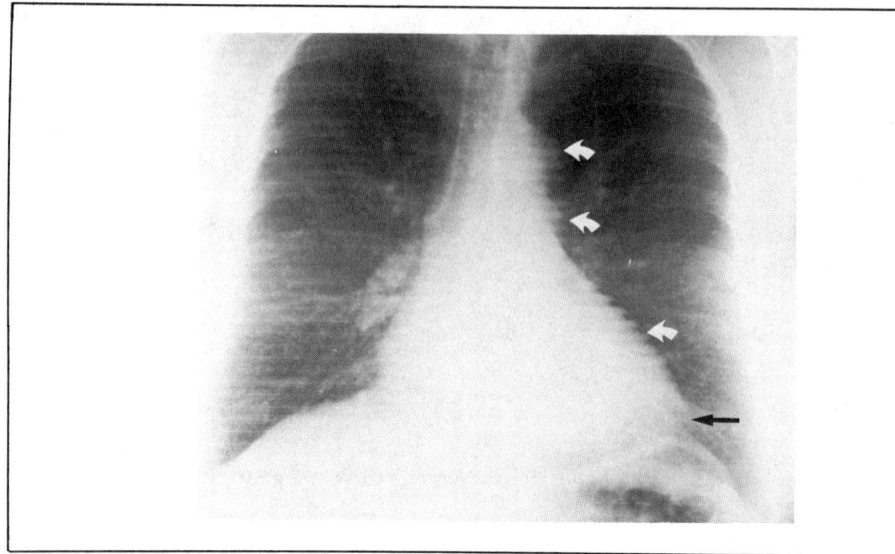

FIGURE 11-12. Roentgenkymography using the interlaced ECG-gated radiographic system. In the frontal view a serrated edge is noted in the region of the aorta, pulmonary artery, and left ventricle (*upper white arrows*). The irregular edge indicates normal motion between systole and diastole. At the lower portion of the left ventricle and the apex (*black arrow*) the heart border is smooth, indicating an area of akinesis and an aneurysm of the left ventricle. This system allows adequate visualization of the lung fields and extracardiac structures; thus an extra film of the lungs is unnecessary. (Courtesy of Robert Dinsmore, M.D., Massachusetts General Hospital, Boston, MA)

Newer Radiographic Examinations

ROENTGENKYMOGRAPHY

The technique of roentgenkymography has undergone several modifications in the course of its development. The newest method is termed an interlaced ECG-gated radiographic system [24]. The core of this method is a sequential x-ray exposure over varied time intervals. These intervals are gated with the electrocardiogram to provide systolic and diastolic exposures. The exposures, an average of 50 msec apart, are interlaced, thus allowing for visualization of cardiac motion without blurring of other soft tissues including the lung (Fig. 11-12). This short interval between exposure overcomes the greatest difficulties with earlier roentgenkymographic methods; previously, all of the film was blurred, so that the kymographic film had to be obtained *in addition* to posteroanterior and lateral chest films. The new technique allows for two separate exposures that will identify cardiac motion but will also provide adequate visualization of other cardiac and pulmonary structures. This method is presently used to evaluate pulsation of the heart to determine abnormalities of ventricular motion and to identify left ventricular aneurysm. The aorta and pulmonary vessels may also be evaluated with this technique, which can provide information in valvular disease and shunt lesions. The major criticism of this method is the lack of truly good indication for

TABLE 11-2. Characteristic Features of Acquired Heart Disease

Lesion	X-Ray Findings	Echocardiographic Findings
NORMAL HEART SIZE OR MILD CARDIOMEGALY		
Aortic stenosis	Dilated ascending aorta; calcified aortic valve	Thickened aortic valve cusps; concentric left ventricular hypertrophy
Systemic hypertension	Dilated ascending aorta and aortic knob	Concentric left ventricular hypertrophy
Mitral stenosis	Pulmonary venous hypertension; left atrial enlargement	Decreased E–F slope; parallel motion of mitral leaflets
Acute myocardial infarction	Pulmonary venous hypertension without cardiomegaly or chamber enlargement	Segmental contractile abnormality
Hypertrophic cardiomyopathy	Inconsistent	Systolic anterior motion of mitral valve; asymmetric septal hypertrophy
Restrictive cardiomyopathy	Pulmonary venous hypertension; left atrial enlargement	Increased left ventricular wall thickness
Constrictive pericarditis	Pulmonary venous hypertension; left atrial enlargement; straightened heart borders	Thickened pericardium; paradoxical septal motion; flat diastolic motion of the posterior left ventricular wall
MODERATE OR MARKED CARDIOMEGALY		
Aortic regurgitation	Left ventricular enlargement; dilated ascending aorta and aortic knob	Diastolic flutter of mitral valve; increased left ventricular dimensions with normal contraction
Mitral regurgitation	Left ventricular enlargement; left atrial enlargement	Left ventricular enlargement; left atrial enlargement; specific etiologic factor (mitral valve prolapse, flail leaflet, rheumatic features)
Tricuspid regurgitation	Right ventricular enlargement; right atrial enlargement	Right ventricular enlargement; right atrial enlargement; paradoxical septal motion
Dilated (congestive) cardiomyopathy	Left ventricular enlargement ± right ventricular enlargement, without proportionate left atrial or aortic enlargement	Marked increase in systolic and diastolic dimension; global decrease in left ventricular contraction
Pericardial effusion	Fat pad sign; differential density sign	Separation of epicardial and pericardial surfaces

From JD Newell et al [4].

the study; for example, the number of ventricular aneurysms is small in relationship to the overall number of chest x-rays. In addition, posteroanterior and lateral views may not be the best projection for visualizing aneurysms. The information gained in valvular and shunt diseases does not warrant the expenditure for equipment in routine practice. A highly specialized, large-volume cardiac radiology practice might provide the best use of this type of equipment, but presently this newer technique has not received wide acceptance.

Intravenous Subtraction Angiography

Angiocardiography and coronary angiography provide detailed anatomic information that is vital for the evaluation of a wide variety of cardiac diseases. Limitations to these procedures include the invasive nature of the procedure itself, the need for a highly skilled operator with broad technical and personnel back-up systems, and the need to introduce contrast materials, which have a low but definable toxic potential. Intravenous subtraction angiography provides the potential for angiocardiographic evaluation in a relatively noninvasive manner with radiographic images which are only slightly less refined than standard angiocardiography. This system will not presently rival coronary angiography but can be used to identify the patency of coronary artery bypass grafts. Standard contrast materials must be used, but their introduction is by intravenous rather than arterial injection.

At this writing a number of rival systems are under development and are available from a variety of manufacturers [25–27]. "Digital subtraction angiography" and "digital vascular imaging" are the names of two such systems, all of which are based on the principle of computer application to the long-used methods of photographic subtraction of radiographic images. High-speed computers allow for digitalization of high-resolution fluoroscopic images of vascular structures before and after the intravenous introduction of standard radiographic contrast materials. The computer is able to subtract the contrast-free cardiac or vascular image from the image with contrast. The result is an image of the heart or blood vessel without the overlapping soft tissue and bony densities.

In the practice of subtraction angiography a number of inherent difficulties tend to degrade the final image. In order to adequately visualize a vascular structure, a 7 to 8 percent difference between the pre- and postcontrast pictures is necessary. In practice, this is accomplished with a superior vena caval contrast injection. The earliest clinical trials have been directed toward the visualization of the great vessels in the neck, renal arteries, and pelvic vessels. The application to the heart has not been fully explored. Ventriculograms, which provide estimates of end-systolic and end-diastolic volumes and thus ejection fraction for both the right and left ventricle, are well within the capabilities of the system. Gross wall motion abnormalities can also be detected. The identification of graft patency is also possible with present systems, as is reasonable visualization of central pulmonary arteries. The substitution of this method for selective pulmonary and coronary angiography is beyond the capabilities of present models. The greatest limitation to imaging is patient body motion as well as respiratory and vascular motion. Some of the motion abnormalities can be corrected by computer manipulation of the imaging data, but inherent limitations exist related to the present capabilities for data processing as a function of overall cost. The final limitation is in the quality of television images, which is the weakest link in the imaging system of all fluoroscopy-based methods. At present, this method is being widely tested in clinical practice. Many changes will be forthcoming, but the application of this technique is a reality.

Computed Tomography

Computed tomography (CT) is a revolutionary imaging technique that incorporates a finely columnated x-ray beam and a circular array of detectors to track the passage of x-rays through the object of interest. A high-speed computer is able to take this large amount of data and reconstruct an anatomic picture based on the differences in x-ray transmission. These differences are termed attenuation coefficients. Current advances in computed tomography hardware and software have resulted in a fourth generation unit. Present generation scanners are capable of performing a CT scan in 2 seconds or less, and reconstructing an image in 30 to 60 seconds. There are two major advantages to computed tomography. First, computed tomography uses photofluorescent detectors and photocell quantification that provide a density resolution of 0.5 percent, compared to 3 to 5 percent using standard radiography techniques. The greatly increased density resolution provided by computed tomography allows the detection of lesions whose density differs only subtly from that of normal tissue. The second unique advantage of computed tomography is its cross-sectional tomographic image display, which is free of the limitations due to interposed air or bone. This imaging format supplements all previous imaging methods. Limitations to the use of CT, especially for the heart, are the spatial and time resolutions of computed tomography, which are less than that available for standard radiographic methods. These are factors that have initially limited its use to the non-moving structures of the body.

Initially, CT investigation of myocardial infarction in an animal model was conducted using excised hearts [28]. The results indicated that there were identifiable differences between normal and infarcted myocardium, but the differences were at the 1 percent level. This original differentiation was only possible in the excised heart because of the degradation caused by motion artifact in the beating heart. The addition of intravenous contrast makes the difference between normal and infarcted myocardium far more obvious [29]. During the first pass of contrast

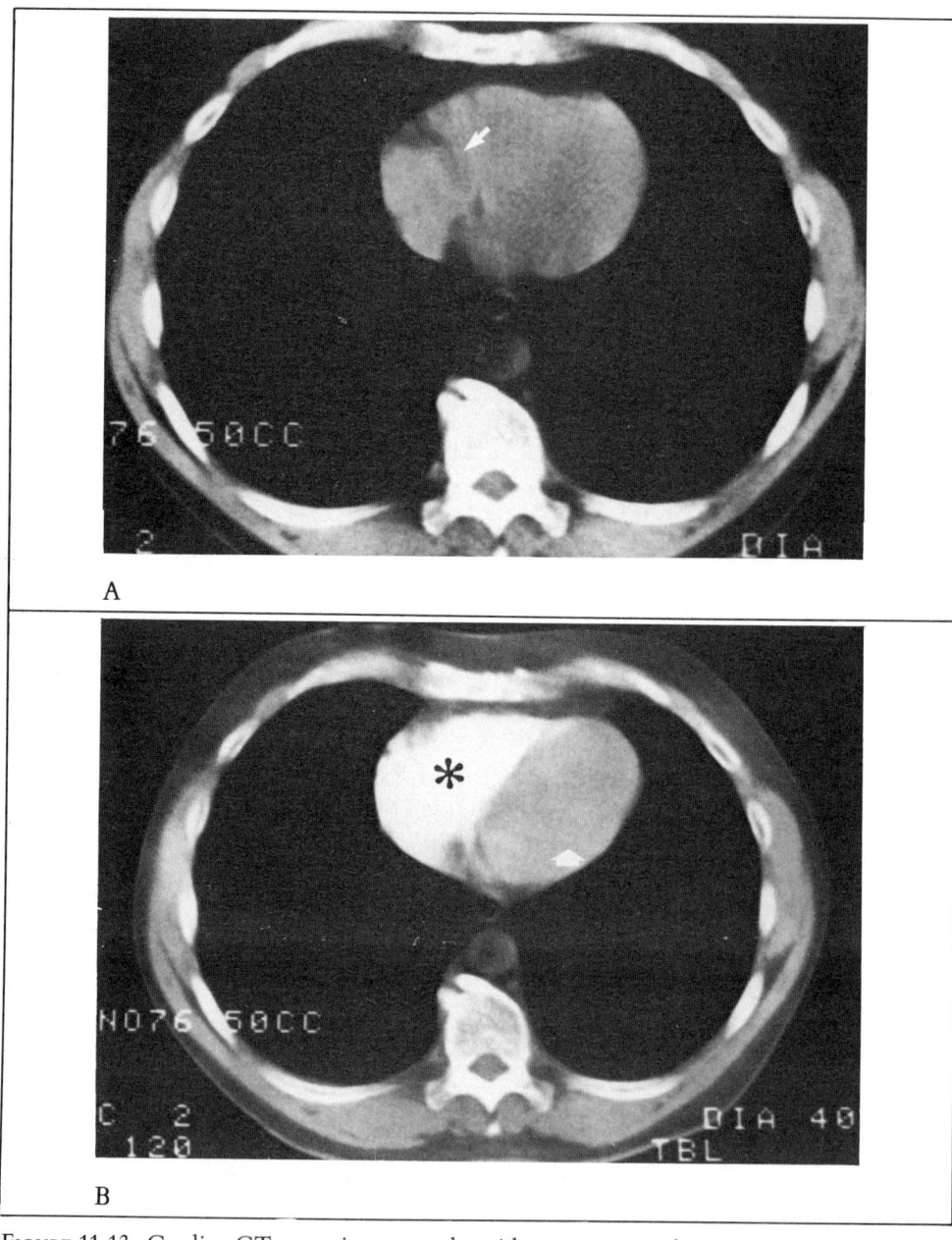

FIGURE 11-13. Cardiac CT scans in ungated rapid sequence, with contrast enhancements. (A) Precontrast: There is no evident difference between the density of blood pool and myocardium. Fat in the right atrioventricular groove does provide some anatomic differentiation (*arrow*). (B) Fifteen seconds after injecting 50 ml of Renografin-76 into a peripheral vein: The right atrium and right ventricle are opacified by the contrast (*asterisk*), but contrast has not yet reached the left side of the heart (*arrowhead*). Differentiation of right atrium and right ventricle cannot be made on this ungated scan owing to motion artifact blurring the atrial-ventricular interface. (C) Six seconds after (B): Contrast now opacifies all four chambers of the heart. The interventricular septum (*black*

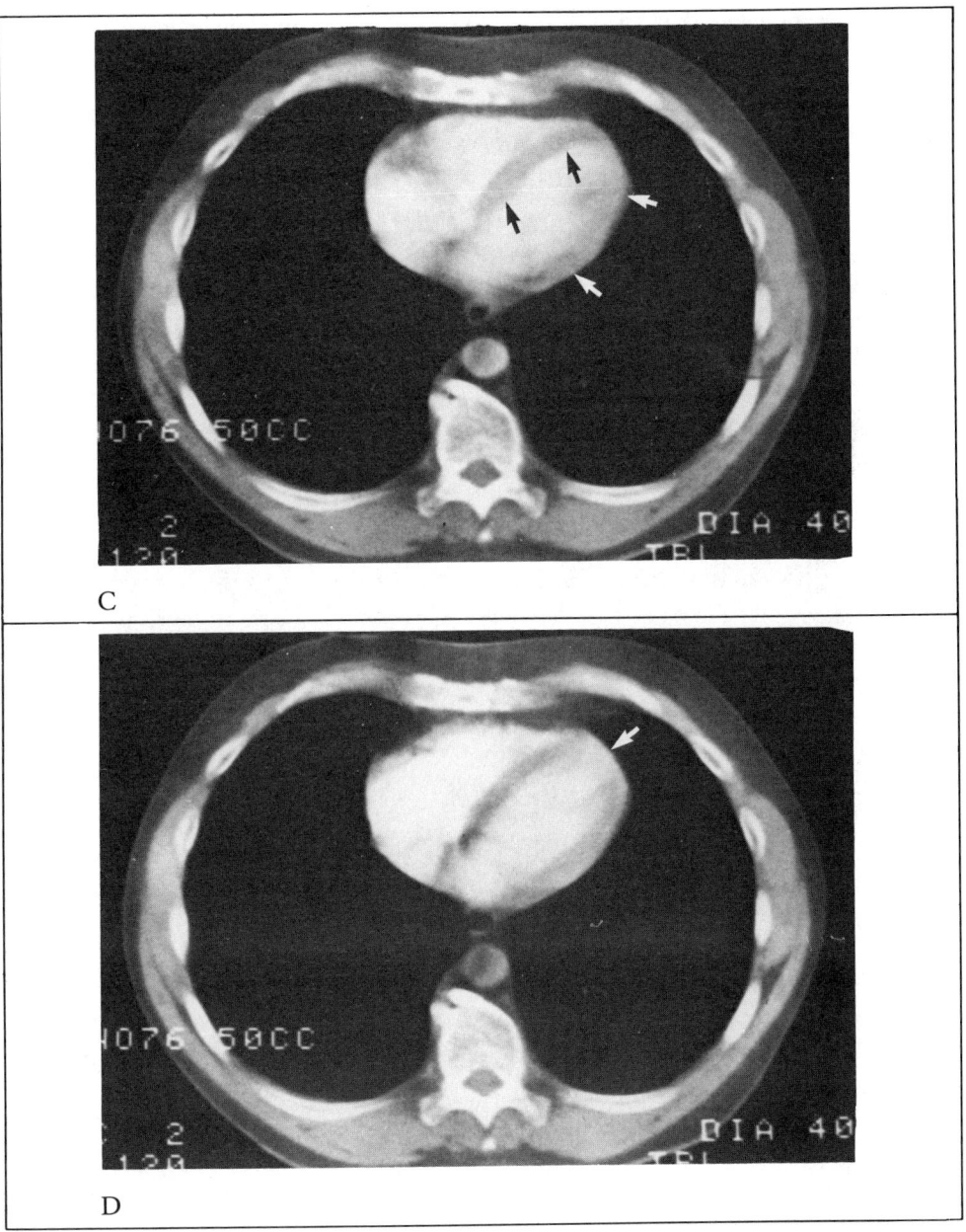

arrows) and the left ventricular free wall (*white arrows*) are readily identifiable. Some differentiation between right atrium and right ventricle is provided by the prominent fat plane between the two. (D) Six seconds after (C): The interventricular septum and free wall are well seen because of the contrast enhancement in the ventricular chambers. The anterior lateral aspect of the left ventricular free wall (*arrow*) is not well seen in (C) or (D). The patient sustained an anterior myocardial infarction four months prior to this study; the lack of delineation of the myocardium in this position is indicative of ventricular thinning at the site of the previous infarction.

through the myocardium, an infarct is seen as an area of reduced attenuation coefficient relative to the normal myocardium (Fig. 11-13). The infarcted tissue then accumulates contrast during the 10 minutes after a contrast bolus injection. This delayed accumulation can last for several hours. The infarct may accumulate contrast in either a generalized manner or only in its periphery, leaving a central area of lucency. Even with the use of intravenous contrast, motion artifacts continue to interfere with visualization of infarcted myocardium. Current research is being directed toward ECG gating of the CT scanner and to scanners that can perform scans in the 15 to 25 millisecond range [30, 31].

Computed tomography also has a proven capability of diagnosing aortic dissection, a diagnosis which may enter into the differential diagnosis of myocardial infarction [32].

Prime areas for future research with millisecond scanners (or once ECG gating of CT scanners is a reality) will be the capability of the CT scanner to evaluate ongoing changes associated with myocardial infarction. Computed tomography may provide a rapid and simplified evaluation of various forms of infarct limitation therapy, thus allowing a wider range of potential agents to be tested quickly. Computed tomography has the potential, therefore, to rapidly assess the status of patients with complex problems and to provide vital information for the management and follow-up of such patients.

Dynamic Spatial Reconstruction

The introduction and practical application of computed tomography to imaging of the head and body led to the previously outlined investigations of computed tomography of the heart. A second area of investigation based on these concepts has evolved a new generation of high-speed electronic whole-body computed tomography termed the dynamic spatial reconstruction system (DSR) [33, 34]. Designed to provide accurate dynamic visualization of any structure, this system will be capable of imaging rapid changes in shape, dimensions, and perfusion of the heart. It features stop action of 1/100 sec with rapid sequencing of images at 60/sec and 240 simultaneous volume images 1 mm thick, which result in a full character reconstruction of the heart and different structures in multiple consecutive cycles. This reconstruction will allow true three-dimensional radiographic visualization of the heart (Fig. 11-14).

The main advantage of dynamic spatial reconstruction over standard computed tomography is the decrease in time from 2 to 20 seconds for a series of images to 0.01 second per scan. The system further differs from computed tomography in that the x-ray detector is fluoroscopic in nature and is coupled with a high-resolution television scanning system, which is then linked to a high-speed computer

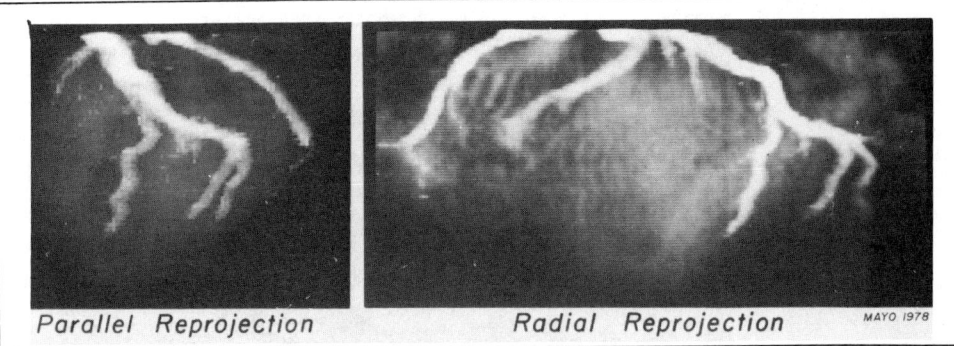

FIGURE 11-14. Dynamic spatial reconstruction (DSR). Two methods of image reconstruction are illustrated. The density of the myocardium in this model, using an isolated canine heart with contrast in the coronary artery, has been dissolved by computer prior to reprojection. Parallel reprojection (*left*) presents a two-dimensional representation of the structure on a parallel plane in the same manner as the standard radiograph. Radial representation (*right*) represents the image as if projected onto the surface of a cylinder surrounding the volume of interest for each image. For the parallel reconstruction, the right coronary artery is seen to the left, while the circumflex and septal arteries are superimposed centrally. The left anterior descending artery is ligated. For the radial projection, the right coronary artery is to the right, the septal artery is centrally located, while the circumflex artery is to the left. DSR will also allow the volume to be rotated to any angle desired. (From LD Harris et al: *J Comput Assist Tomog* 3:439, 1979.)

for image reconstruction in any plane. The final product is a multidimensional CT image of the scanned volume.

Presently in the design stage, the system has many limitations, not the least of which are very high cost and enormous space requirements. Although years will be required for final refinement and practical use, the DSR system represents the most advanced application of computer principles to dynamic imaging of the heart.

NUCLEAR MAGNETIC RESONANCE

Nuclear magnetic resonance (NMR) is a property of many nuclei in which the nuclei resonate at a detectable frequency when placed in a uniform magnetic field and then stimulated with a pulse of radiofrequency (RF) energy. Appropriate atomic elements, such as hydrogen, carbon 13, nitrogen 15, fluorine 19, sodium 23, and phosphorus 31 will absorb a small increment of energy, which they will then emit after cessation of the RF pulse, establishing the basis for detection, analysis, and ultimately imaging of the object in question using computer assistance [35, 36].

Lauterbur, a pioneer in NMR, and his colleagues demonstrated that NMR could be used to differentiate between normal and ischemic myocardium in animal experiments in which ischemia was induced by coronary artery ligation

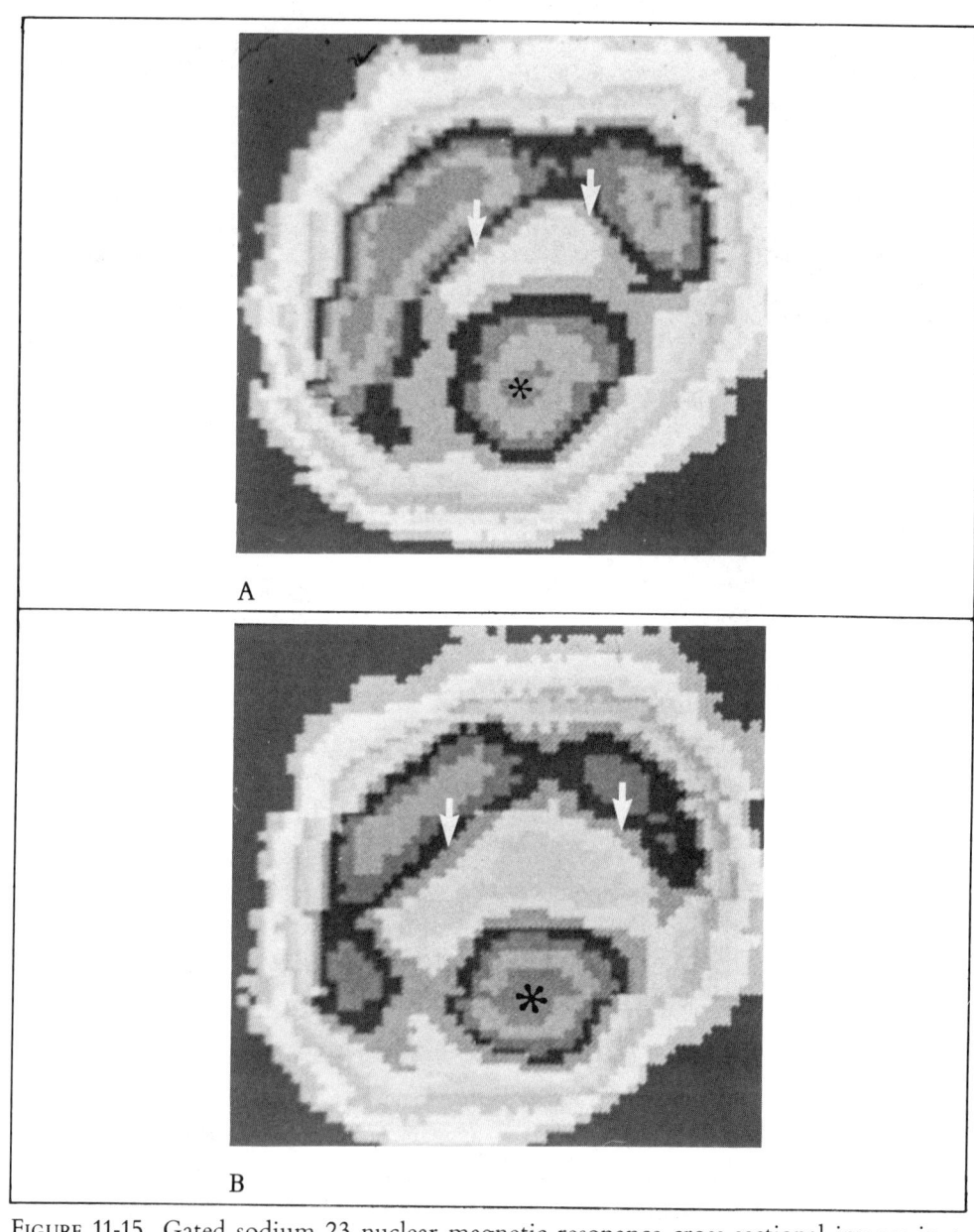

FIGURE 11-15. Gated sodium 23 nuclear magnetic resonance cross-sectional images in a perfused beating rat heart. (A) Diastole. (B) Systole. In each frame, the asterisk indicates the region of the left ventricular chamber, filled with perfusate. The lighter area above the left ventricle represents the left ventricular wall. The darker area beyond the left ventricular wall represents perfusate surrounding the heart. The differences in wall thickness between systole and diastole are well visualized. Wall thickness, ventricular volume, and other parameters are easily obtainable. (Adapted from JL DeLayre et al: *Science* 212:935, 1981. Copyright 1981 by the American Association for the Advancement of Science.)

[37]. Phosphorus in compounds such as adenosine triphosphate and creatinine phosphate have a direct relationship to myocardial function and ischemic changes. Phosphorus 31 can be detected (although not imaged in tissues at this time), giving useful information concerning normal cardiac function, in addition to detecting ischemic changes [38]. Sodium 23 also has potential as a marker for imaging the myocardium, as illustrated in Figure 11-15 and detailed in the work of DeLayre and associates, who provided imaging and cardiac function measurement in isolated perfused and beating rat hearts using sodium 23 NMR imaging in a gated fashion [39]. While the most significant experiments to date have used animal models, there is little doubt that NMR imaging will be usefully applied to man in the future [36].

NMR imaging, particularly of moving structures such as the heart, still requires extensive development. At present, the greatest limitation of the method lies in the time needed for scanning; with seconds required for each measurement (using any available nuclei), repeated measurements and a statistical reconstruction by a computer are necessary for the imaging process. This data build-up presents the greatest technical challenge in NMR imaging. These problems overcome, NMR will be useful in the identification and follow-up of infarcts as well as in studying the biochemical interactions that make up normal and abnormal cardiac function.

Conclusion

Cardiac imaging has advanced rapidly in the last two decades. The standard radiographic techniques still provide a wide range of anatomic and functional information at low cost. Newer modalities such as the various modifications of cardiac CT scanning and NMR promise to further enhance our ability to image and diagnose normal and abnormal cardiac anatomy and function.

References

1. Williams FH: A study of the adaptation of the x-rays to medical practice. Medical and Surgical Reports of the Boston City Hospital, 1897, pp 1–59
2. Kerley PD: Radiology in heart disease. *Br Med J* 2:594, 1933
3. Milne EN: Physiological interpretation of plain radiograph in mitral stenosis, including review of criteria for radiological estimation of pulmonary arterial and venous pressures. *Br J Radiol* 36:902, 1963
4. Newell JD, Higgins CB, Kelley MJ: Radiographic-echocardiographic approach to acquired heart disease: Diagnosis and assessment of severity. *Radiol Clin N Am* 18:387, 1980
5. Baron MG: Radiological and angiographic examination of the heart. In Braunwald E (ed): *Heart Disease.* Philadephia: WB Saunders, 1980, p 147

6. Cooley RN, Schreiber MH: Radiology of the heart and great vessels. In Robbins LL (ed): *Golden's Diagnostic Radiology*. 3rd ed. Baltimore: Williams & Wilkins, 1978
7. Danzer CS: The cardio-thoracic ratio: An index of cardiac enlargement. *Am J Med Sci* 157:513, 1919
8. Sherman RS, Bertrand CA, Duffy JC: Roentgenographic detection of cardiomegaly in employees with normal electrocardiograms. *Am J Roentgenol* 119:493, 1973
9. Glover L, Baxley WA, Dodge HT: A quantitative evaluation of heart size measurements from chest roentgenogram. *Circulation* 47:1289, 1973
10. Keats TE, Enge IP: Cardiac mensuration by the cardiac volume method. *Radiology* 85:850, 1965
11. Hammermeister KE, Chikos PM, Fisher L, Dodge HT: Relationship of cardiothoracic ratio and plain film heart volume to late survival. *Circulation* 59:89, 1979
12. Chikos PM, Figley MM, Fisher L: Correlation between chest film and angiographic assessment of left ventricular size. *Am J Roentgenol* 128:367, 1977
13. Baxley WA, Dodge HT, Sandler H: A quantitative angiocardiographic study of left ventricular hypertrophy and the electrocardiogram. *Circulation* 37:509, 1968
14. Dash H, Lipton MJ, Chatterjee K, Parmley WW: Estimation of pulmonary artery wedge pressure from chest radiograph in patients with chronic congestive cardiomyopathy and ischemic cardiomyopathy. *Br Heart J* 44:322, 1980
15. McHugh TJ, Forrester JS, Alpert L, Zion D, Swan HJC: Pulmonary vascular congestion in acute myocardial infarction: Hemodynamic and angiographic correlation. *Ann Intern Med* 76:29, 1972
16. Harrison MB, Conte PJ, Heitzman ER: Radiological detection of clinically occult cardiac failure following myocardial infarction. *Br J Radiol* 44:265, 1971
17. Margolis JR, Chen JTT, Kong YH, Peter RH, Behar VS, Kisslo JA: The diagnostic and prognostic significance of coronary artery calcification. *Radiology* 137:609, 1980
18. Langou RA, Huang EK, Kelley MJ, Cohen LS: Predictive accuracy of coronary artery calcification and abnormal exercise test for coronary artery disease in asymptomatic men. *Circulation* 62:1196, 1980
19. Bream PR, Elliott LP: Prosthetic valve evaluation by angled cineradiography. Presented at the 66th Scientific Assembly and Annual Meeting of the Radiological Society of North America, November 1980, Dallas, Texas
20. Higgins CB, Lipton MJ: Radiography of acute myocardial infarction. *Radiol Clin N Am* 18:359, 1980
21. Battler A, Karliner JS, Higgins CB, Slutsky R, Gilpin EA, Froelicher VF, Ross J Jr: The initial chest x-ray in acute myocardial infarction: Prediction of early and late mortality and survival. *Circulation* 61:1004, 1980
22. Cascade PN, Kantrowitz A, Wajszczuk WJ, Rubenfire M: The chest x-ray in acute left ventricular power failure: An aid to determining prognosis of patients supported by intraaortic balloon pumping. *Am J Roentgenol* 126:1147, 1976
23. Lachman AS, Roberts WC: Calcific deposits in stenotic mitral valves: Extent and relation to age, sex, degree of stenosis, cardiac rhythm, previous commissurotomy and left atrial body thrombus from study of 164 operatively excised valves. *Circulation* 57:808, 1978

24. Dinsmore RE, Wernikoff RE, Miller SW, Pohost GM, Block PC, Potasio MS: Evaluation of left ventricular free wall asynergy due to coronary artery disease: Use of interlaced ECG-gated radiographic system. *Am J Roentgenol* 132:909, 1979
25. Ovitt TW, Christenson PC, Fisher HD III, Frost MM, Nudelman S, Roehrig H, Seeley G: Intravenous angiography using digital video subtraction: X-ray imaging system. *Am J Roentgenol* 135:1141, 1980
26. Kruger RA, Mistretta CA, Houk TL, Kubal W, Riederer SJ, Ergun DL, Shaw CG, Lancaster JC, Rowe GG: Computerized fluoroscopy techniques for intravenous study of cardiac chamber dynamics. *Invest Radiol* 14: 279, 1979
27. Meaney TF, Weinstein MA, Buonocore E, Pavlicek W, Borkowski GP, Gallagher JH, Sufka B, MacIntyre WJ: Digital subtraction angiography of the human cardiovascular system. *Am J Roentgenol* 135:1153, 1980
28. Lipton MJ, Higgins CB: Evaluation of ischemic heart disease by computerized transmission tomography. *Radiol Clin N Am* 18:557, 1980
29. Hessel SJ, Adams DF, Judy PF, Fishbein MC, Abrams HL: Detection of myocardial ischemia in vitro by computed tomography. *Radiology* 127:413, 1978
30. Berninger WH, Redington RW, Doherty P, Lipton MJ, Carlsson E: Gated cardiac scanning: Canine studies. *J Comput Asst Tomog* 3:155, 1979
31. Boyd DP, Gould RG, Quinn JR, Sparks R, Stanley JH, Herrmannsfeldt WB: A proposed dynamic cardiac 3-D densitometer for early detection and evaluation of heart disease. *IEEE Trans Nucl Sci* 26:2724, 1979
32. Egan TJ, Nelman HL, Herman RJ, Malave SR, Sanders JH: Computed tomography in the diagnosis of aortic aneurysm dissection of traumatic injury. *Radiology* 136:141, 1980
33. Robb RA, Ritman EL: High speed synchronous volume computed tomography of the heart. *Radiology* 133:655, 1979
34. Ritman EL, Harris LD, Kinsey JH, Robb RA: Computed tomographic imaging of the heart: The dynamic spatial reconstructor. *Radiol Clin N Am* 18:547, 1980
35. Partain CL, James AE, Watson JT, Price RR, Coulam CM, Rollo FD: Nuclear magnetic resonance and computed tomography. *Radiology* 136:767, 1980
36. Goldman MR, Pohost GM, Ingwall JS, Fossel ET: Nuclear magnetic resonance imaging: Potential cardiac applications. *Am J Cardiol* 46:1278, 1980
37. Lauterbur PC, Dias MHM, Rudin AM: Augmentation of tissue water proton spin-lattice relaxation rates by in vivo addition of paramagnetic-ions. In Dutton PL, Leigh JS, Scarpa A (eds): *International Symposium on Frontiers of Biological Energetics: Electrons to Tissues*, Vol 1. New York: Academic Press, 1978, p 752
38. Fossel ET, Morgan HE, Ingwall JS: Measurement of changes in high-energy phosphates in the cardiac cycle by using gated ^{31}P nuclear magnetic resonance. *Proc Natl Acad Sci* 77:3654, 1980
39. DeLayre JL, Ingwall JS, Malloy C, Fossel ET: Gated sodium-23 nuclear magnetic resonance images of an isolated perfused working rat heart. *Science* 212:935, 1981

Chapter 12

Blood Tests

Samuel Z. Goldhaber and Thomas W. Smith

Blood tests aid in confirming clinical suspicions about the presence or extent of cardiac disease but cannot serve as adequate substitutes for a careful history, physical examination, and clinical judgement. If ordered haphazardly, they can be costly and misleading. Used wisely, blood tests can be most helpful in the evaluation of specific disorders as well as the optimal utilization of medications that have a narrow range of efficacy and safety. Unexpected results should be followed up with repeat blood sampling and determination to decrease the possibility of laboratory or processing error. In this chapter we will focus on several blood tests to diagnose and evaluate acute myocardial infarction and lipid disorders, but we will also discuss briefly blood tests used in a wide variety of cardiovascular disorders, such as diabetes and hypertension. Finally, we will consider tests that measure serum levels of certain commonly used cardiac medications: antiarrhythmic agents, digitalis glycosides, and antianginal agents.

Acute Myocardial Infarction

Prior to the routine clinical use of cardiac enzyme assays, serial white blood cell counts and erythrocyte sedimentation rates were obtained for indirect assessment of myocardial necrosis. Peak values of 12,000 to 14,000 white blood cells per cubic millimeter were often seen on the third to fifth day after infarction, followed by a rapid return to normal [1]. Unfortunately, this simple blood test lacks both sensitivity and specificity. Small infarctions are not necessarily associated with leukocytosis, and elevated white blood cell counts can be caused by a wide range of disorders. The erythrocyte sedimentation rate (ESR) is normal for several days after infarction and then gradually increases, with a peak in the second week after infarction. During the ensuing 1 to 2 weeks, the ESR gradually returns to normal [1]. Compared to leukocytosis, the ESR is an equally nonspecific marker of disease and becomes elevated so late in the course of myocardial infarction as to be virtually useless clinically.

The introduction of cardiac enzyme measurements to the clinical laboratory has led to major advances in the early and accurate identification of myocardial necrosis. The three cardiac enzymes most frequently assayed are creatine kinase (CK) (previously referred to as creatine phosphokinase or CPK), serum glutamine oxaloacetic transaminase (SGOT), and lactic dehydrogenase (LDH). Each enzyme has a particular time course for release into the vascular compartment from irreversibly damaged heart cells during acute myocardial infarction [2] (Table 12-1).

Isoenzymes are different gene products that catalyze the same overall reaction but differ in their dependence on substrate concentration and/or in their kinetics. They are usually identified in the laboratory by different electrophoretic patterns. CK isoenzymes consist of dimers of M and B subunits and include MM (present in skeletal muscle and heart), BB (present chiefly in brain), and MB (present mainly in heart muscle, with very small amounts in tongue, diaphragm, and small intestine). The five common LDH isoenzymes are named in order of rapidity of migration toward the anode in an electrophoretic field. LDH_1, the fastest migrating LDH isoenzyme, is found primarily in heart tissue. The cardiac isoenzymes of CK and LDH can be assayed routinely and provide additional specificity. Over the past few years, advances in techniques for rapid assay of CK-MB have made this isoenzyme especially useful in helping the physician determine whether infarction has occurred.

We shall review briefly the rationale and laboratory methods for cardiac enzyme assays, using CK as our example. CK is abundant in heart, skeletal muscle, and brain, but unlike SGOT and LDH, only trace amounts are present in erythrocytes and liver. CK catalyzes the following reaction:

$$\text{Creatine phosphate} + \text{ADP} \xrightarrow{\text{CK}} \text{creatine} + \text{ATP}$$

CK transfers a high-energy phosphate from creatine phosphate to adenosine diphosphate (ADP), forming creatine and adenosine triphosphate (ATP). For assay purposes, the ATP thus formed is linked to the reduction of NADP to NADPH as shown in the following two reactions:

$$\text{ATP} + \text{glucose} \xrightarrow{\text{hexokinase}} \text{glucose 6-phosphate} + \text{ADP}$$

$$\text{Glucose 6-phosphate} + \text{NADP} \xrightarrow{\text{glucose 6-phosphate dehydrogenase}} \text{6-phosphogluconate} + \text{NADPH}$$

Absorbance spectrophotometry is used to measure the increase in optical density at 340 nm when NADP is reduced to NADPH. Conditions are maintained such that the first of these three reactions is rate-limiting, and the change in optical

TABLE 12-1. Time Course of Release of Cardiac Enzymes During Acute Myocardial Infarction

Enzyme	Becomes Elevated (hr)	Peaks (hr)	Returns to Normal (days)
CK	6–8	24	3–4
SGOT	8–12	18–36	3–4
LDH	24–48	72–144	8–14

CK = creatine kinase, SGOT = serum glutamic oxaloacetic transaminase, LDH = lactic dehydrogenase.
From JS Alpert, E Braunwald [3].

density provides a measure of CK activity. One international unit of CK is that amount of enzyme that utilizes 1 μmole of creatine phosphate substrate per second. For each micromole of creatine phosphate consumed, 1 μmole of NADP is reduced to NADPH [2].

Because CK is present in other tissues (particularly skeletal muscle), CK elevation is not specific for myocardial necrosis. However, three CK isoenzymes can be separated by conventional electrophoresis in cellulose acetate strips. The BB isoenzyme predominates in brain and moves rapidly toward the anode. The MM isoenzyme, found in heart and skeletal muscle, moves much less rapidly. MB, found in myocardium, migrates toward the anode at a rate intermediate between the BB and MM isoenzymes. The CK isoenzyme bands are visualized by fluorescence of the NADPH generated in the sequence of reactions outlined above. By the early 1970s, it was recognized that CK isoenzymes could increase the diagnostic specificity of CK for acute myocardial infarction [4]. The presence of CK-MB isoenzyme can be assessed qualitatively, or quantitatively if more precision is desired [5]. Rapid separation of CK isoenzymes has been accomplished with batch absorption on glass beads [6]. In addition, a radioimmunoassay for CK isoenzymes has been developed that can rapidly measure CK-MB. This method for CK-MB determination is also highly specific, with the capability of detecting CK-MB despite a 25,000-fold excess of CK-MM [7].

Because of the time course of cardiac enzyme release (Table 12-1) [2], standard practice is to obtain serial cardiac enzyme determinations for patients suspected of acute myocardial infarction. To avoid missing early elevations of cardiac enzymes, a reasonable protocol is to order baseline CK, CK-MB, SGOT, and LDH measurements. CK, CK-MB, and SGOT measurements can be repeated at 8 and 16 hours after the baseline tests. Then, daily enzyme determinations should suffice until the diagnosis of infarction is confirmed or excluded.

For patients admitted several days after possible infarction, elevated LDH cardiac isoenzymes may be particularly useful in suggesting the diagnosis, despite CK and SGOT levels that have returned to normal. LDH isoenzymes can be separated by ion exchange chromatography or by electrophoresis. An elevated

$LDH_{1:2}$ isoenzyme ratio is typical of myocardial infarction and was 96 percent sensitive and 97 percent specific in a recent study [8]. Despite this high degree of accuracy, CK-MB is even more sensitive and specific earlier in the course of myocardial infarction.

A major advantage of CK-MB over total CK is that CK-MB is not usually elevated following intramuscular injection, noncardiac surgery, and exercise. The height of the CK-MB rise can be related to infarct size [9]. Recently, a group of Danish investigators suggested that serial CK-MB determinations may be sufficiently accurate to replace all standard enzyme tests for patients with acute infarction [10]. In their study, CK-MB was positive within 17 hours after admission in all patients with confirmed acute myocardial infarction. They found that CK-MB was more effective than total CK, aspartate aminotransferase, LDH, and electrocardiographic criteria for diagnosing acute infarction.

CK-MB is highly sensitive, and its absence in the serum virtually excludes the diagnosis of acute infarction following coronary artery bypass grafting [11]. Despite the utility of the CK-MB test, its specificity is not as great as its sensitivity. CK-MB may also be elevated without acute infarction following electrical countershock or in patients with hypothyroidism, muscular dystrophy, polymyositis, myocarditis, and chronic dilated cardiomyopathy. Except for myocarditis, these conditions are usually clinically evident, so that an elevated CK-MB in the absence of other symptoms and signs of acute infarction can be appropriately discounted as an incidental finding.

Thus, the proper selection and timing of cardiac enzyme determinations can be of value in establishing an early and accurate diagnosis of acute infarction. As the costs of coronary care units increase, cardiac enzyme measurements should allow clinicians to make optimal use of these expensive and limited facilities.

Lipid Disorders

Unequivocal evidence has demonstrated an increased risk of coronary heart disease in persons younger than age 50 who have an elevated total cholesterol level [12]. However, evidence for elevated triglyceride levels as an independent risk factor for coronary heart disease is inconclusive [13].

During the past few years, much attention has been focused on the partition of total cholesterol levels into the various lipoprotein fractions, especially low-density lipoproteins (LDL) and high-density lipoproteins (HDL). Each lipoprotein has a particular combination of lipids (cholesterol, triglyceride, and phospholipid) and protein. The major lipoproteins can be classified according to density (weight per volume) or according to electrophoretic mobility (discussed subsequently). From highest to lowest density, the lipoproteins are: HDL, LDL, intermediate density lipoprotein (IDL), very low density lipoprotein (VLDL), and chylomicrons. Large-scale lipid studies in patients under age 50 from Tromso, Norway [14] and in both young [15] and old [16] adults from Framingham, Massachusetts, have shown that HDL cholesterol has a strong inverse association with coronary heart disease and LDL cholesterol has a weaker positive association with coronary heart disease.

Physicians frequently order tests of blood lipids to help predict the presence or risk of development of atherosclerosis in asymptomatic patients. Characteristics associated statistically with increased HDL levels include a lean body habitus, no cigarette smoking, alcohol consumption, exercise, and low dietary consumption of sucrose and starch [17]. Although the reduction of total serum cholesterol or LDL levels and the augmentation of HDL levels have not been proven to reduce the incidence of coronary heart disease, lipid screening can identify some patients at increased risk for myocardial infarction and can also help diagnose five specific types of hyperlipoproteinemia. The hyperlipoproteinemias can occur as primary disorders or can be secondary to other disease states. Specific dietary and drug treatments can be prescribed for each type of hyperlipoproteinemia if clinically indicated.

The five types of hyperlipoproteinemia (Table 12-2) [18] can often be deduced from observing a plasma sample after overnight refrigeration and then measuring total cholesterol and triglycerides. A creamy supernatant (caused by the least dense of the lipoproteins) with a clear infranatant is due to an elevated level of chylomicrons and is usually diagnostic of a rare disorder, type I hyperlipoproteinemia. Chylomicrons are 90 percent triglyceride, 5 percent cholesterol, and 5 percent phospholipid and protein. Clear plasma with an elevated cholesterol level is characteristic of type IIa hyperlipoproteinemia, which is due to elevated LDL levels. LDLs are 50 percent cholesterol, 25 percent protein, 15 percent phospholipid, and 10 percent triglyceride. Turbid plasma is caused by elevated levels of VLDL or IDL and is usually observed in types IIb, III, IV, and V hyperlipoproteinemia. A creamy top layer of chylomicrons is also present in type V and sometimes in the type III pattern. In the fasting state, VLDL is the primary triglyceride-carrying lipoprotein and is composed of 60 percent triglyceride, 18 percent phospholipid, 12 percent cholesterol, and 10 percent protein [18].

HDL can be measured by adding heparin and manganese to the plasma sample (after the chylomicron supernatant, if present, is removed). Heparin and manganese will precipitate both LDL and VLDL, leaving only HDL in solution. LDL cholesterol levels can then be approximated by applying the following formulas, which are valid only for triglyceride values less than 400 mg/dl:

TABLE 12-2. Patterns of Hyperlipoproteinemia

Type	Abnormality	Usual Age of Expression	Plasma Appearance	Clinical Manifestations
I	↑Chylomicrons	Infancy and childhood	Creamy supernatant, clear infranatant	Pancreatitis, eruptive xanthomas, hepatosplenomegaly
IIa	↑LDL	At birth, if genetic	Clear	Premature atherosclerosis, corneal arcus, xanthelasma; in familial forms, tendon and tuberous xanthomas
IIb	↑LDL, ↑VLDL	At birth, if genetic	Turbid	Milder forms may have glucose intolerance, obesity, in addition to premature atherosclerosis
III	LDL/VLDL of abnormal composition	Third decade; often after menopause in women	Turbid	Glucose intolerance, xanthomas, premature vascular disease, especially peripheral vascular disease
IV	↑VLDL	Usually third decade or later	Turbid	Glucose intolerance, obesity
V	↑VLDL, ↑Chylomicrons	Adulthood	Creamy supernatant, turbid infranatant	Pancreatitis, eruptive xanthomas, hepatosplenomegaly, obesity, hyperuricemia

LDL = low-density lipoprotein, VLDL = very low-density lipoprotein.
From RI Levy [18].

$$VLDL = \frac{\text{total triglycerides}}{5}$$

$$LDL = \text{total cholesterol} - (VLDL + HDL)$$

Patients with very low levels of HDL are sometimes said to have a "type VI" lipid abnormality [19]. As discussed previously, low HDL levels are strongly correlated with an increased risk of coronary heart disease.

For more detailed analysis, the lipoproteins can be separated into discrete bands by electrophoresis, based on their various electrical charges. Negatively charged lipoproteins move toward the anode, while positively charged lipoproteins remain at or near the origin. From the origin, HDL migrates farthest toward the anode and forms an alpha band. LDL does not migrate quite as far as HDL and forms a beta band. VLDL remains closer to the origin and forms a prebeta band. A broad beta band, intermediate between the prebeta (VLDL) and beta (LDL) bands, is found in type III hyperlipidemia. Chylomicrons remain at the origin.

It is important to recognize that lipid values normally increase with age in typical U.S. populations. The Lipid Research Clinics Program of the National Heart, Lung, and Blood Institute has established a range of normal values (from 10th to 90th percentiles) for plasma lipids and lipoproteins based on measurements on approximately 7,000 people [20] (Table 12-3). However, it must be emphasized that values in the 10th to 90th percentiles depend greatly on the population being studied. The range of normal values in Table 12-3 is based on the United States population, which has a very high incidence and prevalence of atherosclerotic cardiovascular disease. It is quite possible that many lipid values "within the normal range" are, in a biologic sense, elevated and abnormal. Other factors can influence lipid levels. Chylomicrons will normally appear in blood up to 10 hours after a meal. Change in diet and weight, certain drugs, and illness can cause major changes in lipid levels. For example, total cholesterol and LDL levels may decrease by 60 percent in the first few days after myocardial infarction. When abnormal lipoprotein patterns are diagnosed after confounding factors have been excluded, causes of secondary hyperlipoproteinemia should be sought. These include hypothyroidism, nephrotic syndrome, myeloma, acute intermittent porphyria, liver disease, diabetes mellitus, and alcoholism [21].

Most asymptomatic patients with lipid abnormalities detected by lipid screening will have type II or IV hyperlipidemia [22], with elevated cholesterol or triglyceride levels, respectively. The finding of an elevated cholesterol but normal triglyceride level will usually indicate type IIa hyperlipoproteinemia. Most individuals with type IIa hyperlipoproteinemia in the general population have a polygenic hypercholesterolemia that puts them on the upper end of the bell-shaped curve for the general population. A few of these individuals, however, will have heterozygous familial hypercholesterolemia, which is an example of a single gene mutation that produces both hypercholesterolemia and atherosclerosis. It is inherited as an autosomal dominant trait, with rare homozygotes (1 in 1 million persons) much more severely affected than heterozygotes (1 in 500 persons). Patients with familial hypercholesterolemia generally have higher cholesterol levels than those with polygenic hypercholesterolemia. Those with familial hypercholesterolemia, both homozygotes and heterozygotes, will usually develop tendinous

TABLE 12-3. Normal Values (10th–90th Percentiles), by Age and Sex, for Plasma Lipids and Lipoproteins (mg/dl)

Age	Plasma Cholesterol		Plasma LDL		Plasma HDL		Plasma Triglycerides	
	Male	Female	Male	Female	Male	Female	Male	Female
5–9	131–183	135–189	69–117	73–125	43–70	38–67	34–70	37–103
10–14	132–191	131–191	73–123	73–126	40–71	40–64	37–94	44–104
15–19	123–183	126–198	68–123	66–129	34–59	38–68	43–125	40–112
20–24	126–197	132–220	73–138	65–141	32–57	37–72	50–146	42–135
25–29	137–223	142–217	75–157	75–148	32–58	39–74	51–171	45–137
30–34	152–237	141–215	88–166	77–146	32–59	40–73	57–214	45–140
35–39	157–248	149–233	92–176	81–161	31–58	38–75	58–250	47–170
40–44	161–251	156–241	98–173	84–165	31–60	39–79	69–252	51–161
45–49	171–258	162–256	106–185	89–173	33–60	41–82	65–218	55–180
50–54	168–263	171–267	102–185	94–186	31–58	41–84	75–244	58–190
55–59	172–260	182–278	103–191	97–199	31–54	41–85	70–210	65–229
60–64	170–262	186–282	106–188	105–191	34–69	44–87	65–193	66–210
65–69	174–275	179–282	104–199	99–205	33–74	38–85	61–227	64–221
70+	160–253	181–268	100–182	108–189	33–70	38–82	71–202	68–189

LDL = low-density lipoprotein, HDL = high-density lipoprotein.
Data from *LRC Population Studies Data Book. Vol I: The Prevalence Study.* U.S. Dept. of Health and Human Services NIH Publication 80-1527, Washington, DC, July, 1980.

xanthomas. These patients are at greatly increased risk for premature coronary disease and constitute about 5 percent of all patients who have a myocardial infarction [23].

Thus, lipid levels can provide the physician with both diagnostic information on hyperlipoproteinemia and predictive information on the risk for coronary heart disease. For an asymptomatic patient, it is probably reasonable to measure total cholesterol, total triglycerides, and HDL levels. Of these three measurements, the strongest predictor of coronary heart disease will be a low HDL level. If HDL levels are low, or LDL levels are calculated to be elevated from the formula given above, then intervention including dietary recommendations and/or drug treatment may be worthwhile [18-21, 24]. In addition, the plasma of patients with abnormal lipid screening tests should be examined to determine the pattern of hyperlipoproteinemia. Lipoprotein electrophoresis may occasionally be necessary for further clarification. After causes of a secondary hyperlipoproteinemia have been excluded, family screening should be undertaken to uncover possible familial forms of hyperlipoproteinemia.

Miscellaneous Disorders

In addition to diagnosing myocardial infarction and lipid disorders, blood tests can be used to help diagnose a wide range of abnormalities related to the cardiovascular system. This section will highlight a few of the more common disease states in which blood tests are helpful (Table 12-4) but will not attempt to catalog all possible blood tests related to cardiovascular abnormalities.

DIABETES MELLITUS

The Framingham study has found that both insulin- and noninsulin-dependent diabetics have an increased morbidity and mortality from all cardiovascular causes. When all associated risk factors (such as higher lipid levels, hypertension, and marked obesity) were accounted for, the relationship between diabetes and increased cardiovascular disease persisted, especially in women from age 35 to 54 [25]. The Coronary Drug Project studied fasting plasma glucose levels in 2,770 male survivors of myocardial infarction placed in the placebo group of its investigation. After adjusting for baseline characteristics, multivariate analysis showed an increased mortality of borderline statistical significance in patients with fasting glucose levels greater than or equal to 140 mg/dl [26]. Based on these studies, determination of a fasting glucose level may help to assess a patient's risk of cardiovascular disease. If the fasting glucose level is substantially elevated, then the diagnosis of glucose intolerance is established. In such cases there is no reason to proceed with an oral glucose tolerance test (OGTT). If the fasting glucose level is

TABLE 12-4. Tests Useful in Diagnosis of Disorders Related to the Cardiovascular System

Disorder	Screening Test(s)	Additional Tests
Diabetes mellitus	Random glucose level	Fasting glucose level, oral glucose tolerance test
Thyroid dysfunction		
Hyperthyroidism	Thyroid hormones T4, T3, and T3 resin uptake test (T3RU)	
Hypothyroidism	Thyroid hormone T4 and T3 resin uptake test (T3RU), and thyroid-stimulating hormone (TSH)	
Hypertension		
Renovascular causes	Blood urea nitrogen, creatinine	Rapid sequence intravenous pyelogram
Pheochromocytoma	24-hour urine for creatinine, metanephrines, and catecholamines	
Mineralocorticoid excess	Serum potassium	
Cushing's syndrome	Overnight dexamethasone suppression test	
Cardiomyopathy		
Hemochromatosis	Plasma iron, total iron-binding capacity (TIBC), ferritin	
Toxin-induced	Heavy metals	
Löffler's endocarditis	Eosinophil count	
Infectious etiology	Bacterial and fungal cultures, viral titers	
Rheumatic diseases		
Acute rheumatic fever	Antistreptolysin-O titer (ASLO), C-reactive protein, erythrocyte sedimentation rate (ESR)	Anti-DNAse B, antihyaluronidase, antistreptozyme slide agglutination test (ASTZ)
Systemic lupus erythematosus	Antibodies to nuclear antigens (ANA)	Lupus erythematosus prep
Systemic lupus erythematosus (during flare)	Total hemolytic complement (CH50) and complement components C3, C4	

TABLE 12-4. (Continued)

Disorder	Screening Test(s)	Additional Tests
Rheumatoid arthritis	Latex fixation	
Congestive heart failure		
Hepatic dysfunction	Liver function tests	
Occult thyroid disease	Thyroid function tests	
Beriberi	Thiamine	
Paget's disease	Alkaline phosphatase	
Anemia	Complete blood count (CBC)	
Metabolic disorders	Serum electrolytes (Na, K, Cl, CO_2, Ca, Mg), arterial blood gases, pH	

at the upper limit of normal or only slightly elevated, the practical information gained from an OGTT should exceed the patient's additional time, expense, and discomfort. Often, a modestly elevated fasting glucose level will be sufficient indication for a physician to recommend modest restriction in carbohydrate and caloric intake, regardless of an OGTT.

THYROID DYSFUNCTION

Thyroid dysfunction frequently has profound cardiovascular effects. Hyperthyroidism may cause palpitations, tachycardia, hypertension, and abnormal left ventricular function. Hypothyroidism frequently causes cardiac dilatation, bradycardia, and exertional dyspnea. Certain patients present clinical findings that should compel the physican to order thyroid screening tests. Attempts to treat a cardiac problem caused by occult thyroid disease will often be unsuccessful until the primary thyroid disorder is diagnosed and controlled. Atrial fibrillation with a rapid ventricular response that does not respond appropriately to conventional doses of digitalis glycosides indicates the possibility of hyperthyroidism.

The normally functioning thyroid gland secretes the active thyroid hormones T3 and T4, which in blood are almost entirely bound to plasma proteins. Thyroxine-binding globulin (TBG) has a high binding affinity for T4. A T3 resin uptake test (T3RU) is frequently used to assess indirectly the concentration of unoccupied binding sites on TBG. Apathetic hyperthyroidism in elderly patients or T3 hyperthyroidism (with a normal T4) may make establishing the diagnosis of hyperthyroidism especially difficult unless serum T3, T4, and resin T4 uptake are all determined [27]. Congestive heart failure can be a manifestation of hyperthyroidism or hypothyroidism. Particularly challenging therapeutically is the patient with severe angina pectoris and hypothyroidism [28]. In such patients, thyroid replacement must be done slowly and cautiously to minimize the exacerbation of chest pain. If suspected, hypothyroidism can usually be diagnosed on the basis of a low serum T4 and elevated thyroid-stimulating hormone (TSH). A more complete discussion of thyroid dysfunction, including clinical findings, laboratory tests, and patient management [29], is outside the scope of this chapter.

Hypertension

Blood tests are not needed to diagnose hypertension. However, blood tests may be invaluable in diagnosing a specific etiology of hypertension in the minority of patients who do not have essential hypertension. For routine management of essential hypertension, renin-sodium profiling [30] has been advocated by Laragh and Sealey [31], but its usefulness is controversial [32]. Patients with low-renin essential hypertension have a greater fall in blood pressure with diuretic therapy than patients with normal renin levels [33], while patients with high-renin essential hypertension respond particularly well to beta blockade [34].

After the diagnosis of hypertension is established, a number of simple laboratory tests will be useful to screen for specific causes of secondary hypertension and to serve as baselines prior to treatment with diuretics. Renal status can be evaluated with a urine analysis, and serum (blood) urea nitrogen (BUN) and serum creatinine determinations. A serum potassium level will screen for mineralocorticoid-induced hypertension and will also be useful as a baseline prior to initiating diuretic therapy. For patients with hypertension under age 25 or with the abrupt onset of severe hypertension after age 50, further tests for causes of secondary hypertension are warranted. In such patients, particularly if an abdominal bruit is heard, renovascular hypertension should be screened for with a rapid sequence intravenous pyelogram, radioisotope renogram, or saralasin test [35]. Pheochromocytoma can usually be excluded with normal 24-hour urine levels for creatinine, metanephrines, and catecholamines. Cushing's syndrome can be conveniently investigated with an overnight dexamethasone suppression test [36].

Cardiomyopathy

As with hypertension, blood tests are not necessary to make the diagnosis of cardiomyopathy. A full discussion of the cardiomyopathies and blood tests that may be useful in determining their etiologies can be found elsewhere [37]. Nevertheless, in some patients with cardiomyopathy of unknown etiology, it may be worthwhile to look for an elevated plasma iron, normal or low total iron-binding capacity, and markedly elevated serum ferritin level—abnormalities found in hemochromatosis. A heavy metal screen may identify toxic cardiomyopathy due to arsenic, cobalt, lead, or mercury. An abnormally high number of eosinophils may point to Löffler's endocarditis. Finally, if an infectious etiology is suspected, appropriate viral titers, bacterial cultures, or fungal cultures may be warranted. Thus, certain blood tests can occasionally offer important etiologic, therapeutic, and prognostic information about cardiomyopathy.

STREPTOCOCCAL INFECTION

Blood tests can determine antibody levels useful in the diagnosis of recent streptococcal infection. Antistreptococcal antibodies reach a peak titer shortly after the onset of acute rheumatic fever. The antistreptolysin-O (ASLO) titer is the most extensively used antibody test. Anti-DNAse B tends to remain elevated longer than other antistreptococcal antibodies. Antihyaluronidase is also frequently used to document recent streptococcal infection. An antistreptozyme (ASTZ) slide agglutination test is very sensitive and therefore provides evidence useful in excluding the diagnosis of acute rheumatic fever. During the acute rheumatic flare, C-reactive protein (CRP) and the ESR are acute phase reactants and serial measurements may be useful guides to the effectiveness of therapy and to the possibility of relapse [38].

SYSTEMIC LUPUS ERYTHEMATOSUS

Systemic lupus erythematosus (SLE) frequently involves the heart, but the manifestations may be subclinical. Antibodies to nuclear antigens (ANA) are present in more than 99 percent of SLE patients. During flares of SLE, total hemolytic complement (CH50) and the complement components C3 and C4 are decreased. The latex fixation test is positive in only 20 percent of patients [39]. However, during the course of subacute infective endocarditis, the latex fixation test becomes positive in about 50 percent of patients after six weeks of illness.

CONGESTIVE HEART FAILURE

The diagnosis of congestive heart failure is usually established on clinical grounds. However, in occult cases liver enzymes may be quite elevated, and the patient may appear jaundiced. In high output congestive heart failure, blood tests may help to elucidate specific etiologies such as hyperthyroidism, beriberi (depletion of thiamine), Paget's disease (elevation of alkaline phosphatase), or anemia.

METABOLIC DISORDERS

Finally, blood tests are useful in diagnosing metabolic disorders that may affect the stability of cardiac rhythm. Electrolyte imbalance and acid-base abnormalities frequently contribute to arrhythmias. In electrolyte screening, calcium and magnesium values should also be determined, since the heart can be exquisitely sensitive to serum calcium and magnesium abnormalities. In addition, hypoxia and acidosis may not be clinically apparent but frequently respond quickly to specific treatment. The correction of metabolic disorders will often make a seemingly resistant arrhythmia become much more manageable.

Blood Tests to Assess Serum Levels of Cardiovascular Drugs

The development of gas-liquid chromatography, mass spectrometry, high-pressure liquid chromatography, and radioimmunoassay methods has permitted the rapid and accurate measurement of a number of cardiovascular drugs [40]. Such measurements have been especially useful in pharmacokinetic studies as well as in individual titration of potent cardiovascular drugs, especially antiarrhythmic agents and digitalis glycosides, which have a narrow range of safety and efficacy.

Gas-liquid chromatography (GLC) separates substances in the vapor phase, usually at 150 to 350°C. GLC relies on a mobile phase, using a carrier gas such as nitrogen or helium, and a stationary phase, using a liquid coated onto an inert material. Many antiarrhythmic drugs, including lidocaine, procainamide, phenytoin, quinidine, disopyramide, and propranolol, have been assayed with GLC. The drug being assayed must be readily volatile and thermally stable. Frequently, GLC is combined with mass spectrometry, which can quantify drug levels to the picogram range after separation by GLC. In the mass spectrometer, the molecules are bombarded with rapidly moving electrons and converted into positive ions. The positive ions move with velocities according to their charge-to-mass ratio and are separated according to their masses as they move toward a negatively charged electrode [41].

High-pressure liquid chromatography (HPLC) has the advantages over GLC of not requiring readily volatile or thermally stable molecules. The speed of analysis, ease of operation, and versatility of HPLC make this technique well suited for routine assays of many cardiovascular drugs [42].

Another method used to measure antiarrhythmic drug concentrations combines immunologic and biochemical techniques. It is known as a homogeneous immunoassay because it is not necessary to separate antigen bound to antibody from unbound antigen [43]. Commercially available enzyme multiplied immunoassay technique (EMIT) systems are available to measure lidocaine, procainamide, quinidine, and disopyramide levels [44]. Serum or plasma is mixed with a reagent containing antibodies to the antiarrhythmic drug, together with the coenzyme nicotinamide adenine dinucleotide (NAD) and substrate for the enzyme glucose 6-phosphate dehydrogenase (G-6-PDh). Drug in the serum or plasma binds specifically to the antibody. A known quantity of the drug coupled to G-6-PDh is then added. The G-6-PDh drug complex combines with remaining unoccupied antibody binding sites, and the enzyme activity is thereby reduced. The residual enzymatic activity is directly related to the drug concentration present in the serum or plasma sample. The G-6-PDh converts NAD to NADH, resulting in an absorbance change that is measured spectrophotometrically using standard laboratory equipment.

Antiarrhythmic Agents

In the emergency treatment of or prophylaxis against ventricular fibrillation or ventricular tachycardia, parenteral drugs are frequently used without blood level monitoring. *Lidocaine* is the intravenous antiventricular arrhythmic drug of first choice and can usually be monitored by therapeutic effect (reduction or abolition of premature ventricular depolarizations) and clinical toxicity (lightheadedness, restlessness, disorientation, tremor, seizure). Based on clinical studies with drug levels, recommended dosage schedules have been devised for bolus [45] and/or continuous infusion therapy [46] (Table 12-5). The dosage of lidocaine should be reduced after prolonged infusion [47], although the extent of reduction is controversial [48]. In patients with advanced heart failure and liver disease, plasma clearance of lidocaine is reduced [49]. Consequently, lidocaine infusion rates should be decreased, although no universally reliable nomogram has been established. Because lidocaine is metabolized by the liver, no dosage reduction is ordinarily needed in patients with renal disease and normal hepatic function. Ochs and coworkers have recently shown that lidocaine clearance during continuous infusion is reduced by coadministration of propranolol [50]. Therefore, patients receiving both propranolol and lidocaine should be monitored especially carefully for lidocaine toxicity. Although blood levels are not needed routinely for safe administration of lidocaine, they may prove useful in situations in which lidocaine clearance is impaired, inadequate therapeutic effect is attained despite high conventional dosages, or clinical toxicity is observed at low or moderate conventional doses in a patient without any known predisposing factors for lidocaine toxicity.

In addition to lidocaine, other antiarrhythmics approved for intravenous use are procainamide, bretylium, and phenytoin. If lidocaine is ineffective in an emergency situation, procainamide has been the conventional drug of second choice for ventricular arrhythmias. Bretylium, which was shown in one study to reverse ventricular fibrillation in the human heart [51], has recently been approved as a second-line emergency antiarrhythmic [52] by the Food and Drug Administration. Phenytoin is generally considered a third-line antiarrhythmic drug. It usually does not impair atrioventricular conduction and therefore has gained a role in the treatment of ventricular arrhythmias due to digitalis toxicity. Each of these drugs has established therapeutic blood levels, dosage ranges, and pharmacokinetics (Table 12-6). Although quinidine is approved for intravenous use and can be administered safely intravenously [53], it is generally used as an oral antiarrhythmic agent and therefore is included in our discussion of oral antiarrhythmic drugs.

For the past 30 years, *procainamide* has been used to treat cardiac arrhythmias. By 1971 it was found that plasma concentrations correlated well with therapeutic

TABLE 12-5. Lidocaine Dosage Regimens

Therapeutic range: 2–6 μg/ml

Dosage excreted unchanged in urine: <5%

Loading dose: 1–2 mg/kg by slow intravenous infusion (up to 50 mg/min)
> or
> 100 mg given over 2 min at 10-min intervals
> or
> 50 mg over 1 min, given 4 times, 5 min apart
> or
> 20 mg/min infused for 10 min

Maintenance dose: 2–4 mg/min for 24 hours

To raise concentration acutely: 50 mg bolus over 1 min and simultaneously increase infusion rate to no more than 5 mg/min

Reduce dosage and consider ordering serum levels in patients who have lidocaine infusions >24 hr and/or heart failure, liver disease, coadministration of propranolol

---

and toxic effects. The usual effective concentration range is 4 to 10 μg/ml. Toxic manifestations are rare with concentrations less than 12 μg/ml but are common with concentrations greater than 16 μg/ml. In most patients, procainamide doses of 50 mg/kg per day produce therapeutic levels. Three-hour dosage intervals prevent fluctuation of procainamide levels greater than 50 percent [54, 55].

Recently, high-dose procainamide therapy was reported to be effective in the treatment of recurrent inducible ventricular tachyarrhythmias in 16 patients using doses of 500 to 1500 mg given orally every 4 hours. Unfortunately, two of these patients developed gastrointestinal toxicity and four developed a lupus-like syndrome [56]. However, new sustained-release procainamide preparations tested recently maintained therapeutic levels for 8 hours after each dose [57]. A third modification of conventional procainamide therapy has been administration of procainamide's major metabolite, N-acetylprocainamide (NAPA), which is currently undergoing clinical trials and is not yet released for general use. The mean plasma concentration associated with efficacy in one study was 14 μg/ml. Side effects, primarily gastrointestinal, occurred at a mean concentration of 22 μg/ml. The antiarrhythmic response to procainamide did not predict the response to NAPA. A major advantage of NAPA over procainamide is NAPA's longer half-life. Although the development of a positive ANA has been reported in one patient on NAPA therapy for more than six months [58], NAPA has not been implicated in causing a lupus syndrome during chronic outpatient therapy [59]. NAPA, like procainamide, is excreted in part by the kidney; half-lives of both NAPA and procainamide can be tripled or quadrupled in patients with renal failure [60].

TABLE 12-6. Antiarrhythmic Drugs Approved for Intravenous Use

Dosage Information	Lidocaine	Procainamide	Bretylium	Phenytoin
Therapeutic range (µg/ml)	2–6	4–10	0.5–1.5	10–18
Usual loading dose*	1–2 mg/kg over several minutes	Up to 1000 mg at up to 50 mg/min	5 mg/kg initially, up to 30 mg/kg over 45–90 minutes	Up to 1000 mg at up to 50 mg/min
Usual maintenance therapy*	2–4 mg/min	1.5–6.0 gm/day	5–10 mg/kg, up to 30 mg/kg/day	200–400 mg/day
Dosage interval	Continuous infusion	3–4 hr	6–8 hr, up to 30 mg/kg/day	12–24 hr
Side effects	CNS	Hypotension with loading dose, GI, lupus-like syndrome (chronic)	Hypotension	CNS, asystole
Decrease dosage with	Prolonged infusion CHF, liver disease	Renal disease	Renal disease	Liver disease

*These values represent first approximations only; adjustments will often be required based on close monitoring of clinical status.
CNS = central nervous system, GI = gastrointestinal, CHF = congestive heart failure

Monitoring peak procainamide and NAPA levels for toxicity and trough levels for therapeutic efficacy may be useful in the management of patients with clinically important ventricular arrhythmias. As is true with any antiarrhythmic agent, drug level monitoring becomes more important in patients who have apparent toxicity or lack of therapeutic response with conventional doses of the drug. In addition, it may be worthwhile to obtain procainamide levels for certain patients with renal impairment (since dosage adjustments may be necessary) and for those taking sustained-release procainamide (especially trough levels).

As indicated above, *bretylium* can be effective acutely in controlling recurring ventricular tachycardia or fibrillation resistant to other antiarrhythmic agents. In emergency situations such as cardiopulmonary resuscitation, an initial dose of 5 mg/kg can be given, with repeated doses of 10 mg/kg after 15 to 30 minutes, up to a maximum of 30 mg/kg. For maintenance therapy, bretylium should be given in doses of 5 to 10 mg/kg every 6 to 8 hours, up to 30 mg/kg per day. Alternatively, a 1 to 2 mg/min constant infusion can be administered, but hypotension may result from this method of administration.

During a resuscitation attempt, there is obviously no time to use bretylium blood levels as a guide to therapy. The most common side effects are postural and supine hypotension. Bretylium is excreted unmetabolized in the urine. Therefore, lower maintenance doses should be used for patients with renal impairment. Therapeutic plasma concentrations are relatively low, 0.5 to 1.5 μg/ml, compared to more commonly used antiarrhythmic agents. There is only sparse clinical experience using bretylium levels to help regulate intravenous therapy [61].

Phenytoin is used sufficiently infrequently for cardiac arrhythmias that not a single study on phenytoin was included among 89 key references recently compiled on antiarrhythmic drugs [62]. Nevertheless, oral phenytoin was recently shown to suppress ventricular arrhythmias in six young ambulatory patients who had undergone previous surgery for congenital heart disease. The effective serum concentration averaged 16 μg/ml [63]. The therapeutic range is generally considered to be 10 to 18 μg/ml. Phenytoin is metabolized by the liver and has a widely varying half-life [64]. When administered intravenously, it should be given at a maximum rate of 50 mg/min, with a loading dose of up to 1000 mg. Faster rates of intravenous administration have been shown to cause asystole.

The antiarrhythmic drugs we have discussed above are approved for intravenous use and are frequently prescribed for urgent clinical situations. Because assay of antiarrhythmic blood levels usually requires at least several hours, dosage decisions must often be based on clinical signs of toxicity or efficacy without the benefit of confirmatory laboratory blood tests. However, even when antiarrhythmic blood levels are readily available, much caution must be exercised in their interpretation. Generally, the mean and two standard deviations of clinically effective therapeutic blood levels for a large number of patients are calculated to establish the therapeutic range. However, any individual patient may have an effective blood level that is above or below the established therapeutic range. Despite a nominally subtherapeutic or toxic blood level of antiarrhythmic drug, no firm conclusions should be drawn unless the laboratory values are correlated with what is occurring clinically. These same principles are equally important in the interpretation of blood levels of digitalis glycosides, as discussed below.

In less urgent situations, oral rather than intravenous antiarrhythmic agents will generally be used to control atrial or ventricular arrhythmias. Because the arrhythmia of concern may occur only intermittently, ambulatory electrocardiographic monitoring (see Chap. 3) may be necessary in addition to direct clinical observation to judge the efficacy of therapy. In chronic outpatient antiarrhythmic regimens, peak and trough blood levels may be of particular importance in both the assessment of patient compliance and the optimal prescribing of dosage and drug interval.

The timing of plasma antiarrhythmic drug determinations is of utmost importance. If a toxic effect is suspected, a peak level of the antiarrhythmic drug should be obtained. For frequently used oral antiarrhythmic drugs, this peak level usually occurs 1 to 2 hours after dosing. If lack of efficacy is suspected, then the minimal blood level (trough level) of the antiarrhythmic drug should be obtained just before the next dose of medication is due. If the trough level is below the standard therapeutic range and the peak level is not in the toxic range, then the dosing interval can be shortened and/or the dosage can be increased. Alternatively, in such circumstances a long-acting preparation of an antiarrhythmic agent can be used, such as quinidine gluconate instead of quinidine sulfate [65].

Acute drug testing is sometimes used in the management of patients who have recurrent malignant arrhythmias [66–68]. One aspect of acute drug testing utilizes peak and trough drug levels after a single large oral dose of an antiarrhythmic drug and attempts to correlate drug levels with a continuous recording of the patient's cardiac rhythm. However, one problem with this approach is that spontaneous variation in cardiac rhythm complicates the evaluation of drug response [69]. Several investigators have suggested that "therapeutic" blood levels of antiarrhythmic agents may protect against recurrent symptomatic ventricular tachycardia or fibrillation even if asymptomatic premature ventricular depolarizations are not predictably suppressed [70, 71]. Other investigators employ serial electrophysiologic testing in combination with monitoring blood levels of antiarrhythmic drugs to predict an effective drug regimen [72].

Quinidine, procainamide, disopyramide, and propranolol are the oral antiarrhythmic agents most frequently used in the United States at this time (Table 12-7). In the treatment of chronic ventricular arrhythmias, *quinidine* is often used as the drug of first choice. It is also frequently effective in treating supraventricular arrhythmias. The therapeutic plasma concentration of quinidine is 2 to 6 μg/ml. Usual oral doses are 300 to 500 mg four times per day. If a rapid oral loading dose is necessary, 600 to 1000 mg can be given [73]. Quinidine is metabolized primarily by the liver and its dosage must be reduced in patients with liver disease or congestive heart failure [74]. Hepatic biotransformation and renal excretion of quinidine also decrease with age and therefore dosage reductions should be made in elderly patients [75]. In patients whose clearance of quinidine is likely to be impaired, blood levels may be especially useful.

Disopyramide was approved by the Food and Drug Administration in 1978 for oral administration in the treatment of ventricular arrhythmias [76]. It was advertised heavily as being equally effective as quinidine and procainamide in suppression of ventricular arrhythmias but with fewer side effects. Now that more experience has accumulated with disopyramide, it is apparent that this drug does have several undesirable features. In addition to a high incidence of anticholinergic side effects, it exerts a negative inotropic effect on the heart and may precipitate con-

TABLE 12-7. Frequently Used Oral Antiarrhythmic Agents

Dosage Information	Quinidine	Procainamide	Disopyramide	Propranolol
Therapeutic plasma concentration range (μg/ml)	2–6	4–10	2–5	0.02–1.00
Loading dose (mg)*	600–1000	500–1000	200–400	Given intravenously in 0.5–1.0 mg increments to avoid first-pass hepatic extraction
Maintenance dose (mg/day)*	1200–2000	2000–9000	400–800	Usually 40–160 but up to 1000
Usual dosage interval (hr)	6	3–4	6	6
Time of peak concentration after oral dose (hr)	1.0–1.5 for sulfate; 3–4 for gluconate	45–90 min for standard capsule; up to 4 hr for sustained capsule	1–2	1.0–1.5
ECG changes	↑QRS, ↑QT	↑WRS, ↑QT	sl. ↑QT	↑PR; ↓ventricular response in AF
Common side effects	GI	GI, lupus-like syndrome	Anticholinergic, CHF	Neurologic, CHF, may exacerbate bradyarrhythmias in sick sinus syndrome
Reduce dosage and consider measuring blood levels in patients with	Liver disease, CHF, age > 60 yr	Renal disease	Renal disease	Liver disease

*These values represent first approximations only; determination of proper dosages requires close and frequent observation of the patient, using ambulatory monitoring techniques as needed.
AF = atrial fibrillation, sl. = slight, GI = gastrointestinal, CHF = congestive heart failure.

gestive heart failure in as many as 50 percent of patients with a past history of cardiac decompensation [77]. Intravenous administration of disopyramide produces coronary vasoconstriction and increases myocardial oxygen consumption [78], both of which may jeopardize patients with ischemic heart disease. The therapeutic plasma concentration range of disopyramide is 2 to 5 μg/ml, and the average maintenance dose is 150 mg every 6 hours. Disopyramide is excreted chiefly by the kidney and the dose should be reduced in patients with renal disease. Unfortunately, blood levels do not seem to predict reliably which patients will develop congestive heart failure from disopyramide.

Propranolol is used to treat supraventricular tachyarrhythmias and can also be effective against some ventricular arrhythmias, especially those triggered by exercise or emotional upset. Daily doses of 40 to 160 mg are frequently effective, and the drug is usually well tolerated. Propranolol is metabolized by the liver and the dosage should be decreased in patients with liver disease. Propranolol usually has a wide margin of safety and blood tests are rarely needed when this drug is used as an antiarrhythmic agent [79–81]. When used as an antianginal agent, blood tests may be useful (see below, Antianginal Agents).

A variety of additional antiarrhythmic agents are currently being evaluated for safety and efficacy [82]. For most of these drugs, effective therapeutic concentration, loading dose, maintenance dose, dosage interval, onset of action, ECG changes, side effects, and metabolism have been elucidated. Table 12-8 lists five of these experimental drugs (amiodarone, aprindine, ethmozin, mexiletine, tocainide) and verapamil. As with other antiarrhythmic drugs, blood levels will be most useful when conventional doses produce an apparent subtherapeutic or toxic effect. Treatment with a given agent should not be regarded as ineffective unless blood levels in the usual therapeutic range have been documented at the time cardiac arrhythmias occur.

Digitalis Glycosides

The introduction of radioimmunoassay to the clinical laboratory has permitted sensitive and specific measurement of very small quantities of certain drugs, especially digitalis glycosides and propranolol. The basic principle underlying drug radioimmunoassay specificity is that a given drug will have a unique structural configuration that will interact with a specific antibody binding site. Requirements for this type of assay procedure include an antibody population of requisite affinity and specificity, a radioactively labeled form of the drug or substance to be measured (radioligand), and a means of separating antibody-bound and free forms of the radioligand. Unlabeled drug in the sample to be assayed competes with radiolabeled drug (added *in vitro*) for a limited number of specific antibody binding sites (also added *in vitro*). A standard curve is generated using known amounts of unlabeled

TABLE 12-8. Investigational Antiarrhythmic Agents

Dosage Information	Amiodarone	Aprinidine	Ethmozin	Mexiletine	Tocainide	Verapamil[†]
Therapeutic plasma concentration range (µg/ml)	?	1–3	0.5–1.0	0.5–2.0	3.5–10.0	?
Oral loading dose (mg)[*]	—	100 mg q6h, day 1; 75 mg q6h, day 2; 50 mg q6h, day 3	—	400–600	400–600	—
Maintenance dose (mg/day)[*]	200–800	50–150	300–750	600–900	1200–2400	240–480
Usual dosage interval (hr)	24	8–12	6–8	8	8	6–8
Time of peak concentration after oral dose (hr)	4–6	2	2	1–2	1.0–1.5	1–2
ECG changes	↑QT	↑PR, ↑QRS, ↑QT	—	—	—	—
Side effects	Corneal deposits, thyroid dysfunction, neurologic dysfunction, bluish skin discoloration, pulmonary fibrosis	Cerebellar, GI, agranulocytosis, CHF	Neurologic, GI, cardiovascular	Neurologic, GI, cardiovascular	Neurologic, GI, cardiovascular	Neurologic, GI, AV block, CHF
Reduce dosage and consider measuring blood levels in patients with	—	Liver disease	Liver disease	Liver disease	Liver disease, renal disease	Liver disease

[†]Recently approved.
[*]These values represent first approximations only; determination of proper dosages requires close and frequent observation of the patient, using ambulatory monitoring techniques as needed.
GI = gastrointestinal, CHF = congestive heart failure, AV = atrioventricular.

drug incubated with constant known amounts of both radioligand and antibody. The amount of radioactivity bound to the antibody after incubation is inversely related to the concentration of unlabeled drug being assayed. Unknown sample concentrations are determined by comparison with the known drug concentrations on the standard curve. The radioimmunoassay allows accurate measurement of drug concentrations in the nanogram to picogram range [83].

In general, serum cardiac glycoside concentration measurements are indicated when the state of digitalization is difficult to assess, or when a toxic or subtherapeutic effect is suspected (Table 12-9). Misuse of digitalis levels occurs most commonly when the physician interprets all levels within a narrow range as therapeutic and all other levels as either toxic or subtherapeutic [84]. Substantial overlap in therapeutic and toxic levels occurs among different patients and even in an individual patient if clinical circumstances change.

Since digoxin, ouabain, and deslanoside are excreted principally via the kidneys, impairment of renal function will result in higher serum concentrations at any given dosing level than with normal renal function. Although various formulas and nomograms for adjusting digoxin dosage in renal insufficiency provide useful first approximations to dosage, it is often worthwhile to determine serum levels in patients with renal insufficiency during dosage adjustments. Digitoxin is metabolized primarily by the liver and the usual dosage may need to be decreased in patients with liver disease [85].

Patients undergoing cardiac surgery are frequently digitalized preoperatively or are on chronic digitalis therapy. Perioperatively, these patients are susceptible to rapid changes in renal and hepatic function. In the early postoperative period, dosing is often irregular and the usual clinical clues to digitalization status, such as history and electrocardiogram, may be exceedingly difficult to interpret. Therefore, serum cardiac glycoside levels are often useful in the assessment of body content of digitalis and in the determination of optimal dosing regimens.

A recent important finding related to digoxin use is that the concurrent administration of quinidine increases the serum digoxin level and has been reported by Leahey and colleagues to precipitate overt digoxin toxicity in some instances [86]. Indeed, one wonders how many cases of "quinidine syncope" or sudden death in patients receiving quinidine may in fact have been caused or contributed to by digoxin toxicity. Unfortunately, the magnitude of any individual patient's increase in digoxin level or clinical response to the combination of digoxin and quinidine cannot be predicted by the patient's age, sex, type of heart disease, or initial serum digoxin level. Because the effect of quinidine on digoxin levels is variable but potentially important, management of patients on maintenance digoxin in whom quinidine is to be started (or the quinidine dosage changed)

TABLE 12-9. Indications for Ordering a Serum Cardiac Glycoside Level

Assessment of the state of digitalization
  Fluctuating renal function (especially during digoxin or ouabain dosage adjustments)
  Irregular dosage schedules (e.g., cardiac surgery)
  Digoxin-drug interactions (especially quinidine)
Assessment of suspected toxicity
  Neurologic or gastrointestinal symptoms
  Cardiac arrhythmias (especially enhanced automaticity of an ectopic focus plus impaired conduction)
  Accidental or suicidal ingestion
Assessment of inadequate therapeutic response
  Noncompliance
  Impaired absorption
    Gastrointestinal abnormality
    Drug-digoxin binding
    Poor bioavailability
  True resistance to therapeutic effects (e.g., occult thyrotoxicosis, mitral stenosis)

should often include monitoring of digoxin levels until the new steady-state equilibrium is established [87]. Experimental studies in dogs show that other drugs including aspirin and ibuprofen can also cause appreciable increases in serum digoxin levels [88], but clinical studies are lacking. Simultaneous administration of oral quinidine and intravenous digitoxin has recently been reported to cause a rise in serum digitoxin levels and to decrease the total body clearance of digitoxin [89]. However, this observation is controversial [90, 91], and further study of quinidine-digitoxin interaction is needed.

Assessment of timing and magnitude of digitalis dose, renal function, hepatic function, and body mass will permit a first approximation of the body burden of digitalis. When a patient on digitalis develops fatigue, visual changes, nausea, vomiting, or cardiac rhythm abnormalities, a toxic response should be suspected, and a cardiac glycoside level will probably be useful. Certain metabolic abnormalities, including hypokalemia, hypomagnesemia, hypercalcemia, and severe acid-base imbalance, predispose to digitalis toxicity. In addition to metabolic abnormalities, underlying heart disease is an important variable in determining individual patient sensitivity to digitalis. Myocardial ischemia, myocardial infarction, and advanced cardiomyopathy may increase the heart's sensitivity to digitalis glycosides. Particularly in such patients, a digoxin level in the usual "therapeutic" range of 1 to 2 ng/ml cannot exclude toxicity in the presence of symptoms or signs consistent with digitalis excess. Certain noncardiac disorders, including hypothyroidism and pulmonary disease [92] are also associated with an increased incidence of digitalis toxicity at any given serum cardiac glycoside concentration. Conversely, in the absence of clinical symptoms or signs of toxicity, a slightly elevated digitalis level (such as a digoxin level in the 2–3 ng/ml range) should not dictate withholding digitalis when such levels are required for adequate control of the ventricular response to a supraventricular tachyarrhythmia.

A special subset of patients with digoxin toxicity includes those with massive overdosage due to suicidal or accidental ingestion. It is now possible to reverse advanced and potentially lethal digoxin intoxication with purified Fab fragments of digoxin-specific antibodies [93]. To date, 10 patients have been treated, and Fab fragments are available in a collaborative clinical trial in 15 major medical centers throughout the United States. Serum digoxin concentration measurements should be used initially to document the magnitude of the digoxin overdose and to assist in estimating the dose of digoxin-specific Fab fragments needed to counteract the digoxin ingested. While of investigative interest, serum digoxin concentrations after Fab fragment administration reflect bound, inactive digoxin and are not clinically useful.

A frequently encountered clinical problem is failure to achieve an adequate therapeutic response in a patient on a conventional dose of digitalis. The clinician must decide whether the dose is inadequate (as, for example, due to noncompliance with the regimen prescribed, or to impaired absorption) or whether there are reasons why the patient may be "resistant" to usual doses and serum levels of digoxin (e.g., occult thyrotoxicosis or mitral stenosis). In a compliant patient with a low serum digoxin concentration despite usually adequate dosage, the digitalis level may serve as a clue to other disorders or to digitalis binding in the gut to nonabsorbable substances. Hyperthyroidism tends to cause relatively low serum digitalis levels, in addition to true resistance to control of the ventricular response to supraventricular tachyarrhythmias. Malabsorption syndromes and preparations of digitalis with poor bioavailability may lead to low serum digitalis values and inadequate digitalization. Certain drugs, including cholestyramine, colestipol, kaolin and pectin, and certain antacids, will bind digoxin in the gut and result in clinical and laboratory evidence of subtherapeutic digitalization [94].

Thus, a serum cardiac glycoside concentration measurement may provide valuable information when a patient appears to have an inadequate therapeutic response to a conventional dosage regimen of digitalis. If no underlying problem is found, a low digitalis level accompanied by an inadequate therapeutic effect indicates the need to increase the digitalis dosage.

A common pitfall in the interpretation of serum digoxin levels is encountered when blood for analysis is drawn within 4 hours after oral or parenteral administration of digoxin. Under these circumstances, distribution from the plasma or "central" compartment to the periphery is incomplete, and serum concentrations are higher than they will be after equilibrium with tissues is established. Generally, it is necessary to wait at least 4 hours after the last previous dose before obtaining serum for digoxin concentration measurement. Misinterpretation of a relatively high level in a sample obtained prematurely can lead to unfortunate delays in treatment or to inadequate digitalization.

Another potential problem in the radioimmunoassay of digitalis is prior radioisotope administration for nuclear medicine tests. Residual radioactivity in blood samples can result in falsely high or low apparent serum digitalis concentration values unless special measures are taken to deal with this problem. The digitalis assay laboratory should be notified of such potential technical problems.

A few patients have been reported who degrade digoxin to inactive dihydro metabolites. These patients may require larger than usual doses of digoxin to achieve a desired therapeutic effect. The extent to which the dihydro metabolite will be measured as "digoxin" will vary with the specificity of a particular antibody population used in the radioimmunoassay, and cannot be predicted easily [95, 96].

We do not advocate measuring "routine" serum cardiac glycoside levels in patients with a satisfactory therapeutic response to a conventional dosage regimen. However, when a digitalis level is ordered with an appropriate question in mind and the results are interpreted in the full clinical context, this test provides valuable information with benefits far outweighing costs.

Antianginal Agents

Propranolol and *nitrates* provide the foundation for contemporary medical treatment of angina pectoris. The conventional parameters used to guide dosage, in addition to therapeutic response, are heart rate in the case of propranolol and blood pressure (or the onset of intolerable headache) for nitrates. It is fortunate that heart rate provides a convenient clinical index of the extent of beta-adrenergic blockade in view of the very wide (up to 30-fold) variability in plasma concentrations of propranolol among patients on a given dosage regimen. However, under special circumstances, measurement of blood levels of these drugs may be useful. A propranolol plasma concentration of about 250 ng/ml should completely block the effects of endogenous catecholamines during exercise. In some patients, despite large doses of propranolol (e.g., 160 mg qid), the resting heart rate is not substantially lowered and symptoms of angina are not alleviated. A study of such patients demonstrated levels two to three times higher than the predicted adequate therapeutic concentration. These data suggest that in some patients, resting heart rate is inadequate to assess the effective level of beta blockade. In such patients, propranolol is probably a therapeutic failure and is being administered in

TABLE 12-10. Average Charge for Selected Blood Tests at Three Boston Teaching Hospitals (1981)

Category	Test	Charge ($)
Myocardial necrosis	Creatine kinase (CK)	8
	CK-MB	25
	Serum glutamic oxaloacetic transaminase (SGOT)	7
	Lactic dehydrogenase (LDH)	7
	LDH isoenzymes	14
Lipid disorders	Cholesterol	6
	Triglycerides	6
	High-density lipoprotein (HDL)	12
	Lipoprotein electrophoresis	31
Miscellaneous disorders	Glucose	6
	Thyroid hormone T4, T3 resin uptake	15
	Thyroid hormone T3	23
	Thyroid-stimulating hormone (TSH)	25
	Renin	29
	Complete blood count (CBC)	7
	Plasma iron	9
	Total iron-binding capacity (TIBC)	10
	Trace metals screen	12
	Antistreptolysin-O titer (ASLO)	12
	Erythrocyte sedimentation rate (ESR)	6
	Antinuclear antibody (ANA)	17
	Latex fixation	16
	Thiamine	18
	Alkaline phosphatase	6
	Electrolyte	11
	Arterial blood gases (ABG)	30
Antiarrhythmic therapy	Lidocaine	12
	Procainamide	22
	Quinidine	15
Glycoside therapy	Serum digoxin level (SDL)	33

inappropriately high doses [97]. However, other investigators believe that it is premature to use propranolol levels as a therapeutic guide in the management of coronary artery disease [98].

The individual response to a particular dose of nitrates is very unpredictable. When used intravenously, an indwelling arterial catheter is frequently placed for continuous hemodynamic monitoring. Usually, intravenous nitroglycerin is titrated according to arterial blood pressure. For patients with congestive heart failure, the pulmonary capillary wedge pressure is often monitored for additional assessment of nitrate effect. Recently, accurate blood assays for nitroglycerin have been developed. In addition to yielding valuable information on pharmacokinetics in various disease states, such assays may provide a more rational basis for nitrate therapy in individual patients in the future [99].

Conclusions

The utilization of blood tests to diagnose cardiovascular disorders and to assay plasma concentrations of cardiovascular drugs has progressed rapidly during the past decade. Advances in assay methodology and improvements in clinical laboratory instrumentation have been responsible for this progress. When used appropriately, blood tests can be a relatively inexpensive (Table 12-10) and noninvasive method to obtain important clinical information. However, an isolated blood test result should never be used as the sole criterion for establishing a diagnosis or for determining the efficacy or toxicity of a cardiovascular medication. Above all, no laboratory test should diminish the essential role of clinical observation and followup by a vigilant physician well versed in cardiovascular medicine and in clinical pharmacology.

References

1. Roven RB: The clinical laboratory in heart disease. In Halsted JA (ed): *The Laboratory in Clinical Medicine.* Philadephia: WB Saunders, 1976, p 278
2. Alpert JS, Braunwald EB: Pathological and clinical manifestations of acute myocardial infarction. In Braunwald E (ed): *Heart Disease.* Philadelphia: WB Saunders, 1980, p 1331
3. Rosalki SB: Improved procedure for serum creatine phosphokinase determination. *J Lab Clin Med* 69:696, 1967
4. Klein MS, Shell WE, Sobel BE: Serum creatine phosphokinase (CPK) isoenzymes after intramuscular injections, surgery, and myocardial infarction. *Cardiovasc Res* 7:412, 1973
5. Roberts R, Henry PD, Witteeveen SAGJ, Sobel BE: Quantification of serum creatine phosphokinase isoenzyme activity. *Am J Cardiol* 33:650, 1974
6. Henry PD, Roberts R, Sobel BE: Rapid separation of plasma creatine kinase isoenzymes by batch absorption on glass beads. *Clin Chem* 21:844, 1975
7. Roberts R, Sobel BE, Parker CW: Radioimmunoassay for creatine kinase isoenzymes. *Science* 194:855, 1976
8. Vasudevan G, Mercer DW, Varat MA: Lactic dehydrogenase isoenzyme determination in the diagnosis of acute myocardial infarction. *Circulation* 57:1055, 1978

9. Ahumada G, Roberts R, Sobel BE: Evaluation of myocardial infarction with enzymatic indices. *Prog Cardiovasc Dis* 18:405, 1976
10. Grande P, Christiansen C, Pedersen A, Christensen MS: Optimal diagnosis in acute myocardial infarction: A cost-effectiveness study. *Circulation* 61:723, 1980
11. Raabe DS, Morise A, Sbarbaro JA, Gundel WD: Diagnostic criteria for acute myocardial infarction in patients undergoing coronary artery bypass surgery. *Circulation* 62:869, 1980
12. Kannel WB, Castelli WP, Gordon T: Cholesterol in the prediction of atherosclerotic disease. *Ann Intern Med* 90:85, 1979
13. Hulley SB, Rosenman RH, Bawol RD, Brand RJ: Epidemiology as a guide to clinical decisions: The association between triglyceride and coronary heart disease. *N Engl J Med* 302:1383, 1980
14. Miller NE, Thelle DS, Forde OH, Mjos OD: The Tromsö heart study: High-density lipoproteins and coronary heart disease. A prospective case-control study. *Lancet* 1:965, 1977
15. Wilson PW, Garrison RJ, Castelli WP, Feinleib M, McNamara PM, Kannel WB: Prevalence of coronary heart disease in the Framingham offspring study: Role of lipoprotein cholesterols. *Am J Cardiol* 46:649, 1980
16. Gordon T, Castelli WP, Hjortland MC, Kannel WB, Dawber TR: High density lipoprotein as a protective factor against coronary heart disease: The Framingham study. *Am J Med* 62:707, 1977
17. Heiss G, Johnson NJ, Reiland S, Davis CE, Tyroler HA: The epidemiology of plasma high-density lipoprotein cholesterol levels: The lipid research clinics program prevalence study-summary. *Circulation* 62(Suppl IV):IV-116, 1980
18. Levy RI: Hyperlipoproteinemia and its management. *J Cardiovasc Med* 5:435, 1980
19. Witztum JL: Diagnosis and treatement of hyperlipidemia. *Hosp Med* 14:60, 1978
20. Levy RI, Feinleib M: Risk factors for coronary artery disease and their management. In Braunwald E (ed): *Heart Disease*. Philadelphia: WB Saunders, 1980, p 1251
21. Levy RI (Moderator): Dietary and drug treatment of primary hyperlipoproteinemia. *Ann Intern Med* 77:267, 1972
22. Frederickson DS: It's time to be practical. *Circulation* 51:209, 1975
23. Goldstein JL, Brown MS: Genetics and cardiovascular disease. In Braunwald E (ed): *Heart Disease*. Philadelphia: WB Saunders, 1980, p 1706
24. Lipid-lowering drugs. *Med Letter* 22:65, 1980
25. Garcia MJ, McNamara PM, Gordon T, Kannel WB: Morbidity and mortality in diabetics in the Framingham population. Sixteen year followup study. *Diabetes* 23:105, 1974
26. Coronary Drug Project, Baltimore: The prognostic importance of plasma glucose levels and of the use of oral hypoglycemic drugs after myocardial infarction in men. *Diabetes* 26:453, 1977
27. Williams GH, Braunwald E: Endocrine and nutritional disorders and heart disease. In Braunwald E (ed): *Heart Disease*. Philaphia: WB Saunders, 1980, p 1828
28. Levine HD: Compromise therapy in the patient with angina pectoris and hypothyroidism. *Am J Med* 69:411, 1980

29. Ingbar SH, Woeber KA: Diseases of the thyroid. In Isselbacher KJ, Adams RD, Braunwald E, Petersdorf RG, Wilson JD (eds): *Principles of Internal Medicine.* New York: McGraw-Hill, 1980, p 1694
30. Laragh JH: Vasoconstriction-volume analysis for understanding and treating hypertension: The use of renin and aldosterone profiles. *Am J Med* 55:261, 1973
31. Laragh JH, Sealey JE: Renin-sodium profiling: Why, how, and when in clinical practice. *J Cardiovasc Med* 2:1053, 1977
32. Mitchell JR (Moderator), NIH Conference: Renin-aldosterone profiling in hypertension. *Ann Intern Med* 87:596, 1977
33. Vaughan ED Jr, Laragh JH, Gavras I, Buhler FR, Gavras H, Brunner HR, Baer L: Volume factor in low and normal renin essential hypertension. *Am J Cardiol* 32:523, 1973
34. Esler M, Julius J, Zweifler A, Randall O, Harburg E, Gardiner H, DeQuattro V: Mild high-renin essential hypertension: Neurogenic human hypertension? *N Engl J Med* 296:405, 1977
35. Hollenberg NK, Williams GH, Adams DF, Moore T, Brown C, Borucki LJ, Leung F, Bavli S, Solomon HS, Passan D, Dluhy R: Response to saralasin and angiotensin's role in essential and renal hypertension. *Medicine* 58:115, 1979
36. Williams GH, Jagger PI, Braunwald E: Hypertensive vascular disease. In Isselbacher KJ, Adams RD, Braunwald E, Petersdorf RG, Wilson JD (eds): *Principles of Internal Medicine.* New York: McGraw-Hill, 1980, p 1171
37. Wynne J, Braunwald E: The cardiomyopathies and myocarditides. In Braunwald E (ed): *Heart Disease.* Philadelphia: WB Saunders, 1980, p 1437
38. Stollerman GH: Connective tissue disease of the cardiovascular system. In Braunwald E (ed): *Heart Disease.* Philadelphia: WB Saunders, 1980, p 1737
39. Mannik M, Gilliland BC: Systemic lupus erythematosus. In Isselbacher KJ, Adams RD, Braunwald E, Petersdorf RG, Wilson JD (eds): *Principles of Internal Medicine.* New York: McGraw-Hill, 1980, p 358
40. Elin RJ: Instrumentation in clinical chemistry. *Science* 210:286, 1980
41. Kaye CM: Methods for assaying cardiac drugs. In Hamer J (ed): *Drugs for Heart Disease.* Chicago: Year Book Medical Publishers, 1979, p 21
42. Brown PR, Krstulovic AM: Practical aspects of reversed-phase liquid chromatography applied to biochemical and biomedical research. *Analyt Biochem* 99:1, 1979
43. Bastiani RJ, Phillips RC, Schneider RS, Ullman EF: Homogenous immunochemical drug assays. *Am J Med Tech* 39:211, 1973
44. Engvall E: Enzyme immunoassay ELISA and EMIT. In Van Vunakis H, Langone JJ (eds): *Methods in Enzymology,* Vol 70, *Immunochemical Techniques.* New York: Academic Press, 1980, p 419
45. Wyman MG, Lalka D, Hammersmith L, Cannom DS, Goldreyer BN: Multiple bolus technique for lidocaine administration during the first hours of an acute myocardial infarction. *Am J Cardiol* 41:313, 1978
46. Harrison DC: Should lidocaine be administered routinely to all patients after acute myocardial infarction? *Circulation* 58:581, 1978

47. LeLorier J, Grenon D, Latour Y, Caillé G, Dumont G, Brosseau A, Solignac A: Pharmacokinetics of lidocaine after prolonged intravenous infusions in uncomplicated myocardial infarction. *Ann Intern Med* 87:700, 1977
48. Routledge PA, Stargel WW, Wagner GS, Shand DG: Increased alpha-1-acid glycoprotein and lidocaine disposition in myocardial infarction. *Ann Intern Med* 93:701, 1980
49. Thomson PD, Melmon KL, Richardson JA, Cohn K, Steinbrunn W, Cudihee R, Rowland M: Lidocaine pharmacokinetics in advanced heart failure, liver disease, and renal failure in humans. *Ann Intern Med* 78:499, 1973
50. Ochs HR, Carstens G, Greenblatt DJ: Reduction in lidocaine clearance during continuous infusion and by administration of propranolol. *N Engl J Med* 303:373, 1980
51. Sanna G, Arcidiacono R: Chemical ventricular defibrillation of the human heart with bretylium tosylate. *Am J Cardiol* 32:982, 1973
52. Holder DA, Sniderman AD, Fraser G, Fallen EL: Experience with bretylium tosylate by a hospital cardiac arrest team. *Circulation* 55:541, 1977
53. Woo E, Greenblatt DJ: A reevaluation of intravenous quinidine. *Am Heart J* 96:829, 1978
54. Koch-Weser J, Klein SW: Procainamide dosage schedules, plasma concentrations, and clinical effects. *JAMA* 215:1454, 1971
55. Koch-Weser J: Serum procainamide levels as therapeutic guides. *Clin Pharmacokin* 2:389, 1977
56. Greenspan AM, Horowitz LH, Speilman SR, Josephson ME: Large dose procainamide therapy for ventricular tachyarrhythmia. *Am J Cardiol* 46:453, 1980
57. Giardina E-GV, Fenster PE, Bigger JT Jr, Mayersohn M, Perrier D, Marcus FI: Efficacy, plasma concentrations and adverse effects of a new sustained release procainamide preparation. *Am J Cardiol* 46:855, 1980
58. Lahita R, Kluger J, Drayer DE, Koffler D, Reidenberg MM: Antibodies to nuclear antigens in patients treated with procainamide or acetylprocainamide. *N Engl J Med* 301:1382, 1979
59. Roden DM, Reele SB, Higgins SB, Wilkinson GR, Smith RF, Oates JA, Woosley RL: Antiarrhythmic efficacy, pharmacokinetics and safety of N-acetylprocainamide in human subjects: Comparison with procainamide. *Am J Cardiol* 46:463, 1980
60. Lowenthal DT: Pharmacokinetics of propranolol, quinidine, procainamide, and lidocaine in chronic renal disease. *Am J Med* 62:532, 550, 1977
61. Heissenbuttel RH, Bigger JT Jr: Bretylium tosylate: A newly available antiarrhythmic drug for ventricular arrhythmias. *Ann Intern Med* 91:229, 1979
62. Lucchesi BR: Key references—antiarrhythmic drugs. *Circulation* 59:1076, 1979
63. Garson A Jr, Kugler JD, Gillette PC, Simonelli A, McNamara DG: Control of late postoperative ventricular arrhythmias with phenytoin in young patients. *Am J Cardiol* 46:290, 1980
64. Kumana C, Hamer J: Anti-arrhythmic drugs. In Hamer J (ed): *Drugs for Heart Disease.* Chicago: Year Book Medical Publishers, 1979, p 99
65. Ochs HR, Greenblatt DJ, Woo E, Franke K, Pfeifer HJ, Smith TW: Single and

multiple dose pharmacokinetics of oral quinidine sulfate and gluconate. *Am J Cardiol* 41:770, 1978

66. Lown B: Sudden cardiac death: The major challenge confronting contemporary cardiology. *Am J Cardiol* 43:313, 1979
67. Gaughan CE, Lown B, Lanigan J, Voukydis P, Besser HW: Acute oral testing for determining antiarrhythmic drug efficacy: Quinidine. *Am J Cardiol* 38:677, 1976
68. Lown B, Graboys TB: Management of patients with malignant ventricular arrhythmias. *Am J Cardiol* 39:910, 1977
69. Winkle RA: Measuring antiarrhythmic drug efficacy by suppression of asymptomatic ventricular arrhythmias. *Ann Intern Med* 91:480, 1979
70. Winkle RA, Alderman EL, Fitzgerald JW, Harrison DC: Treatment of recurrent symptomatic ventricular tachycardia. *Ann Intern Med* 85:1, 1976
71. Myerburg RJ, Conde C, Sheps DS, Appel RA, Kiem I, Sung RS, Castellanos A: Antiarrhythmic drug therapy in survivors of prehospital cardiac arrest: Comparison of effects on chronic ventricular arrhythmias and recurrent cardiac arrest. *Circulation* 59:855, 1979
72. Horowitz LN, Josephson MF, Spielman SR, Greenspan AM, Harken AH: New approaches to diagnosing and treating ventricular tachycardia. *J Cardiovasc Med* 5:715, 1980
73. Bigger JT Jr, Hoffman BF: Antiarrhythmic drugs. In Goodman LS, Gilman A (eds): *The Pharmacological Basis of Therapeutics*. New York: Macmillan, 1980, p 768
74. Ochs HR, Greenblatt DJ, Woo E: Clinical pharmacokinetics of quinidine. *Clin Pharmacokin* 5:150, 1980
75. Ochs HR, Greenblatt DJ, Woo E, Smith TW: Reduced quinidine clearance in elderly persons. *Am J Cardiol* 42:481, 1978
76. Koch-Weser J: Disopyramide. *N Engl J Med* 300:957, 1979
77. Podrid PJ, Schoenberger A, Lown B: Congestive heart failure caused by oral disopyramide. *N Engl J Med* 302:614, 1980
78. Kotter V, Linderer T, Schroder R: Effects of disopyramide on systemic and coronary hemodynamics and myocardial metabolism in patients with coronary artery disease: Comparison with lidocaine. *Am J Cardiol* 46:469, 1980
79. Gibson D, Sowton E: The use of beta-adrenergic receptor blocking drugs in dysrhythmias. *Prog Cardiovasc Dis* 12:16, 1969
80. Frieden J, Rosenblum R, Enselberg CD, Rosenberg A: Propranolol treatment of chronic intractable supraventricular arrhythmias. *Am J Cardiol* 22:711, 1968
81. Nies AS, Shand DG: Clinical pharmacology of propranolol. *Circulation* 52:6, 1975
82. Zipes DP, Troup PJ: New antiarrhythmic agents: Amiodarone, aprindine, disopyramide, ethmozin, mexiletine, tocainide, verapamil. *Am J Cardiol* 41:1005, 1978
83. Thorell JI, Larson SM: Fundamentals of radioimmunoassay and other radioligand assays. In Strauss HW, Pitt B (eds): *Cardiovascular Nuclear Medicine*. St Louis: CV Mosby, 1979, p 377
84. Smith TW, Curfman GD, Green LH: The use and misuse of digoxin blood levels. In Hurst JW: *The Heart — Update 1*. New York: McGraw-Hill, 1979, p 75

85. Smith TW: Digitalis glycosides. *N Engl J Med* 288:719, 942, 1973
86. Leahey EB Jr, Reiffel JA, Giardina E-GV, Bigger JT Jr: The effect of quinidine and other oral antiarrhythmic drugs on serum digoxin — a prospective study. *Ann Intern Med* 92:605, 1980
87. Leahey EB Jr: Digoxin-quinidine interaction: Current status. *Ann Intern Med* 93:775, 1980
88. Wilkerson RD, Mockridge PB, Massing GK: Effects of selected drugs on serum digoxin concentration in dogs. *Am J Cardiol* 45:1201, 1980
89. Fenster PE, Powell JR, Graves PE, Conrad KA, Hager WD, Goldman S, Marcus FI: Digitoxin-quinidine interaction: Pharmacokinetic evaluation. *Ann Intern Med* 93:698, 1980
90. Ochs HR, Pabst J, Greenblatt DJ, Dengler HJ: Noninteraction of digitoxin and quinidine. *N Engl J Med* 303:672, 1980
91. Noninteraction of digitoxin and quinidine (Letter). *N Engl J Med* 304:118, 1981
92. Green LH, Smith TW: The use of digitalis in patients with pulmonary disease. *Ann Intern Med* 87:459, 1977
93. Smith TW, Haber E, Yeatman L, Butler VP Jr: Reversal of advanced digoxin intoxication with Fab fragments of digoxin-specific antibodies. *N Engl J Med* 294:797, 1976
94. Brown DD, Spector R, Juhl RP: Drug interactions with digoxin. *Drugs* 20:198, 1980
95. Clark DR, Kalman SM: Dihydrodigoxin: A common metabolite of digoxin in man. *Drug Metab Disp* 2:148, 1974
96. Peters U, Falk LC, Kalman SM: Digoxin metabolism in patients. *Arch Intern Med* 138:1074, 1978
97. Homcy CJ, Rockson SG: The role of propranolol radioimmunoassay in clinical decision making. *Circulation* 62(Suppl 3): 298, 1980
98. Ishizaki T: Plasma propranolol levels in angina pectoris. *Am J Cardiol* 46:701, 1980
99. Abrams J: Nitroglycerin and long-acting nitrates. *N Engl J Med* 302:1234, 1980

Index

Index

Acute myocardial infarction. *See* Myocardial infarction, acute
A-H interval, 274
Ambulatory electrocardiographic monitoring. *See* Electrocardiographic monitoring, ambulatory
Aneurysms, true and false
  radiographic examination of, 311-312
  radionuclide ventriculography and, 190-192
Angiography
  coronary, 1
  digital subtraction, 322
  intravenous subtraction, 322-323
  pulmonary. *See* Pulmonary angiography
Antianginal agents and blood tests, 358-359
Antiarrhythmic agents
  blood tests for serum levels of, 347-353
  investigational, 354
Aortic regurgitation (AR), 125
  and mitral regurgitation in cardiac catheterization, 255
  noninvasive approach to, 147-150
Aortic stenosis
  and cardiac catheterization, 254-255
  with cardiac decompensation, 296
  noninvasive approach to, 142-145
Aortic valve disease and radiographic examination, 315, 316
Aortic valve and root in echocardiography, 103-118
  infective endocarditis, 107-108
  normal and bicuspid, 103-104
  prosthetic, 108
  regurgitation, 106-107
  root aneurysm, 107
  valvular stenosis, 104-106
Apexcardiogram (ACG), 130
  abnormal morphology, 133
  abnormal systolic events, 133
  early to mid-diastolic events, 133-135
  late diastolic events, 134-135
  normal morphology, 130-133
Apexcardiography, 121, 130-135
  in aortic regurgitation, 148-149
  in hypertrophic obstructive cardiomyopathy, 146
  in mitral regurgitation, 152-153
  in mitral stenosis, 151
  in mitral valve prolapse, 154
  in pericardial disease, 156
  in valvular aortic stenosis, 143, 145

Arrhythmias
  diagnosis of suspected, 40-41
  diagnostic procedures for, 2
  mechanisms of reentry versus automaticity, 275-276
Arterial pulse, 122-127
  abnormal carotid pulse morphology, 124-127
  normal carotid pulse morphology, 122-123
Asymmetric septal hypertrophy (ASH), 114-115
Atrial abnormalities on ECG, 8-10
  left, 9-10
  right, 8-9
Atrial enlargement on ECG, 8. *See also* Cardiac radiography; Echocardiography
Atrial pacing, 278
Atrial septal defect
  in the adult and cardiac catheterization, 256
  and echocardiography, 118
Atrium, left, and echocardiography, 110
Automatic internal defibrillator (AID), 285-287

Balke treadmill protocol, 56
Bedside hemodynamic monitoring, 235-253
  complications, 251-252
  data acquisition and interpretation, 248-249
    evaluation of PCWP tracing, 248-249
    transducers and recorders, 248
  determination of cardiac output, 249-250
  indications, 235-241
    intractable pulmonary edema, 239-241
    myocardial infarction complications, 235-239
    vasodilator therapy, 241
  pulmonary artery catheter, 241-248
Beta-adrenergic blocking agent and exercise radionuclide ventriculography, 189
Bigeminal pulse, 126
Blood tests, 333-365
  and acute myocardial infarction, 333-336
  antianginal agents and, 358-359
  assessment of antiarrhythmic agents with, 347-353
  and cardiomyopathy, 342, 344-345
  and cardiovascular drug assessment, 346-353
  and congestive heart failure, 343, 345
  and diabetes mellitus, 341-343
  and hypertension, 342, 344
  lipid disorders, 336-341
  and metabolic disorders, 343, 345
  and streptococcal infection, 345
  and systemic lupus erythematosus, 342, 345

369

370 / Index

Blood tests — *Continued*
   and thyroid dysfunction, 342, 343–344
Blood tests and cardiovascular drug assessment
   enzyme multiplied immunoassay technique (EMIT), 346
   gas-liquid chromatography (GLC), 346
   high-pressure liquid chromatography (HPLC), 346
   homogenous immunoassay, 346
Brachial approach for arterial catheter, 257
Bretylium and serum level blood tests, 349–350
Bruce treadmill protocol, 55–56
Bundle branch reentry (BBR), 276

Cardiac catheterization, 2, 253–263
   complications, 261–263
   indications for, 253–254
   intracardiac pressure waveforms, 260
   method of approach, 257–258
   patient preparation, 257
   postcatheterization care, 260–261
   radiographic procedures and, 293–294
   specific indications for, 254–257
      aortic and mitral regurgitation, 255
      aortic stenosis, 254–255
      atrial septal defect in the adult, 256
      coronary artery disease, 254
      hypertrophic cardiomyopathy, 256
      idiopathic dilated (congestive) cardiomyopathy, 256–257
      mitral stenosis, 255–256
Cardiac catheterization protocol, 258
Cardiac diagnostic procedures
   comparison of, 293–294
   value and limitations of, 1–2
Cardiac enzymes in myocardial infarction, 334–336
Cardiac events, probability of, 74
Cardiac glycoside level, indications for ordering, 356–358
Cardiac lesions and cardiomegaly, 320
Cardiac output, determination of, in bedside hemodynamic monitoring, 249–250
Cardiac radiography
   and cardiac size, 295, 298–302
   and fluoroscopy, 294–310
   frontal and lateral chest radiography, 294–303
   and pulmonary vascularity, 302–303
Cardiac size, radiographic estimates of, 295, 298–302
Cardiac ultrasound. *See also* Echocardiography
   and chest radiograph, complementary role of, 317, 319
   and radiographic procedures, 294
Cardiac volume measurements, 299, 300
Cardiogenic shock and radiographic examination, 313

Cardiomyopathy and blood tests, 342, 344–345
Cardiothoracic ratio, 295, 298–299, 301
Cardiovascular disease states, integrated noninvasive approach to, 142–156
Cardiovascular drugs, blood tests to assess serum levels of, 346–353
Cardiovascular responses to exercise, 52
Cardiovascular system, blood tests for disorders related to, 342–343
Carotid pulse morphology
   abnormal, 124–127
      pulsus parvus et tardus, 124
   normal, 122–123
Carotid pulse tracing (CPT), 122–127, 135
   in aortic regurgitation, 148
   in disease and health, 123
   in hypertrophic obstructive cardiomyopathy, 146
   in mitral regurgitation, 152
   in mitral stenosis, 151
   in pericardial disease, 155–156
   valvular aortic stenosis, 143, 144
Carotid "shudder," 125
Chronic bifascicular disease, asymptomatic, 271
Coanda effect, 125
Computed tomography (CT), 323–324, 326–327
   and radiographic procedures, 294
Congestive heart failure
   and blood tests, 343, 345
   left ventricular abnormality, 179–181
   and radionuclide ventriculography, 189
Coronary angiography, 1
Coronary artery disease, 2
   and cardiac catheterization, 254
   and radiographic examination, 311–313
   and radionuclide ventriculography, 183–187
   and thallium-201 myocardial perfusion imaging, 205–211
Coronary artery distribution beds, image defects in, 222
Coronary bypass surgery
   and radionuclide ventriculography, 190
   and thallium-201 myocardial perfusion imaging, 215–216
Coronary disease diagnosis
   exercise-induced R-wave changes, 68–69
   exercise test performance and, 62–72
Corrected sinus node recovery time (CSNRT), 275
Creatine kinase (CK) or creatine phosphokinase (CPK), 334–336
Cumulative life table survival rates in low and high-risk subgroups, 72

Diabetes mellitus and blood tests, 341–343
Diastolic dysfunction in congestive heart failure, 179

Diathermy, 84
Dicrotic pulse, 126
Digitalis glycosides, radioimmunoassay of, 353–358
Disopyramide
 as oral antiarrhythmic drug, 351–353
 and radionuclide ventriculography assessment, 189
Dizziness or syncope, 271–272
Doxorubicin and radionuclide ventriculography assessment, 189
Drug therapy
 assessment with radionuclide ventriculography, 189
 evaluation of, 45–46
Dynamic spatial reconstruction system (DSR), 324–325, 328

Early repolarization as variation in normal ECG, 7–8, 9
Echocardiogram in mitral stenosis, 255–256
Echocardiographic examination, 88–89
Echocardiography, 2, 83–120
 in aortic regurgitation, 150
 aortic valve and root in, 103–108
 atrial septal defect (ASD) and, 118
 diseases assessed by, 89–103
 B-mode scanning system, 85
 causes of abnormal septal motion and, 116
 Doppler ultrasound, 86, 88
 in hypertrophic obstructive cardiomyopathy, 146
 imaging modes in, 85
 instrumentation for, 84–88
 left atrium and, 110
 left ventricle and, 111–117
 mitral valve disease and, 89–103
 in mitral regurgitation, 153
 in mitral stenosis, 151
 in mitral valve prolapse, 154
 M-mode, 317, 319
  imaging system, 86
 in pericardial disease, 156
 pericardium and, 117–118
 principles of ultrasound, 83–84
 pulmonic valve and, 109–110
 and radiographic procedures, 294
 tricuspid valve and, 108
 two-dimensional (2-D), 86–88
 in valvular aortic stenosis, 143
Effective refractory period (ERP), 274
Eisenmenger's syndrome and radiographic procedures, 303
Ejection fraction (EF), 111–112
 and abnormal afterload, 182
 and exercise studies, 183
 as indicator of LV systolic function, 171–172

 in myocardial infarction, 176–179
 in right ventricular function, 187
 and systolic function, 189
Electrocardiogram (ECG), 1, 2, 135
 normal, variations in, 6–8
 resting, 5–28
  atrial abnormalities, 8–10
  constitutional variables and, 5
  diffuse ST-segment and T-wave abnormalities, 26
  intraventricular conduction defects, 18–19
  myocardial infarction, 19–26
  variations in normal, 6–8
  ventricular hypertrophy, 10–18
 technique variations and, 5–6
Electrocardiographic gating, 165
Electrocardiographic monitoring, ambulatory, 29–50
 clinical indications for, 40–48
 components of system, 30–31
 data analysis and quality control in, 32–35
 future directions of, 49
 optimal duration of monitoring, 29–30
 recorders, 31–32
 report form of components, 36–37
 reproducibility in, 40
 scanners, 32
 studies in normal individuals, 37–40
 ventricular arrhythmias in normal subjects, 39
Electrocardiography, 3–79
 ambulatory electrocardiographic monitoring, 29–50
 exercise testing, 51–79
 resting ECG, 5–28
Electrode placement in ambulatory recording, 32
Electrophysiologic measurements, basic intervals in, 274
Electrophysiologic studies, 271–289
 and cardiac conduction disturbances, 279–281
 complications, 277–278
 equipment and techniques, 277
 indications for, 271–273
 measurements, definitions, and mechanisms, 274–277
 noninvasive, 279
 stimulation protocols, 278–279
 and supraventricular tachycardia, 281–282
 syncope or dizziness, 271–272
 ventricular or supraventricular arrhythmia, 272–273
 ventricular tachycardia and, 282–286
Ellestad treadmill protocol, 55–56
Embolism, acute pulmonary, 18
End-diastolic dimension (EDD), 111
End-diastolic volume in left ventricular function, 171, 173, 176
Endocardial mapping, 284–285

End-systolic dimension (ESD), 111–112
End-systolic volume
  and exercise studies, 185
  in left ventricular function, 171, 173, 176
Enzyme multiplied immunoassay technique (EMIT), 346
Equilibrium-gated
  left ventricular volume measurement, 169–170, 172, 173
  radionuclide ventriculography in assessing right ventricular function, 187
Exercise, physiologic response to, 51–54
Exercise ECG, problems with interpretation of, 73–75
Exercise-induced ST-segment changes, 62–69
Exercise protocols in exercise testing, 55–57
Exercise stress testing
  indications for, 57–58
  terms used in, 59
Exercise test after myocardial infarction, 72–73
Exercise testing, 2, 51–79
  appropriate use of, 58–62
  complications of, 75
  contraindications for, 58
  exercise protocols in, 55–57
  historical perspective of, 54–55
  and physiologic response to exercise, 51–54
Exercise test performance and coronary disease diagnosis, 62–72
  arrhythmias and conduction disturbances, 69–70
  combination of variables, 70–72
  exertional hypotension, 69
  R-wave changes, 68–69
  ST-segment changes, 62–68
External pulse recordings. See Pulse recordings, external

Femoral approach for arterial catheter, 257
First-degree heart block, 279–280
First-pass radionuclide ventriculography, 187
Fluoroscopy of the heart
  evaluation of, 303–309
  four views of the heart with barium, 309–310
Four views of the heart with barium, 309–310
French quadripolar pacing electrodes, 277
Functional refractory period (FRP), 274

Gamma (Anger) scintillation camera, 165, 166–167, 168
  in myocardial perfusion imaging, 205
Gas-liquid chromatography (GLC), and cardiovascular drug assessment, 346
Glucose intolerance, 2

Heart block, types of, and electrophysiologic studies, 279–281
Hemodynamic and angiographic findings, interpretation of, 258–260
Hemodynamic evaluations, 1, 2
Hemodynamic monitoring, bedside. See Bedside hemodynamic monitoring
Hemodynamic values, range of normal resting, 259
Hepatic pulse tracings, 131
High-pressure liquid chromatography (HPLC) and cardiovascular drug assessment, 346
His bundle electrogram (HBE), 274, 275, 279, 283
His-Purkinje system, 274, 276
Holter monitoring, 2
Holter recording, 32, 272–273
H-V interval, 274
Hyperlipidemia, 2
  patterns of, 338
  types of, 337–338
Hypertension and blood tests, 342, 344
Hypertrophic cardiomyopathy (HCM), 114–115, 145–147
  and cardiac catheterization, 256
  and echocardiography, 114–115, 146
  and radionuclide ventriculography, 180–181
Hypertrophic obstructive cardiomyopathy (HOCM), 125–126
  noninvasive approach to, 145–147, 148, 149

Immunoassay, homogenous, and cardiovascular drug assessment, 346
Intracardiac conduction disturbances, evaluation of, 279–281
Intraventricular conduction defects, 18–19
Intraventricular reentry (IVR), 276
Invasive procedures, 233–289
  bedside hemodynamic monitoring, cardiac catheterization, and pulmonary angiography, 235–269
  electrophysiologic studies, 271–289
Ischemic heart disease
  and exercise radionuclide ventriculography, 189
  and thallium-201 myocardial perfusion imaging, 199

Jugular venous pulse (JVP), 127–130
  morphology, abnormal, 129–130
  morphology, normal, 127–129
Jugular venous pulse tracing
  in health and disease, 128
  in hypertrophic obstructive cardiomyopathy, 146

in mitral stenosis, 151
in pericardial disease, 154–155
valvular aortic stenosis, 143

Kerley B lines, interstitial, and radiographic procedure, 294, 302

Lactic dehydrogenase (LDH), cardiac enzyme, 334–336
Left atrial abnormalities on ECG, 9–10
Left bundle branch block, 19
Left ventricular abnormalities
  exercise studies, 183–187
  resting function, 176–183
    abnormal afterload, 182
    congestive heart failure, 179–181
    increased systolic function, 182–183
    myocardial infarction, 176–179
Left ventricular echocardiography, 111–117
  aneurysm, 114
  hypertrophic cardiomyopathy (HCM), 114–115, 146
  interventricular septal motion, 115–117
  septal defect, 115
Left ventricular ejection rate, 174
Left ventricular ejection time (LVET), 137
  factors affecting, 140
Left ventricular end-diastolic pressure (LVEDP), 134–135, 138
Left ventricular end systolic volume, 173
Left ventricular hypertrophy (LVH), 10–11
  point score system in diagnosis of, 10–11
Left ventricular outflow tract (LVOT), 122, 124, 125
Left ventricular preejection period, factors affecting, 137–139
Left ventricular systolic dysfunction in congestive heart failure, 179–180
Left ventricular systolic function
  ejection fraction as measurement of, 171–172, 174, 176
  evaluation of global function of, 170–174
  increased, causes of, 182
  parameters of, 173–174, 180
  regional, 174–176
Left ventricular systolic time intervals, 136
Left ventricular volume
  activity method measurement of, 173
  equilibrium-gated method and, 172, 173, 174
Lidocaine and serum level blood tests, 347, 348, 349
Limb lead criteria for LVH, 10
Lipid(s)
  disorders, 336–341

and lipoproteins, normal values of, 340
Lipoproteins, 336–339
  high-density (HDL), 336–339
  low-density (LDL), 336–339
Lown-Ganong-Levine (LGL) preexcitation syndrome, 273
Lown grading system for VPB's, 33–34, 36

Maximal effort test in exercise testing, 56–57
Maximal rate of carotid rise, 124
Mean velocity of circumferential fiber shortening (mean Vcf), 111–112
Metabolic disorders and blood tests, 343, 345
Mitral regurgitation (MR), noninvasive approach to, 151–154
Mitral stenosis
  and cardiac catheterization, 255–256
  and fluoroscopy, 304–305
  noninvasive approach to, 150–151, 152, 153
Mitral valve disease, radiographic examination of, 313–315
Mitral valve echocardiography
  aortic regurgitation, 94–96, 99
  infective endocarditis, 100–102
  mitral stenosis, 90–93, 96, 97
  normal, 89–90, 92
  prolapse, 96–98
  prosthetic, 102
  regurgitation, 99
  systolic anterior motion (SAM), 102–103
Mitral valve prolapse, noninvasive approach to, 154, 155
Mobitz type I (Wenckebach) second degree heart block, 280–281
Mobitz type II second degree heart block, 281
Modified Åstrand treadmill protocol, 56
Monitoring
  electrocardiographic. See Electrocardiographic monitoring, ambulatory
  optimal duration of, 29–30
  trans-telephonic monitoring, 32
Multicrystal scintillation camera, 167
Myocardial disease, radiographic examination of, 315
Myocardial infarct imaging with technetium-99m-pyrophosphate, 221–227
  clinical applications, 223–227
  imaging technique and interpretation, 223
  pyrophosphate uptake, 221–223, 224, 225, 226
Myocardial infarction
  acute, 333–336. See also Myocardial infarct imaging
    cardiac enzymes in, 334–336
    electrocardiogram in, 19–26

Myocardial infarction, acute — *Continued*
  hemodynamic subsets, 237
  and stroke work index, 237
  acute anterior, 20–22
  anterolateral, 22
  complications
    acute mitral regurgitation, 239
    and bedside hemodynamic monitoring, 235–239
    cardiogenic shock, 235–237
    septal rupture, 237–239
  inferior, 22
  left ventricle abnormalities, 176–179
  and radiographic examination, 311
  true posterior, 22–23
Myocardial ischemia
  and necrosis, 19–26
  transient, diagnosis of, 41, 45
Myocardial perfusion imaging with thallium-201. *See* Thallium-201 myocardial perfusion imaging
Myocardial perfusion study, 2

Nitrates and blood tests, 358–359
Nuclear magnetic resonance (NMR), 325, 329
Nuclear stethoscope, 167

Oxygen debt, 55

Pacemaker
  function, monitoring, 46–47
  indications for, 272
  manually activated overdrive, 285, 287
Percent fractional shortening (%ΔD), 111
Pericardial calcification in chest radiography, 296
Pericardial disease
  noninvasive approach to, 154–156, 157
  radiographic examination of, 317, 318
Pericardium and echocardiography, 117–118
Peripheral systemic arterial catheters, 252–253
Phenytoin and serum level blood tests, 349, 350
Phonocardiogram (PCG), 135, 142
Phonocardiography, 121, 142
  in aortic regurgitation, 147–148
  in hypertrophic obstructive cardiomyopathy, 145
  in mitral regurgitation, 151–152
  in mitral stenosis, 150
  in mitral valve prolapse, 154
  in pericardial disease, 154
  in valvular aortic stenosis, 142
Phosphorus 31 in NMR, 325
P mitrale, 10
Postmyocardial infarction patients, ambulatory monitoring of, 47–48
Precordial lead criteria for left ventricular hypertrophy, 10
Predictive accuracy in exercise stress testing, 58–61
Preejection period (PEP), 137
  left ventricular ejection time ratio, factors affecting, 141
Preexcitation syndromes and electrophysiologic studies, 281–282
Procainamide and serum level blood tests, 347–349, 352
Propranolol
  and blood tests, 358–359
  as oral antiarrhythmic drug, 352, 353
  radioimmunoassay of, 353
  radionuclide ventriculography assessment, 189
  and serum level blood tests, 347, 348
Pseudoinfarction patterns, 23–24
  on ECG, causes of, 24
Pulmonary angiography, 1, 263–267
  contraindications and risks, 264, 266–267
  indications, 263–264
  interpretation of findings, 264
  techniques, 264
Pulmonary artery catheter
  brachial approach, 244–245
  femoral approach, 246–248
  insertion of flow-directed balloon-tipped, 241–244
  internal jugular approach, 245–246
Pulmonary capillary wedge pressure (PCWP)
  in bedside hemodynamic monitoring, 235–236, 238–241, 244, 248–249, 252
  and radiographic procedures, 302–303, 310
  tracing, evaluation of bedside hemodynamic monitoring, 248–249
Pulmonary edema
  intractable, and bedside hemodynamic monitoring, 239–241
  radiographic procedures for, 306–307
Pulmonary embolism, role of scintigraphy in, 265
Pulmonary hypertension and radiographic procedures, 308
Pulmonary time-activity curves, 192–193
Pulmonary vascularity and radiographic procedures, 302–303
Pulmonic valve and echocardiography, 109–110
Pulse
  arterial, 122–127
  hyperkinetic, causes of, 124
  hypokinetic, causes of, 124
  jugular venous, 127–130
Pulse recordings
  arterial, 122–127
  external, 121–130
Pulse tracings with phonocardiographic recording, 1, 2

Pulsus
  alternans, 126
  bisferiens, 125–126
  paradoxus, 126–127
  parvus et tardus, 124
Purkinje system, reentry in, 276

Quinidine as oral antiarrhythmic drug, 351, 352
Quinidine syncope, 355–356

Radiograph, chest
  and cardiac ultrasound, complementary role of, 317, 319
  portable, 310
Radiographic examination of
  aortic valve disease, 315, 316
  cardiogenic shock, 313
  coronary artery disease, 311–313
  mitral valve disease, 313–315
  myocardial disease, 315
  myocardial infarction, 311
  pericardial disease, 317, 318
  specific diseases, 311–317
  true and false aneurysms, 311–312
  valvular heart disease, 313–315
Radiographic examinations, newer
  computed tomography as, 323–324, 326–327
  dynamic spatial reconstruction system (DSR), 324–325, 328
  intravenous subtraction angiography, 322–323
  nuclear magnetic resonance (NMR), 325–329
  roentgenkymography, 319–320, 322
Radiographic system, interlaced ECG-gated, 319
Radioimmunoassay and digitalis glycosides, 353–358
Radioisotopic examination of the heart, 165–232
  myocardial perfusion and infarct imaging, 199–232
  radionuclide ventriculography, 165–199
Radionuclide imaging techniques, 121
Radionuclide studies and radiographic procedures, 294
Radionuclide ventriculogram
  and abnormal afterload, 182
  and cardiac surgery, 190–193
  dyskinetic segment, 176, 177
  and exercise studies in LV abnormalities, 183–187
Radionuclide ventriculography, 164–198
  advantages and disadvantages of, 166
  in assessment of drug therapy, 189
  in congestive heart failure, 179–180
  in diagnosing myocardial infarction, 176–179
  equilibrium-gated method of, 169–170, 171, 172
  first pass methods of, 168–169, 172
  and increased systolic function, 182–183

  regional function in, 174–176
  right ventricular function in, 187–189
  technetium-99m, 168, 169
  techniques, 166–170
    imaging instruments, 166–168
Rapid filling wave, 132, 134
Recorders
  continuous, 31
  event, 31
Recording, continuous versus continuous monitoring, 28
Rectilinear scanner, 166–167
Refractory periods, 274
Relative cardiac volume (RCV), 299, 300
Relative refractory period (RRP), 274
Repolarization, early, as variation in normal ECG, 7–8, 9
Right atrial abnormalities on ECG, 8–9
Right bundle branch block(s), 18–19
  incomplete in normal ECG, 6
Right ventricular function
  radionuclide ventriculography in, 187–189
  resting and exercise assessment of, 188
Right ventricular hypertrophy, 11–17
  in normal ECG, 6
  type A, 12, 14
  type B, 12, 15
  type C, 12–13, 16
Right ventricular infarction
  myocardial infarct imaging in, 214
  radionuclide ventriculography in, 187–188
Right ventricular systolic time intervals, 141–142
Roentgenkymography, 319–320, 322
R-wave changes, exercise-induced, 68–69

Sensitivity in exercise stress testing, 58–59
Serum blood tests, 1. See also Blood tests
Serum glutamine oxaloacetic transaminase (SGOT), 334–335
Shunt scintigraphy and radionuclide ventriculography, 192–193
Sinoatrial conduction time (SACT), 274–275
Sinus bradycardia, asymptomatic, 271
Sinus node assessment, 274–275
Sinus node recovery time (SNRT), 274
Sodium pertechnetate (NaTcO$_4$), 168
Sodium 23 in NMR, 325, 329
$S_1S_2S_3$ pattern variation in normal ECG, 6
Specificity in exercise stress testing, 58–59
Streptococcal infection and blood tests, 345
Stroke volume
  and exercise studies, 183
  in left ventricular function, 173–174
ST-segment abnormalities, 26
ST-segment changes, exercise-induced, 62–69
ST and T-wave changes, 24–27

Submaximal effort test in exercise testing, 56–57
Supraventricular tachycardias, evaluation of, 280, 281–282
Supraventricular or ventricular arrhythmia, 272–273
Surgery, determining indications for
 chronic valvular heart disease, 192
 coronary bypass, 190, 209
 shunt scintigraphy, 192–193
 ventricular aneurysm, 190–192
Swan-Ganz catheterization, 235, 239, 241, 247, 249, 251
 complications with, 251–252
Syncope or dizziness, 271–272
Systemic lupus erythematosus and blood tests, 342, 345
Systolic dysfunction in congestive heart failure, 179–180
Systolic function
 and drug therapy assessment, 189
 increased, 182–183
Systolic movement on ACG
 bifid motion, 133
 hyperdynamic motion, 133
 sustained motion, 133
Systolic time intervals (STI), 121, 135–142, 174
 alterations in disease states, 139
 in aortic regurgitation, 149–150
 factors influencing, 138
 in hypertrophic obstructive cardiomyopathy, 146
 in mitral regurgitation, 153
 in mitral stenosis, 151
 in mitral valve prolapse, 154
 in pericardial disease, 156
 in valvular aortic stenosis, 143
Systolic wall motion, radionuclide ventriculogram and, 174–176
Systolic wall stress or afterload, 182

Technetium-99m, as imaging agent, 165
Technetium-99m-pyrophosphate
 myocardial imaging with, 221–227
 in right ventricular infarction, 188
Thallium-201 imaging and radionuclide ventriculography, 185–186
Thallium-201 myocardial perfusion imaging
 abnormal resting ECG, 209
 asymptomatic patients, 207–208
 basic principles of, 200
 biologic properties of, 200–204
 cardiomyopathies, dilated, 216–217
 cardiomyopathy, hypertrophic, 217
 clinical experience, 205–217
 coronary artery bypass-graft surgery, 215–216
 coronary artery spasm, 216
 development of, 199
 exercise study
  exercise, 218
  imaging, 218
  interpretation of images, 218–221
  preparation, 217–218
 ideal versus actual biologic properties, 200–201
 instrumentation, 205
 localization of coronary artery disease, 209–211
 myocardial infarction
  diagnosis, 211–212
  localization, 213
  shock, 214–215
  sizing, 213–214
 myocardial infiltrative diseases, 217
 physical properties, ideal versus actual, 204–205
 physiology of initial distribution, 201–202, 204
 postmyocardial infarction rehabilitation, 215
 redistribution phenomenon, 204
 right ventricular pressure or volume overload, 216
 sensitivity and specificity of exercise studies, 206–207
 severe coronary artery disease, 208–209
 severe left ventricular dysfunction, 209
 suspected coronary artery disease, 205–206
Thyroid dysfunction and blood tests, 342, 343–344
Total electromechanical systole (Q-A$_2$), 137
Trendscription, 30, 31, 33
Tricuspid valve and echocardiography, 108
T-time, 124
T-wave
 abnormalities, 26
 morphology variation in normal ECG, 6
 and ST-wave changes, 24–27

Ultrasound, 1. See also Echocardiography
 principles of, 83–84
Upstroke time (U-time), 124
Urokinase-Pulmonary Embolism Trial and ECG, 18

Valvular aortic stenosis, noninvasive approach to, 142–144, 149
Valvular heart disease
 diagnostic procedures for, 2
 radiographic examination of, 313–315
Vascular imaging, digital, 322
Vasodilator therapy, bedside hemodynamic monitoring, 241
Ventricular aneurysm and radionuclide ventriculography, 190–192
Ventricular hypertrophy, 10–18
 combined, 17
 left, 10–11

right, 11–17
Ventricular, left. *See specific entry under* Left ventricular
Ventricular pacing, 278
Ventricular premature beats (VPBs), 29–34, 47–48
Ventricular, right. *See specific entry under* Right ventricular
Ventricular septal defect (VSD), congenital, 115
Ventricular or supraventricular arrhythmia, 272–273
Ventricular tachycardia (VT)
  evaluation of, 282–286
  symptomatic, 273
v wave, abnormalities of the, 129–130

Wenckebach (Mobitz type I) second degree heart block, 280–281
Wolff-Parkinson-White (WPW) preexcitation syndrome, 273

x descent, abnormalities of the, 129

y descent, abnormalities of the, 130